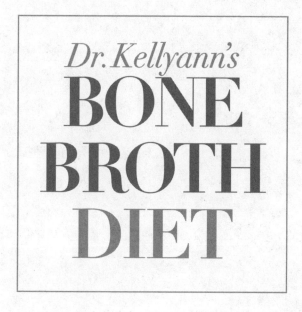

Dr. Kellyann's
BONE
BROTH
DIET

Dr. Kellyann's
BONE
BROTH
DIET

— Lose Up to —
15 POUNDS,
4 INCHES—
and Your Wrinkles!—
in **JUST 21 DAYS**

KELLYANN PETRUCCI, MS, ND

RODALE.

NEW YORK

This book is intended as a reference volume only, not as a medical manual. The information given here is designed to help you make informed decisions about your health. It is not intended as a substitute for any treatment that may have been prescribed by your doctor. If you suspect that you have a medical problem, we urge you to seek competent medical help.

While the author has made every effort to provide accurate telephone numbers, internet addresses, and other contact information at the time of publication, neither the publisher nor the author assumes any responsibility for errors or for changes that occur after publication. Further, publisher does not have any control over and does not assume any responsibility for author or third-party websites or their content.

Published in the United States by Rodale Books, an imprint of Random House, a division of Penguin Random House LLC, New York.

rodalebooks.com

RODALE and the Plant colophon are registered trademarks of Penguin Random House LLC.

Originally published in hardcover and in different form in the United States by Rodale, an imprint of Random House, a division of Penguin Random House LLC, New York, in 2015. Some charts and text were originally published in *Dr. Kellyann's Cleanse and Reset* (New York: Rodale Books, 2019).

Library of Congress Cataloging-in-Publication Data is on file with the publisher.

ISBN 978-0-593-23398-6
Ebook ISBN 978-0-593-23399-3

Printed in the United States of America

Illustrations courtesy of Dr. Kellyann Petrucci, MS, ND and Best of Organic, LLC
Photographs by Jennifer Bonde
Book design by Christina Gaugler
Cover design by Anna Bauer Carr
Cover photograph by Keith Major

5th Printing

Revised Edition

To my father, John, who listens to me go on and on in life,
when all he really wants to do is play golf. He taught me to trust the timing
in life. To keep it right, do the work—and you will not be denied.

To Mother El, a beautiful artist who gave me
any bit of creative juice I have.

And to my boys, my oxygen.

You sure had to endure a lot with me as your momma. The late nights with
the laptop, the trips, and the 24/7 pull. But you always understood. You
both had a front-row seat to watch your momma go for it even when it
didn't make sense. Thank you for always giving me a wonderful grounding
pad that I could look forward to. I am beyond proud of you both!

CONTENTS

FOREWORD xi

ACKNOWLEDGMENTS xiii

Part I: The Fundamentals of the Bone Broth Diet: Fat-Burning Foods, Liquid Gold, and Intermittent Fasts

Chapter 1 My 21-Day Challenge to You: Lose the Weight—
and the Wrinkles! 3

Chapter 2 The Basics of the Bone Broth Diet 12

Chapter 3 Your Intermittent Fasting Secret to Success: "Liquid Gold" 30

Chapter 4 Metabolic Magic for Your Nonfasting Days:
Foods That Melt Off Fat and Erase Wrinkles 45

Chapter 5 My Bone Broth Lifestyle Plan—or
How to Keep Those Pounds Off FOREVER 78

Part II: Recipes, Meal Plans, and Batch-Cooking Tips

Chapter 6 Fabulous Recipes for Beautiful Bone Broth
(Plus Intermittent-Fasting-Day Snacks) 93

Chapter 7 Fat-Blasting Entrées and Soups for Your Nonfasting Days 116

Chapter 8 Luscious Sides, Condiments, and "Extras" for Your
Nonfasting Days 221

Chapter 9 Making It Easy: Meal Plans and Tips for Batch Cooking 291

Chapter 10 Mouthwatering Meals for Your Bone Broth Lifestyle Plan 302

Part III: Optimizing Your Results with Exercise, Stress Reduction, and Lifestyle Changes . . . Plus My Top Ten Beauty Tips!

Chapter 11 Add More Fat-Burning Power with Exercise 317

Chapter 12 Live Long and Stay Healthy by Making Smart Choices 326

Chapter 13 Get Slimmer by Lowering Your Stress 338

Chapter 14 Develop a Positive Mind-Set to Keep Extra Pounds Off 350

Chapter 15 Look Drop-Dead Gorgeous with My Top Ten Beauty Tips 361

SPREAD THE WORD! 369

APPENDIX: MEASUREMENT TRACKER AND CARB COUNTER 371

NOTES 377

INDEX 385

FOREWORD

I WISH I COULD say my first bone broth experience happened many years ago in my kitchen. After all, colleagues have long raved about this healing food (or drink, depending on how you view it), and I've read numerous trustworthy blogs proclaiming its well-earned superfood status.

But that first experience didn't happen in my kitchen. Truthfully, simmering bones all day just seemed tedious and unappealing, so for years I avoided what seemed a herculean task.

As someone who regularly keeps her pulse on arising nutrition trends—I was eating kale decades before it became the "it" food—I'm a little embarrassed to say that my first broth encounter occurred a few years ago at a Manhattan hole-in-the-wall, which smartly called this suddenly trendy concoction the world's first comfort food.

Therein lie its contradictions. While lately a hot health trend, bone broth carries a reputation as one of the oldest, most nourishing medicinal foods. Perfectly at home in the slow-food movement, broth also makes the ultimate fast food. It takes minutes to prepare but keeps you full for hours. And while seemingly complex to create, making bone broth—as I eventually discovered—actually proves quite simple.

On that cold New York day, I finally understood bone broth's appeal, its accolade-deserving nourishing goodness more satisfying than a hot cup of coffee. I felt full for hours afterward, with a newfound energy I attributed to the city's energy but more likely came from the delicious broth.

Abundant nutrients mean bone broth carries an impressive health-benefits résumé. Its ability to crush hunger and cravings makes it the perfect fat-loss contender, so it was only a matter of time before someone designed a bone broth–centered eating plan.

Thankfully, my esteemed friend and colleague Dr. Kellyann Petrucci embraced this task, and she totally nailed it. I've worked with this rock star practitioner for years, witnessing firsthand how she has helped thousands of people transform their bodies and their lives.

From her two decades' experience coupled with impeccable research comes *Dr. Kellyann's Bone Broth Diet.* (I suggested she change it to "Bone Broth Miracle" because the transformation becomes that amazing.)

This easy-to-implement 21-day plan accommodates the most hectic schedule. Twice a week, you'll center a mini-fast on bone broth, which provides deep, nourishing nutrition that stifles hunger as you effortlessly burn fat, reduce inflammation, and reclaim your awesome.

Banish any negative connotation about *fast* here. You've heard about intermittent fasting's benefits, yet you know someone who becomes, shall we say, less than pleasant during those fasting hours. Well, Dr. Kellyann's twice-weekly bone broth fast provides all of intermittent fasting's benefits without hunger, deprivation, or other miseries. Win-win!

The other 5 days every week, you'll eat delicious, satisfying, nutrient-dense foods that have a naturally low impact on blood sugar. You'll eliminate food intolerances (potentially forever) and nasty additives like artificial sweeteners (definitely forever).

Forget bland, boring "diet" foods. Dr. Kellyann designed this decadent, delicious repertoire of abundant gourmet recipes (including, yes, desserts) for busy, short-on-time, sometimes kitchen-phobic people.

These nutrient-rich, hunger-busting foods help balance hormones, create glowing skin, detoxify, heal the gut, reduce inflammation, and blast stubborn excess weight. You'll discover a newfound energy and feel like you've turned back the clock about a decade. (Hey, mirrors don't lie.)

Dr. Kellyann knows that fat loss and glowing health demand more than the right diet; hence, four effective exercise options (including my favorite—burst, or interval, training) coupled with a get-results plan that incorporates things such as stress control, optimal sleep, and cultivating the right mind-set for success.

Within these pages, you'll find techniques for implementing this program in real-life situations, troubleshooting your concerns, getting back on the wagon after you've crashed, and strategic tracking to stay the course.

That last one especially becomes important because, ultimately, you want to maintain those results. While Dr. Kellyann asks for 21 days—come on, anyone can do 21 days!—an instant body transformation (good-bye forever, stubborn belly fat) coupled with an invigorating "new normal" feeling will help you stay on track. Ultimately, this becomes a way of life, not a diet.

Don't be surprised if bone broth becomes your new favorite food. I'm proud to say I overcame my preparation phobia when I returned from New York, and broth now remains a kitchen staple.

I want you to develop that same broth love, ditch that refuse-to-vacate fat, and become your most vibrant, sexiest, youthful *you*.

Here's to fast, lasting fat loss . . . One sip at a time!

JJ Virgin

ACKNOWLEDGMENTS

To the DKA Squad. You are the reason I get up in the morning. Thank you to each and every one of you. I will never take it lightly that you trust me. I will never take it lightly that you have taken the time to read, watch, or listen to my thoughts, mastery, and life lessons. I will never take it lightly that there is a lot out there to choose from and you've made the decision to spend your resources on my products. I will never take it lightly that every once in a while, we all need someone to help pull us out of the tunnel when we feel aimless or unsure. You can count on me. Thank you for making my life mission filled with so much joy. I'm planting my BIG Italian kiss on each and every one of you.

To the DKA Team. How lucky am I to somehow be a part of the most creative and futuristic company in the industry? I am truly grateful for your support and belief in the DKA brand. I admire and respect all of you, and I'm always sending you my love (I hope you can feel it). Special thanks to Jenna, Krystle, Jordan, and Kendall for sticking with me through the marathon. So glad to have you by my side.

To Jodi. You are the bionic woman in every sense of the word. You have handled all the strife and turbulence with nothing but grace and ease. Most important, I trust you with my life—literally—and for that I am without words. I hope you know how much I love you, and you truly are my rock.

To Cody. I was captured by your no-formalities, let's-get-it-done approach from day one. I knew you would make magic happen, and boy did you ever. Thank you for being so bullish and acquiring the DKA brand. Most of all for doing it with your whole heart and commitment to the bigger picture . . . the mission. The mission to help millions. You are a phoenix and I thank God for the gift of being in your center orbit.

To Alison. How many years has it been, well let's just say it started out with Dummies and ended with the *New York Times* . . . HA! I could not have done it without you. Thank you for always being my quiet warrior.

To Ashley. Thank you for always being there for me, encouraging, inspiring, and creating a beautiful DKA landscape. But most of all for keeping every little thing—including me—in order. I treasure you.

To Kaylan. Your creativity has always been awe-inspiring, and so is your incredible commitment. Thank you for charging all of the elegant words I've had the privilege of commanding.

To Vincent. I don't think there is a more heart-centered doctor on the planet. You're not only a brilliant researcher and physician, but you are grounded in truth and selflessness. You should be a model for many to follow. You know what you did for me, and I am forever grateful.

To JJ. You are an inspiration to me in a million ways. What I'm most grateful for is that you have tucked me under your wing for all these years. Thank you for cherishing me even when I was at my very lowest and when everything looked so dismal. You have my back, and I have yours. We are lifers.

To Celeste. Okay, Harvard, you are so brilliant, and I love kicking ideas around with you. Thank for not only caring about my publishing career—but about me. You have shown your colors so many times, and I thank you for lifting me when I needed it and telling me to shut up when I needed it. You're the best!

To Marnie, Katherine, and the gang at Penguin Random House. Thank you for embracing me and my voice and putting my words into print. You have been such a help in empowering me to get my message to so many, and I truly thank you. More to come . . .

To Rachel. You are a rare find, my friend. You dialed in to me straightaway and so unselfishly mentored me through the ups and down of business and life. Thank you for being solid in who you are and what you know I stand for. For investing in me as a person and not just DKA. I truly value you, and you mean the world to me.

To Mitchell. I can only think it was divine intervention that you and I managed to meet up after years of friendship to create such a powerful daily mastermind. I love our conversations, filled with life strategy, business best practices, inspiration, and hope. Thank you for being such a trusted confidant. I appreciate your effusive, I'm-in-no-matter-what perspective with all things DKA. Looking forward to catching a show with you someday in New York City.

To Lynn. I cannot express how lucky I am. You reached out to me all those years ago when I was just getting started. You have shared your beautiful home, family, and design brilliance with me so unselfishly. With you, it's always about friendship and never agenda. I love you and Larry and look forward to every visit, where the conversation, wine, and beautiful food are always free-flowing. Thank you for providing me with a safe haven, my love always.

To Nicole. You are a treasure trove of intellect, humor, and business knowhow. Your creativity is like an avalanche that just keeps getting bigger all the time. You know who you are, and your wisdom and guidance have meant so much to me. I feel so lucky you choose to share your friendship and insights with me. Oh, and Nicole . . . you're so damn funny. Love you always.

To Jasmine. For black hair to blonde. You have stood beside me and listened, laughed, and had nothing but positivity to share. Thank you for your beautiful work. You are one of my inner-orbit people always.

To Katie. Whenever I think of you, I smile. You have such amazing energy that everyone can't help but love you. Thank you for always making me beautiful and always saying "Kellyann, it will *all* pay off." The sexy doctor adores you.

To Marci. You are family. You take care of my needs that go well beyond fashion. You are the kindest, sweetest energy I have ever known. I hope you know you are truly precious to me.

To Cindy. You are a master of your domain, and I enjoy working with you so much. Each of your recipes is filled with an abundance of your healthy light and undaunted experience. We have been together forever, and, for us, it only gets better. Thank you for filling my plate and my soul.

To Kevin. Thank you for giving me the greatest gifts in my life and for making them the center of your world. You are such a wonderful human being, and I'm so glad our sons have so many of your attributes. Thanks for never faltering in your belief of DKA.

To Kathy. You have had such a positive influence on my life, both personally and professionally. You really pulled through for me on this book. Thank you so much for volunteering your help, encouraging me at every step of the way, and forgiving me when I had "book brain"!

PART I

THE FUNDAMENTALS OF THE BONE BROTH DIET:

Fat-Burning Foods, Liquid Gold, and Intermittent Fasts

CHAPTER 1

My 21-Day Challenge to You:
Lose the Weight—
and the Wrinkles!

NEW YORK CITY IS my home. And I love to eat—hey, I'm Italian!—so when I'm out on the town, I hit every place from Le Bernardin to the Pearl Oyster Bar.

But back in 2015, when I was strolling around the city, I did a double-take when I walked past Brodo in the East Village and saw its menu: bone broth. Just *bone broth*. Turkey broth. Pasture-fed beef broth. Amish chicken broth.

I was amazed to see that New Yorkers were discovering the food I'd been prescribing for years—and suddenly they couldn't get enough of it. People were abandoning Starbucks in droves for their daily fix of bone broth, and chic restaurants all over the city were selling it faster than they could make it.

And it wasn't just a New York craze. Celebrities like Shailene Woodley and Gwyneth Paltrow got hooked on their daily fix of bone broth; morning talk-show hosts raved about it; and foodies everywhere started making it in their own kitchens.

As it turned out, that was just the beginning. The craze has since become a full-blown revolution. Today, you'll find bone broth in grocery stores and on restaurant menus everywhere. And from NFL players to the Kardashians, everyone's drinking it.

I'm thrilled to see the bone broth movement catch fire, because as a doctor who's been prescribing bone broth for decades, here's what I know: Bone broth isn't just broth. And it isn't just soup. It's concentrated healing. This broth, made from meat, poultry, or fish bones and simmered until it turns into nutrient-rich "liquid gold," is one of the world's oldest and most powerful medicinal foods.

Millions of people are discovering that there's more to bone broth than meets the eye. That's because this magical food strips weight off your body and takes years off your age. When you combine the power of bone broth intermittent fasts with a core diet of fat-burning foods, you will drop pounds like crazy—and at the same time, you'll erase wrinkles and under-eye bags.

In fact, if you're willing to commit to just 21 days on this diet, I promise you this: You will transform your body.

How do I know this? It's my job. I'm a naturopathic physician and a certified nutritional consultant with more than 20 years of clinical experience, and my specialty is transforming people. What's more, I'm really good at it. Over the course of my career, I've helped thousands of people lose weight and become healthy, sexy, and energetic again. My success stories include everyone from 450-pound patients who lost all of their excess weight to Hollywood celebrities who need to have perfect bodies and faces for the big screen. And bone broth is a key to my transformations.

....

Jenny showed up in my office weighing 180 pounds. As soon as I said hi, she started to cry.

Why? Because she was sure I couldn't help her. "Nobody has," she said. She told me she went on her first diet at 13, and 20 years later—after Weight Watchers, Nutrisystem, and a dozen other diets—she weighed more than ever. Now she was borderline diabetic. And after watching her mother die from complications of diabetes, she was terrified that it would happen to her.

Jenny knew she needed to lose weight. But every diet she'd tried left her weak, trembly, and hungry. She'd lose 5 or 6 pounds right away, but she could never keep the momentum. After the first few days, her cravings would grow so strong that she couldn't do anything except obsess about food. After a week or two, she'd crash, bingeing on ice cream and pizza. And then she'd feel disgusted with herself.

She'd seen me on TV, and she wanted to believe that I could help. But she'd been burned too often to really think I could.

So I didn't promise her anything. Instead, I simply described my program. And then I said, "Just give me 3 weeks."

She did. At the end of that time, she'd lost 20 pounds. Six months later, she now weighs 130 pounds. She's not prediabetic anymore. She looks like she's 25, and she feels like a teenager.

Just 6 months ago, Jenny looked matronly. Nobody noticed her when she walked by. Men ignored her. Women dismissed her as "no competition." Instead of being the center of attention, she was on the sidelines. And instead of posing for pictures, she was hiding behind the camera. In essence, she was invisible.

Now, however, Jenny looks hot—from her slim figure to her glowing skin. The first time she came to my office, she was wearing a plus-size flowered muumuu—that classic "overweight old lady" dress. On her last visit, she wore skinny jeans and a halter top. Invisible? Not this girl. Not ever again.

....

Why was Jenny able to lose weight so quickly on my program, after decades of struggling? Because I took the pain and fear out of dieting. When I showed her that she never had to starve in order to lose weight—and that, in fact, she could eat *well*—I gave her the information she needed to transform her body and her life.

Now Jenny has enough confidence and energy to light up a room. And when she walks through a door, heads turn.

MY SECRET WEAPON FOR FAST, HUNGER-FREE WEIGHT LOSS: BONE BROTH

I've been guiding weight-loss transformations like Jenny's for more than two decades. However, it took me a while to discover the most powerful weapon in my weight-loss arsenal.

Early in my career, I quickly established a track record of success. But I wanted to do even better for my patients—and, in particular, I wanted to achieve the biggest results in the shortest time for patients struggling with obesity.

Many of the people I work with merely want to lose a dress size or a pants size, but others are dangerously overweight. They're diabetic, they have heart disease, they have sleep apnea, and they can barely move. So they need to drop weight fast.

As any weight-loss expert will tell you, fasting is the quickest way to jump-start weight loss (even though it's difficult or impossible for many people—more on my easy and painless solution for this shortly!). Unlike mere calorie restriction, fasting sends your metabolism into hyperdrive (I'll talk more about this in Chapter 3). That's why I've always encouraged my obese or even mildly overweight patients to fast at least 1 or 2 days a week. Besides cutting down on calories, here are some of the reasons fasting jump-starts weight loss.

■ **It optimizes hormones.** Fasting causes your levels of insulin to drop and your levels of another hormone called glucagon to rise. Think of glucagon as the mirror image of insulin. While insulin packs on fat, glucagon pulls fat out of cells (I'll get into this in Chapter 3).

- **It makes levels of human growth hormone surge.** This hormone burns fat and builds lean muscle, sculpting the core, arms, and legs.

- **It cleanses the body.** Think of the fluid around your cells—your cellular matrix—as similar to the water in a fish tank. When it's filled with sludge, the cells are sludgy, too. Fasting cleanses your cellular matrix, removing debris that makes cells sluggish.

So fasting works. And it works immediately. But here's the problem: Fasting can be hard.

Over time, I found that while many people can handle total fasts with ease, many others can't. They get hungry and shaky. They start having headaches. They can't focus at work or at home. They get anxious, and they start obsessing constantly about food. So they give up.

No way was I going to let this happen to my patients. For many of them, I'm the "last chance" doctor—and I wasn't about to let them down. And while I knew my patients could lose weight over time without fasting, I also knew that they needed to see immediate results. Both emotionally and physically, they had to get a quick win.

So I had to find an answer. I needed to create a program that would give these dangerously overweight patients—and all of my patients, including those who need to lose only a few pounds—the immediate benefits of fasting without the drawbacks.

And then it hit me: *bone broth.*

I was already prescribing bone broth as a core part of my weight-loss program because it's a high-octane fat burner. So I thought: Why not combine the power of easy intermittent fasts with the power of bone broth?

When I began doing this, I discovered that my patients got all of the benefits of full fasting without the pain. They lost weight and, as a bonus, took years off their skin.

I'd found the missing key.

Why? Because here's what bone broth does.

- **It fills you up—without adding pounds.** Bone broth is rich, complex, hearty, and soul satisfying. It has virtually zero carbs and very few calories, so it's sin-free and you can indulge in it as much as you want. Translation: no hunger, even when you're fasting.

- **It's packed with the building blocks of collagen.** Collagen blasts wrinkles, so you can take years off your face at the same time as you lose weight. (I'll talk more about this in Chapter 3.)

- **It detoxifies your body.** Like fasting, bone broth helps cleanse your cellular matrix, energizing and de-aging your cells.

- **It heals your gut.** If you're battling extra pounds, I'm guessing that you also have digestive problems—constipation, diarrhea, gas, or even all three. That's because weight gain and digestive problems often stem from a common source: a sick gut. The gelatin and other nutrients in bone broth help heal the gut (something I'll talk about in Chapter 3), curing digestive problems while they facilitate weight loss.

- **It heals your joints.** One reason people become overweight is that as they get older, their joints develop wear and tear and it becomes harder to move. So they exercise less and they sit more. Bone broth gives you a generous supply of nutrients that help heal your joints. (I'll tell you more about this in Chapter 3 as well.)

- **It's anti-inflammatory.** One of the most important scientific findings of the century is that inflammation underlies obesity. To understand why, you need to understand the difference between *acute* and *chronic* inflammation.

  Acute inflammation—for instance, the inflammation you experience when you have a cold or the flu—typically is a good thing, because it helps your body fight off infections and repair tissues. But if you develop chronic low-grade inflammation, that's a whole different story. Chronic inflammation damages your cells, and it leads to biochemical changes that make you put on weight. Fat cells are inflammatory, so when you add pounds, a vicious cycle—inflammation leading to weight gain, leading to more inflammation—begins. This sets the stage for insulin resistance and other metabolic changes that cause you to put on even more weight, develop more inflammation, and so on.

  When you break this cycle by healing inflammation with nutrients like those concentrated in bone broth—such as the amino acid glycine, one of the most powerful anti-inflammatory nutrients on the planet—the pounds start to fall off. Remember this rule: *Anything that increases inflammation puts weight on you, while anything that decreases inflammation takes weight off.* In addition, dry, rough skin and acne—which are outward signs of internal inflammation—will start to clear up.

When my patients do twice-a-week intermittent fasts combining the power of fasting with the fat-melting qualities of bone broth, the effect is stunning. They can't believe how little sacrifice they need to make, how little they're tempted to eat the junk they used to crave, and how fast they see results.

For more facts on bone broth and the magic it can do for you, go to my Resources page at drkellyann.com/resources.

My patients love my plan for another reason: They get to spend the other 5 days of the week eating fabulous food . . . and they still lose weight. Why? Because I show them how to throw out the foods that are making them fat and aging their skin—and add the foods that will make them thin and reverse their wrinkles.

MY SECOND KEY TO WEIGHT LOSS: PEELING OFF POUNDS WITH FAT-BURNING FOODS

On the Bone Broth Diet, my patients spend only 2 days each week intermittent fasting. They spend the other 5 days eating an amazing variety of foods—from

BONE BROTH DIET DEVOTEES

Lora Probert

BEFORE   AFTER

Lora, who was part of my test group in Detroit, had asked her doctor for a referral to a therapist because she couldn't handle her intense food cravings. She wanted to lose weight, but when food was in front of her, she told me, "I had to eat it. If I saw it, I wanted it. It was a real struggle."

When she started the Bone Broth Diet, Lora didn't believe me when I said she'd eventually lose those cravings. But she did. During the diet, she went to four birthday parties and didn't have any urge to eat the cakes, cupcakes, or pizza.

"That to me has been really, really amazing," she says. "That I feel like I have control over my food and I'm not missing the chocolate and the cake and the ice cream. It's been life changing for me."

frittatas and stews to soups, chili, and steaks. At first they're a little worried because they feel like they're overindulging—but then they see that the numbers on the scale are dropping fast.

Why? Because they're getting rid of the foods that made them fat and replacing them with foods that accelerate fat-burning.

To understand why eliminating certain foods and adding others is so critical to losing weight, you need to know the real reason people get fat. Many doctors will tell you that it's because their patients are lazy, they're weak, or they have low willpower. But none of this is true. In reality, most people gain weight because they're doing exactly what their doctors tell them to do.

If you're one of these people, here's what you're doing.

- You're dutifully eating lots of high-carb foods like whole wheat bread, sugary low-fat yogurt, cereal, rice, and pasta. So what's the problem? To digest foods like these, your body has to churn out massive amounts of insulin. Eventually, your cells stop responding to this insulin. (This is called insulin resistance, and I'll talk more about it throughout the book). When this happens, you store more fat. In addition, a high-carb diet causes your brain to become resistant to leptin, a hormone that tells you when you're full, so you're always hungry (more on this on page 52).

- You're also following your doctor's orders by eating a diet that contains fats like canola oil and corn oil. In the process, you're loading your body with inflammatory omega-6 fatty acids and depriving it of anti-inflammatory omega-3 fatty acids. The result: sick cells and rapid weight gain.

- In addition, you're eating tons of soy—again, on the advice of your doctor. You've probably been led to believe that soy is a health food—but in reality, it's a hormone disruptor that may cause your thyroid, the "conductor" of your body's hormones, to become underactive. And hypothyroidism, in addition to making you feel sluggish and miserable, is a leading cause of obesity. In addition, soy (and particularly processed soy) has other dangerous effects I'll talk about in Chapter 4.

- Finally, you're following your doctor's advice to strictly limit egg yolks and meat and to skimp on the healthy fats in foods like cocoa, coconut, and avocado. As a result, you're missing out on crucial fat-burning and anti-inflammatory nutrients like the choline in eggs, the conjugated linoleic acid (CLA) in beef, the lauric acid in coconut oil, the anti-inflammatory phytosterols in avocado, and the polyphenolic antioxidant compounds in cocoa.

I'll talk more about all of this in later chapters. For now, the message you need to know is that your weight gain isn't your fault. It's the fault of doctors who continue to hand out diet advice that's decades out of date and actively harmful. This is why nearly 90 percent of diets fail.

To me, that statistic is astonishing—and completely unacceptable. As a weight-loss transformation expert, I need to have a success rate close to 100 percent. Otherwise, I'd be out of a job. And worse yet, my patients would still be overweight, sick, and miserable.

So I won't offer you a traditional diet plan that's never worked and never will. Instead, I'll show you how to center your 5 nonfasting days on real foods that have powerful fat-burning properties. These are the natural foods your body is meant to eat—and when you eat them, you will lose weight. And that's not all: These foods are natural de-agers as well.

Here's what these foods do.

- **They cause your insulin levels to drop rapidly.** Insulin packs on fat—something I'll talk about at length later. When you eat foods that minimize insulin spikes, you begin to lose that fat. In particular, you'll get rid of that "muffin top" or "beer belly" fat around your abdomen.

- **They normalize your leptin levels.** When your leptin levels are optimal (see page 52), your brain can tell when you're full. Result: those constant food cravings become history.

- **They nourish and rejuvenate your body.** These foods push nutrition into your cells, smoothing your skin, energizing your body, and speeding your metabolism. At the same time, they provide nutrients (for instance, glycine—see Chapter 3) that help pull toxins out of your body, cleansing it of harmful substances that age you and put pounds on.

- **They're anti-inflammatory.** These foods are rich in anti-inflammatory nutrients like omega-3 fatty acids, choline, vitamins, and phytosterols, which heal sick and inflamed cells, making them "bounce." And when your cells bounce, you burn off weight fast and your skin—which is highly sensitive to internal inflammation—becomes radiant.

- **Several of them are lipotropic.** Lipotropic foods help carry fat away from your liver, burning extra calories and shaving off pounds.

When you eat these foods 5 days a week, you'll quickly flip your body's fat-burning switch from off to on. And when that happens, the stubborn pounds that wouldn't come off will start to disappear.

MY CHALLENGE TO YOU: GIVE ME 3 WEEKS

If you've tried dozens of diets without success, I know that you're probably skeptical about trying new ones—and I understand where you're coming from (especially since standard low-calorie and low-fat diets actually make you gain weight, not lose it). I know that emotionally and physically, it can be tough to commit to another diet. I also know that if you've tried total fasts and felt miserable, the word *fast* is a little scary. And if you haven't tried bone broth yet, it may sound a little . . . well . . . crazy.

But here is my promise to you: *This program will work.* I know because in my practice I see it work every day. And it won't just make you thinner; it'll also take years off your face.

So give me 3 weeks.

That's all I asked of Jenny, the patient I talked about earlier. And it's all I'm asking of you.

Here's my challenge: Whether you're battling an extra 15 pounds or an extra 200 pounds, decide that it's time to take your life back. It's time to feel healthy, young, and sexy again. And it's time to stop feeling fat, tired, and invisible.

That ends right now . . . with me.

"What gets measured gets managed," as the saying goes. So before you get started, check out the Bone Broth Diet measurement tracker in the Appendix (see page 371) or on the Resources page of my website: drkellyann.com /resources.

CHAPTER 2

The Basics of the Bone Broth Diet

IN THIS CHAPTER, I'M going to give you a quick overview of the Bone Broth Diet. I promise I'll get to that in a minute. However, before we talk about what you'll do on this diet, I want to talk about three things I don't want you to do. That's because I know how many times diets have failed you in the past—and I want you to know that this one is different.

....

Charlie, a former college soccer player, came to me because at 30, he was getting a beer belly. After two failed diets, he figured he'd just learn to learn to live with it. But his wife saw me on TV and insisted that he come to see me.

"So tell me what to count," Charlie said right off the bat.

"What?" I asked.

He sighed. "Just tell me what to count. You know—calories, carbs, fat grams, whatever. I'll do it."

I laughed. "Nothing. You're not going to count anything. You're just going to eat."

He looked bewildered. And he said, "No, really. What am I supposed to count?"

....

I'm guessing that, like Charlie, you equate dieting with counting calories, grams of fat, or carbs or with endlessly weighing out tiny portions on a scale. (Some of my patients' former doctors even ordered them to take their scales to restaurants.) What's more, I'm betting that you also equate dieting with eating dry, tasteless food. And finally, I'm sure you equate dieting with being desperately hungry and not being able to eat. If so, here's how my diet is different.

- I don't want you to count calories.
- I don't want you to count grams of fat.
- I don't want you to count carbs (you'll control them naturally).
- I don't want you to force yourself to eat idiotic, tasteless "diet" foods like dry toast, egg-white omelets, and fat-free yogurt. Instead, I want you to eat real food.
- I don't want you to ever, ever say, "I'm starving, but I can't eat right now."

Okay? No counting. No tasteless diet food. And even more important: no starving. One of the worst things about ill-conceived approaches like low-calorie and low-fat diets is that they drive people into desperate hunger—and that absolutely guarantees failure.

On this diet, you'll have five or six meals of bone broth on your mini-fast days. On nonfasting days, you'll have three full meals plus two snacks. And if you get hungry anyway, there are "extras" you can grab. So promise yourself right now: "If I get really hungry, I will eat."

Good. And now I have just one more thing I want you to say to yourself. And that is: "If I do cheat and eat something that's not on my diet, I won't hate myself and feel like I'm a loser. I'll just move on to the next moment in my life and start the diet over."

Why am I stressing this? For two reasons.

First, stuff happens. Believe me, I know this firsthand. If you carefully plan your 3-week diet and then things go wrong—you total your car, lose out on a promotion, or go through a breakup—then it's possible that you're going to give in to the temptation to console yourself with pizza or a carton of ice cream. And I totally get that, because I've been there.

If this happens, beating yourself up afterward won't make anything better. Here's what I want you to understand: Stress hormones are made from fat and sugar. So when you stress more, guess what your body naturally craves—sugar and fat. Of course, eating crappy food will just cause you more stress . . . and that stress will tempt you to overeat again and again.

There's another good reason to avoid beating yourself up if you eat a candy bar or drink a soda. One big key to why this diet works is that it cuts out sugar and sugary carbs. But here's the thing: If you have a sweet tooth, there's a good chance you're actually addicted to these foods. If that's the case, it might take you a few tries to wean yourself. (I'll talk more about this in Chapter 4.)

And you know what I have to say about that? It's perfectly fine. Think of sugary foods as that bad lover you keep going back to. Eventually, you'll break free. I have confidence in you.

If you give in to temptation and break your diet because you had a bad day or the Sugar Demon got to you, here's what I want you to do: Simply realize that you're a beautifully imperfect human being, and sometimes you're going to screw up. And guess what: That's perfectly fine, as long as you don't stay stuck in your screwup. So just say *next*, move on to the next moment in your life, and start your 3-week clock over again. (I'll talk a lot more in Chapter 14 about the power of *next*.)

So okay. There are your ground rules: No counting. No eating tasteless non-food or starving. No beating yourself up if you slip up.

Now let's get down to the basics.

IS THE BONE BROTH DIET RIGHT FOR YOU?

The Bone Broth Diet is an extraordinarily safe and healthy diet. In fact, I believe it's the healthiest diet on the planet. My patients love what it does for their waist-lines, their skin, and their well-being.

However, there are two situations in which I don't recommend this diet: if you're pregnant or if you're nursing. Millions of pregnant women do fast on religious holidays, and there's no evidence that it's harmful—but until we're absolutely sure it's fine, don't do it.

In addition, if any of these conditions apply to you, check with your doctor before starting the diet.

Diabetes. The Bone Broth Diet is an outstanding choice for people with diabetes, and I've used variations of it to reverse diabetes and metabolic syndrome in many patients. (Metabolic syndrome, a precursor to diabetes, is a group of symptoms including large waist size, elevated blood glucose levels, high blood pressure, and unhealthy cholesterol levels.) However, because this diet can swiftly lower your blood sugar levels, your doctor will need to monitor you very closely if you're diabetic to make sure you don't experience dangerous hypoglycemia. Start this diet only if your doctor is on board and agrees to carefully supervise you.

Other chronic health problems. The Bone Broth Diet frequently reduces or even eliminates symptoms of autoimmune disorders, gastrointestinal disorders, and many other conditions. Just make sure to get the nod from your doctor if you have any chronic health problems like these. Also, ask your doctor if intermittent fasting will affect your medications, if you're taking any.

An eating disorder. If you have any history of an eating disorder such as bulimia, anorexia nervosa, or orthorexia, make sure your doctor says that it's okay for you to follow this or any other diet plan.

An acute illness or injury. One of the reasons fasting works so well is that it challenges your body. But if you're already being challenged by an infection or injury, this isn't the time to add more stress.

Finally, while this diet can be beneficial for overweight children, be sure to get a doctor's permission before putting any child under the age of 18 on it.

HOW LONG WILL YOU WANT TO STAY ON THE BONE BROTH DIET?

The Bone Broth Diet is basically a 3-week program for taking off weight fast. That's why I'm giving you 3 weeks' worth of recipes and meal plans. However, you can stay on this diet as long as you want. I have patients who've lost more than 100 pounds by staying on it for months. If you want to stick with it longer than 3 weeks, you can rotate back through the recipes and menu plans I've outlined, or you can get creative and make up your own recipes. After 21 days, you'll know which foods to eat and which to avoid, so it'll be easy to get adventurous in the kitchen.

My advice is to initially commit to the Bone Broth Diet for 3 weeks. At the outset of the diet, weigh yourself and take your measurements. (You'll find a handy measurement tracker in the Appendix and on the Resources page on my website, drkellyann.com/resources.) When you're finished, see if you've lost all of the weight and inches you wanted to lose.

If you're excited about your results but you want to shed still more weight, then stick with the diet longer. Once you're happy with what the scale says, you can use my maintenance program to keep the weight off and keep your skin looking young. (I'll tell you more about this program in Chapter 5.)

If you're following the 3-week plan and you do have a "beautifully imperfect" moment at any point, simply start your 3-week clock again. This diet is so easy and so rewarding that spending a little extra time on it won't seem like punishment. I pretty much live on this diet, and I never feel deprived.

Now, one final note. More than 90 percent of people start losing weight right away on this diet. Typically, they lose at least 15 pounds in 3 weeks. Every once in a while, however, it takes a little longer. (I'll discuss some reasons for this later in this chapter.) So if you hit or even pass the 2-week mark and the inches aren't falling off as fast as you'd like, hang in there. As my next story shows, the payoff can be huge.

....

Drew's wife, Pam, called me from a hospital parking lot, crying. Doctors had just told Drew that he was diabetic. At nearly 500 pounds, he had a sky-high blood sugar level (around 350, three times the normal level). Pam, a nurse, knew that Drew was at terribly high risk for diabetic complications or even death.

I told Pam, "I can help." Immediately, I put Drew on an earlier version of my Bone Broth Diet. Because he was so overweight, I expected the pounds to fall off like crazy. But I was startled when hardly anything happened for the first 3 weeks. The numbers didn't budge. I'd actually never seen anything like it before.

Luckily, Drew was determined because he knew his life was at stake. So he stuck it out, and at the end of week 3, bam!—the magic happened. I don't know what it was about that 3-week mark, but suddenly his pounds melted away. In addition, his blood sugar and bad cholesterol levels dropped like a rock. And it kept on happening, week after week.

Overall, Drew lost 212 pounds in a little over a year. He's no longer diabetic, and at the age of 59, he told me, "I feel like I'm 29."

By the way, Pam, who'd been worried only about helping Drew lose weight and get healthy, got two surprises of her own when she went on the diet to support him. First, she lost 40 pounds herself, going from a size 10 to a size 4. In addition, her skin became so beautiful that people asked her if she'd had plastic surgery.

....

What's the moral? If you're one of those rare people like Drew and you're getting close to the 3-week mark without losing many pounds, promise me that you'll stick it out. Once your transformation starts, there'll be no stopping it!

WHAT RESULTS CAN YOU EXPECT ON THE BONE BROTH DIET?

In my experience, patients lose anywhere from 10 to 15 pounds when they spend 3 weeks on the diet. However, that's anecdotal evidence—even though I've seen the same results in thousands of people. So to confirm my own findings, I set up three independent trials run by different clinicians in three different cities: Detroit, Los Angeles, and New York City. The participants in the trials stayed on the diet for 21 days, and here is what the data showed.

- Participants lost up to 15 pounds and up to 4 inches in their measurements.
- Their wrinkles and "double chins" diminished, their skin tone evened out, and their acne healed.
- They felt healthier. Two participants no longer required insulin after the diet, one was able to radically decrease her insulin dose, and one person's shingles cleared up.
- They slept better.
- They felt better emotionally. As one participant put it, "I feel happy again."

You can read participants' testimonials and see photos of their results throughout the book. You can find many of these success stories at drkellyann .com/success-stories. Since that time, thousands more people have done the diet, and I have testimonial after testimonial from people who took off their extra pounds and—better yet—are keeping the weight off effortlessly for the first time in their lives.

WHY DOES THE BONE BROTH DIET ERASE WRINKLES?

Most diets actually wreck your skin. That's because they pull water, healthy fats, and other nutrients out of your skin cells, weakening and aging these cells. But on this diet, at the same time as you're losing weight, you'll be losing wrinkles and getting your "glow" back.

Does that sound too good to be true? If so, it's because you've been conditioned to think that the only way to erase wrinkles is from the outside in—with injections, creams, or surgery. But that's not correct. In reality, the best way to erase wrinkles permanently is to do it from the inside out.

Think of your skin cells as healthy, bouncy balls. As you age, they start to lose their bounce and get tired and flabby. (Picture rows and rows of soccer balls slowly deflating.) As a result, your skin matrix becomes weak, rapidly accelerating the formation of wrinkles. At the same time, if you're eating a diet high in inflammatory grains and sugar and deficient in healthy fats and other key nutrients, your skin gets dry, flaky, rough, and sick—and dry, sick skin wrinkles quickly and deeply.

When you drink bone broth, you'll mainline the building blocks of collagen straight to your cells, "reinflating" them. It's better than Botox because it lasts. Remember, Botox's job is to paralyze the muscles to prevent wrinkles. It doesn't and never will build or replace collagen.

On the Bone Broth Diet, you'll build strong and resilient skin cell walls with healthy fats, and you'll reverse inflammation with anti-inflammatory foods. Plus, you'll load your body with nutrients that protect against photoaging (for instance, the potent anthocyanins in berries).

If you want evidence of how powerful the wrinkle-blasting effects of food are, I'm proof. I'm over 50 years old, I've never had surgery or used Botox, and I always get compliments on my skin. I don't say this to try to impress you, but to impress upon you that you can have beautiful skin at any age. It all happens with food.

HOW THE BONE BROTH DIET WORKS

Are you ready to start losing weight and have younger, healthier skin? Then let's get down to the basics of this diet.

On the Bone Broth Diet, you'll have 2 bone broth fast days per week. The other 5 days, you'll eat three full meals and two bone broth snacks each day. Here's an example.

Becky's Diet

Remember: You can pick any 2 nonconsecutive days for your fast days.

SUN	MON	TUES	WED	THURS	FRI	SAT
Mini-Fast Day	Nonfasting Day	Nonfasting Day	Mini-Fast Day	Nonfasting Day	Nonfasting Day	Nonfasting Day
6 cups of bone broth (or 5 cups plus a 7:00 p.m. snack)	3 meals of "yes" foods per day plus 2 bone broth snacks	3 meals of "yes" foods per day plus 2 bone broth snacks	6 cups of bone broth (or 5 cups plus a 7:00 p.m. snack)	3 meals of "yes" foods per day plus 2 bone broth snacks	3 meals of "yes" foods per day plus 2 bone broth snacks	3 meals of "yes" foods per day plus 2 bone broth snacks

How will your mini-fast days work?

You can pick any days you want for your mini-fast days, and they don't need to fall on the same days each week. Just separate your 2 mini-fast days with at least 1 or 2 nonfasting days. For instance, try doing one on Sunday and the other on Thursday.

On your fast days, you have your choice of two plans.

Plan 1: Bone broth all day. You can have up to 6 cups during the day. This is 300 to 500 calories' worth per day. (You'll find easy gourmet recipes for bone broth in Chapter 6.)

Plan 2: Bone broth until 7:00 p.m., followed by a light snack or a Bone Broth Diet– approved shake. I've carefully designed these light snacks (you'll find a list in Chapter 6) to be filling without interfering with your goal of transforming your body into a fat-burning machine.

For more information on Bone Broth Diet–approved shakes, see the Resources page on my website, drkellyann.com/resources.

Which fasting plan is right for you?

I'm unique and so are you, so what works for me might not work for you. That's why I'll give you choices whenever I can. I call this your *personal play.*

Now, I prefer not to eat anything solid on fast days, because the act of chewing can trigger my brain to think that a big meal is coming. That's why I always stick to Plan 1 myself. But some people have trouble making it through the night without a little solid food before bedtime. If that sounds like you, give Plan 2 a try instead. (And if you change your mind, you can always switch plans on your next fast day.)

Plan on beginning a fast when you wake up on your fast day and ending it 24 hours later. Basically, you'll skip a breakfast, lunch, and dinner, replacing them with bone broth (and with a 7:00 p.m. snack if you choose Plan 2).

Do you want to know more about intermittent fasting? Check out "The Truth about Intermittent Fasting" on my Resources page at drkellyann.com /resources.

Should you weigh-in every day?

No, no, no! In fact, I'd like you to resolve that the scales are off-limits for the entire 21 days. Ideally, you should weigh yourself only at the start and end of your diet. (Okay—if you can't stand the suspense, weigh yourself at the end of each week. I can tell you, though, that based on my clinical experience, not weighing yourself often yields better results.)

There are two reasons to avoid focusing on the scale. First, lots of things can cause your weight to go up an extra pound or two—for instance, constipation or hormonal fluctuations (especially for women). Paying too much attention to these fluctuations can make you crazy.

And second, I want you to focus on the real goal: healing your cells. Make your cells healthy and all else will follow: weight loss, glowing skin, bright eyes, and vanishing wrinkles.

Here's what I tell my patients: Instead of weighing yourself, notice how your clothes fit at the end of each week. That's a good guide to how much weight you're losing.

How will your nonfasting days work?

On these days, as I've noted, you'll eat three full meals and two snacks. There are just two simple keys to success.

- First, you'll choose everything you eat from the "yes" foods I list in Chapter 4. And don't worry. These are really, really good foods. No dry toast, egg-white omelets, or weird stuff, I promise! And you can also have 2 cups of bone broth each day for snacks.

- Second, you'll become aware of what your body needs. So instead of weighing and measuring food, you'll simply eat mindfully rather than mindlessly. This is the beginning of your changing your relationship with food. It will feel liberating to take charge of this relationship. I'll give you some easy guidelines in Chapter 4.

Now, one thing I've learned over time is that some of my patients love to cook, some don't mind cooking, and some don't want to cook at all. So in Part II, you'll find everything from fancy recipes to easy half-hour meals and simple soups to ideas for no-cook meals. Just choose whatever works best for you and your lifestyle.

IMPORTANT! BE PREPARED FOR THE "CARB FLU"

As the Bone Broth Diet begins revitalizing your cells, you're going to feel your "sparkle" coming back. My guess is that by the time you're 2 weeks into the diet, you'll look and feel years younger. However, there's one temporary roadblock you may hit. I call it the *carb flu*.

Right now, if your cells are used to a high-sugar, high-carb diet, switching to real foods can throw them for a loop. They're like lazy kids lying on the couch, shoveling in junk food and playing video games. If you tell these kids, "Get off the couch!" you're going to get some serious attitude.

Similarly, your cells may give you a little lip when you first cut down on carbs. That's because they're used to getting their blood sugar the easy way, and now you're making them work for it.

Here's what's happening at this stage: If you've been eating a typical high-carb diet, you've been burning glucose from your diet for fuel. When you switch to a low-carbohydrate diet, your body will need to switch to fat for its primary fuel. It takes more work to create energy from fat, and your sluggish cells may complain at first. As a result, you may spend 3 to 7 days feeling mildly flulike. I describe the feeling as "tired, cranky, wired, and weird." You want to kick everything and everyone.

This stage isn't fun, but here's the good news: The carb flu phase typically comes just before the "I feel better than I have in years!" phase. In fact, this process is so predictable that I'm including a "what to expect" section later in this chapter. When you know what to anticipate, your temporary symptoms won't trip you up.

Here's a story that illustrates why knowledge is power when it comes to the carb flu. Joan, a 48-year-old woman, came to my office because she needed to lose 50 pounds. But when I told her about the Bone Broth Diet, she said, "No. I'm sorry, Dr. Kellyann. But I tried a low-carb diet before. After a week, I totally crashed. My joints ached and I was miserable. So I know that diet isn't for me."

What I knew, however, is that her former doctor—while he was on the right track diet-wise—let Joan down by failing to tell her that she was experiencing the carb flu. I explained to her that this is a totally normal and very temporary condition, and I asked her if she thought she could tough it out for a few days, explaining that she could ease her symptoms on nonfasting days by increasing her fat intake a little.

Once she knew the score, Joan said yes. And while she did indeed need to weather a mild bout of carb flu, she found that eating half an avocado or a handful of coconut chips made her feel much better. She got over her carb flu in 4 days, and after that she easily stuck with the diet, lost all of her extra weight, and took 10 years off her face.

I'm confident that, like Joan, you'll get through the carb flu just fine when you recognize it for what it is and realize that it's your body making the switch from a lazy state to a fat-blasting state. It's a mildly unpleasant transition, but think of it as a necessary in-between stage as you're transforming your metabolism from "sloth" to "cheetah."

Here's a closer look at the carb flu and related problems that can crop up in the very early days of your diet. Remember: All of this will pass quickly! Just hang tough, because this is a make-or-break time. As I guide life-changing transformations, this is one of the moments when I need my clients to stay strong. Make it past this stage and I promise you: It gets easier. Stay the course right now, and you'll thank yourself later—honest. So keep your eyes on the prize: that slimmer, younger, healthier, more energetic body that you deserve. And keep those carb flu cures close at hand in case you need them.

How You May Feel Early On

EXHAUSTED	"CARB FLU-ISH"	MOODY	ICKY
You might feel a bit low on energy, and that's completely normal. Be patient with yourself during this time, and try to keep your schedule light. If necessary, ease off the intensity of your workouts. Take a nap if you can, and aim to get to bed an hour earlier than usual so your body can rest and adapt. Also, try not to rely too much on caffeine to get you through afternoon slumps. Right now, your body is beginning its transition from using sugar as fuel to burning fat—and that's what will turn you into a super–fat-burning machine.	It's not uncommon, especially if you've typically eaten a diet high in processed carbohydrates and fast food, to feel like you're getting a cold during this time. This is more evidence that your body is transitioning from using sugar as fuel to using fat. So don't be alarmed if you feel tired or foggy headed or get the sniffles. These are signs (and temporary ones!) that your diet is working the way it's supposed to.	Are you feeling short-tempered or moody for no reason? Actually, there *is* a reason: Your brain is throwing a hissy fit because it misses sugar, bread, and all the other foods you're not giving it. Be patient. This will all pass in a few days, so don't give in to your cravings or your moodiness. That moodiness, by the way, is related to your changing blood sugar levels. Eating real foods will eventually regulate your blood sugar and have you smiling again.	While you're making the transition to a super-fat-burning state, you may experience a few other odd symptoms. These can include digestive distress, allergies, and even a little acne. These might get worse before they get better, but they will get better . . . soon! Remember that this is your body removing toxins and healing itself. It's just throwing a small temper tantrum while it does this. At the end of that tantrum, you'll be rewarded with a shrinking waistline, clearer skin, fewer wrinkles, glossier hair, and glowing health.

One good way to cope with the carb flu is to keep a daily journal during your diet, describing how you feel physically, mentally, and emotionally. This will help you spot symptoms of carb flu and identify the point at which your symptoms end and you start to feel energized and revitalized. You can also use your journal to describe your cravings for "cheats" (and to congratulate yourself when you resist them!).

In addition, consider recruiting an ally—someone who can keep you on course if you start to waver. Even better, see if you can find someone who'll go on the diet with you. That way, you can support each other during those carb flu days and celebrate together when they're over.

A DAY-BY-DAY LOOK AT WHAT TO ANTICIPATE ON THE BONE BROTH DIET

This diet is a process. I've experienced this process myself, and I've guided many, many others through it. Based on years and years of experience, I can give you a pretty exact timetable of what most people experience as they go through this process.

Don't make me put my hand on a Bible and swear to this—but this is how the 21 days go for the majority of the participants on the diet. If you don't hit this timeline straight on, and you're following the plan exactly, it doesn't mean you're doing something wrong. Your body may simply be adjusting differently than the average person's. If you have a medical condition or you've been a junk-food junkie for years, you may feel more discomfort, or it may take you more time to achieve that "natural fat-burning" state. Lean into this and let your body just "do you."

If you follow the typical pattern, however, here's what I predict will happen.

DAY 1

Yeah . . . like this is a big deal.

You have your pot of broth cooking, you turned your back on the cookies at work with no effort, and you discovered that putting coconut milk instead of cow's milk in your coffee was easy. And you think, "This is gonna be too easy."

An hour later you may feel a bit nervous. Then excited. Then overwhelmed.

Doc's advice: Stay grounded today. Talk about your feelings with supportive people. And here's a warning: Don't buy into that easy-breezy bill of goods just yet. I say this to protect you.

After all . . . have you met the Sugar Demon?

DAYS 2–7

What did I get myself into? The Sugar Demon is a bitch.

This is the "I feel tired and cranky, and you'd better back off" stage I call the carb flu. You want to take a nap. You want to eat everything and *kick* everything. You wonder why you feel like you're hungover . . . is it the flu? You have achy joints and a headache, and you feel light-headed.

Doc's advice: Resist the urge to say "This isn't working out for me" and hit the eject button.

Understand clearly what's happening. You're engaging in an epic battle, whether you know it or not. Your brain is having a fit because it's not at all happy that it's being deprived of its normal rewards of sweet, salty, fatty junk foods. The Sugar Demon has arrived, and it's going to make you pay.

These days are all about awareness. If you truly understand what's going on here, you can lean into this stage and let your body deal with your new eating choices. Close your eyes (really do this) and see your body regulating your blood sugar, burning stored fat for fuel so you become a natural fat burner, regulating your hormones, relieving inflammation, and healing your gut like nobody's business.

This is what you're allowing your body to do, and you need to honor what's happening here. Cracking open a can of soda is not honoring this. Plus, it's not going to solve anything. You just have to stare the Sugar Demon right in the eye and decide to win.

Doc's advice: Here's a tip that may help. The average craving lasts only about 3 minutes. Distracting yourself is the best Rx. Do something you love for those 3 minutes. Also, remember that eating a small handful of coconut chips, a few olives, or a small piece of avocado will ease your carb flu.

DAY 8

My hangover is gone! But wait . . . Oh. My. God. My clothes feel tight. Dr. Kellyann is dead.

You feel clearheaded, full of energy, and back in the game. You throw on one of your favorite outfits to celebrate. *Grrrrrrr.* Your pants feel tighter than when you started. Talk about a buzz kill.

BONE BROTH DIET DEVOTEES

Nadine Leonardi

This is something that can be part of a life change. I was pleased to see a drop in weight [11 pounds], as nothing else has worked in the past 3 years. Well worth the effort!

Try it—you have nothing to lose but inches and weight. There are no pills or special foods to purchase. It's quite easy.

BEFORE   AFTER

Doc's advice: First of all, this is the shortest of all the phases you'll experience during the 21 days. You may not experience this even a little. But if you do, realize that nothing bad is happening here. Quite the opposite, in fact. Your body is adjusting. Period.

Your body is like any other ecosystem, and right now you are changing that ecosystem for the better. This means that the enzymes that digest your food and the trillions of bacteria that live in your gut are adjusting to new quantities of vegetables—and possibly a new intake of meat—and to living without readily available sugar. This adjustment may lead to temporary bloating, diarrhea, or constipation—or all three. If so, remember that this phase passes very quickly.

DAYS 9–11

I'm just done. I wish I hadn't told my coworkers I was doing this, because I'm tempted to quit.

By now, the excitement is wearing off. You're sick of the damn eggs and broth. You feel like the world is teasing you with its grilled cheese sandwiches and grand slam specials. You start doubting the results.

Doc's advice: Stay the course. This is important. When people throw in the towel, this is usually when they do it.

Here's what I want you to ask yourself: What were you looking for when you started this program in the first place? This phase is all mental, my friend. Food cannot offer you the emotional support you may need or fill any emptiness you feel within. It cannot relieve your stress or empower you in any way. Look for inspiration, and don't give any power to thoughts that will not serve you. You'll pass through this phase quicker than you can say "Give me the #3 supersized, please."

DAYS 12–15

Okay, I'm all in. I get it now. But what's with the dreams?

You're past the ups and downs, you're checking off the milestones, and you're starting to feel stronger, slimmer, and healthier. But wait . . . you're having some weird dreams. About food? Seriously?

Doc's advice: This is totally normal. My patients and I refer to these as guilt-free doughnut dreams. Try to look at it as a creative outlet—a food comedy broadcast in your brain. It has no meaning or significance other than this: Your brain is making one last-ditch effort to get you to remember the good old days of doughnuts and soda.

We have a deep-seated history when it comes to our relationship with food. It's no joke. Your brain is trying to trick you, and it has a whole lot of power to do so. Don't let it. Lead with your heart, not with your head, and remember all the milestones you've already passed. Wake up and laugh.

DAYS 16–18

Okay, whoa. I want to clean my entire house, have sex 24/7, and look at myself in the mirror again.

Now you're starting to see the true value of this program. You have way more energy, you're sleeping better, and you're seeing improvements in your skin and the way your clothes fit. This is when you're finally starting to "hit," as my patients and I say. Even better, everyone else is starting to notice. Yippee!

Doc's advice: Most likely you've flipped the switch at this point. You're now burning stored fat for energy, the inflammation in your body is easing, and you're feeling good. You're bursting with energy, and your cravings for junk are diminishing or even gone.

If you haven't hit yet and the magic isn't happening, it's A-OK. You're not doing anything wrong. Many factors may be in play here. If you have medical issues, you're under massive stress, or you've had poor lifestyle habits for some time, this can affect your timeline.

And that's fine. Earlier, I told you about Drew, who didn't start losing weight until day 18—and then he dropped pounds like crazy and lost more than 200 pounds over time. If you don't follow the norm, just do what Drew did: Trust that you are doing right by your body and hang tight.

BONE BROTH DIET DEVOTEES

Denise Townsend-Gamblin

BEFORE   AFTER

This diet taught me a better way to eat and manage my approach to food. I enjoyed doing this with my daughter . . . preparing meals, finding and testing recipes, shopping for good food together. . . . We loved this program.

I have osteoarthritis in both of my knees. I know it comes from inflammation, and as soon as my knees are swollen or I've done too much, they hurt. They don't hurt now.

Many of my friends have knee problems, and I have already recommended this program to several friends.

I am shocked at how my attitude has changed. I'm not as anxious or concerned. I'm more at peace. I'm more relaxed.

DAYS 19–20

Holy hot stuff, Batman. What happened here?

You look and feel amazing. You're thrilled, and you can't stop looking in the mirror. However, you may be starting to worry about what comes after the 21 days.

Doc's advice: It's perfectly normal to worry about what's next. It's how we're designed.

Here's what you need to know. You've changed your relationship with food. A big part of this change is that you now understand how certain foods make you feel. So when you're done with your 21 days, you'll simply introduce certain foods and see how you do with them. You'll learn how far you can stray from the Bone Broth Diet template without consequence. When you stray too far, you'll know what to do: Just pull back to the foods you know work for you. You're in control now. That's gotta feel good, no? Later in the book, I'll talk more about what comes after day 21.

DAY 21

Today I feel exhilaration at the most primal level.

And you should! Today is your day, and I'm so proud of you. You no

BONE BROTH DIET DEVOTEES

Beverly Deitch

I talked to the nurse practitioner today, and she reduced my insulin from 20 units down to 8. I lost about 9 pounds. Usually I'd fall asleep at some time during the day, but I can't sit still. . . . I have this energy that I didn't have before.

BEFORE

AFTER

longer feel sad, tired, old, and invisible. Instead, you're strong, radiant, beautiful, and energetic. Please write to me and tell me about your success at hello@drkellyann.com. Transformations like yours are the reason I get up in the morning.

Doc's advice: A glass of wine or a shot of potato vodka? Absolutely.

CHAPTER 3

Your Intermittent Fasting Secret to Success: "Liquid Gold"

NOW THAT YOU KNOW the basics of the Bone Broth Diet, I want to talk more about the first element of the diet—your two weekly intermittent fasts. That's because I want you to understand two things.

1. Intermittent fasting is easier than you think.

2. The payoff is huge.

Here's the bottom line: Intermittent fasting is the biggest secret to losing weight. Yes, you can take off pounds simply by following the nonfasting diet plan every day—but if you want to see incredible results in just 3 weeks, you need to add in the intermittent fasts. (I'll explain why later in this chapter.)

Now, I know that right now, the thought of intermittent fasting may make you anxious. But trust me, because I've been down this road with hundreds of patients.

Here's how it typically goes: When I tell my patients about the quick results they'll get from intermittent fasting, many of them believe me and are willing to jump right in. But others are skeptical when I tell them that doing a fast is easy. When I tell these patients that they won't be hungry because they can drink bone broth, they're still skeptical. And when I tell them that they're going to love bone broth—well, I'm pretty sure they think I'm lying.

When these patients leave my office, they aren't happy. And I'm pretty sure they aren't thinking nice thoughts about me.

Then they come back to my office 3 weeks later. They're 15 pounds lighter, and their waistlines are inches smaller. They're radiating energy. Their skin looks 10 years younger. They're so happy, they're actually bouncing. And they say, "You're right. It works."

And then they add, "And you know what? Bone broth is good."

And I say, "I told you so."

By this point, these patients have discovered what gourmets around the world already know: Bone broth is filling, fabulous, and even fun. It truly does satisfy both your psychological cravings and your physical needs. (That's why I call it liquid gold.) And it's the biggest secret to fasting without feeling deprived.

If you haven't tried bone broth yet, you might find all of this hard to believe. If so, I'm guessing that you're picturing that thin, watery broth you get out of a can or carton. But bone broth is nothing like that at all. Even if you're picturing something like the nice, rich broth you get from simmering a chicken on the stove for a couple of hours—think again.

You're about to discover that bone broth is entirely different from the broths you're used to. It's a rich, warm, satisfy-you-down-to-your-toes meal—and that's why in addition to being a hot trend today, it's been a favorite food of every culture on the planet since the dawn of time.

THE WORLD'S FIRST "FAST FOOD"

Back in the old days, families kept a huge cauldron of soup bubbling all day long on the stove or over the fire. In the old, *old* days, bone broth was one of the first foods that primitive people cooked in pots. And even earlier than that, people made broth by throwing bones, water, and heated rocks into the stomachs of animals they'd killed.

In short, bone broth is the original fast food. And it's even more convenient today than it was back in the cavepeople's day.

Why do I call bone broth fast food? Because it takes about 5 minutes to throw the ingredients for a basic bone broth together. (That's less time than it takes to drive to a fast-food restaurant.) After that, your stove, slow cooker, or Instant Pot does all the work. Food just doesn't get any faster or easier than that.

While you'll throw your broth together quickly, it'll cook for hours if you make it on the stovetop or in the slow cooker—so in addition to being a fast food, it's a slow food. As it cooks, it'll envelop your home in a warm, comforting aroma. There's nothing more soothing than a savory bone broth, loaded with onions, carrots, garlic, and spices, simmering slowly and aromatically on a back burner all day. I think it's the ultimate aromatherapy.

And then there's the taste—wow. It's why trendy restaurants from L.A. to Manhattan are selling bone broth faster than they can make it and why they can charge insane prices for it. Turkey bone broth is like Thanksgiving in a bowl. Beef and chicken bone broths are luscious, warm, and mouthwatering. Fish bone broth is subtle and sophisticated.

The reason bone broth is far more complex and full flavored than the broths or soups you're used to is that it cooks for hours and hours. (I cook mine on the stove for at least 6 hours for chicken and up to 48 hours for beef bones.) As the broth simmers away, the bones start to dissolve, releasing amino acids, minerals, vitamins, and other nutrients that provide "deep nutrition." Our bodies crave this nutrition, so bone broth satisfies us on a cellular level in a way that most foods can't.

Here's my prediction: You will love bone broth so much that even when you finish your diet, you'll want to keep making it and eating it forever. And I hope you will—because in addition to tasting heavenly, it does wonderful things for your body. Here's a closer look at those remarkable health benefits I touched on back in Chapter 1.

THE WEIGHT-LOSS, HEALING, AND ANTI-AGING PROPERTIES OF BONE BROTH

When you drink bone broth, you just feel good all over. And on the inside, your cells are celebrating, too. That's because bone broth contains these potent fat-burning and cell-energizing nutrients.

Collagen and gelatin

Do you want to lose weight and have younger-looking skin? Then think *collagen* and *gelatin*.

Collagen is an integral part of bone, containing a large supply of amino acids. When you cook bone broth for a long time, the collagen in the bones turns into gelatin. Here's what that gelatin does for you.

- **Gelatin strengthens your skin.** There's a reason women have used gelatin for centuries to help keep their skin smooth. The nutrients in gelatin provide you with the building blocks of collagen—and collagen is like natural Botox, erasing wrinkles and reversing sagging and stretch marks. For more information on why collagen is your liquid gold, go to the Resources page on my website, drkellyann.com/resources.

- **Gelatin fights inflammation.** Research shows that even basic chicken soup helps quell inflammation by preventing proinflammatory immune cells called neutrophils from moving to an inflamed area.[1] The glycine from the gelatin in bone broth—an amino acid that has so many important jobs that I'll discuss it in another section later—is even more powerful, inhibiting both local and systemic inflammation. And remember my formula from Chapter 1: *Less inflammation equals faster weight loss.* Lowering inflammation also reduces symptoms of autoimmune disorders, which is why my patients with arthritis, celiac disease, and psoriasis swear by the healing powers of bone broth.

■ **Gelatin heals your gut.** Researchers speculate that gelatin stabilizes your gut mucosa by decreasing damage from excess acid or increasing protective mechanisms such as gastric mucosal bloodflow.[2] Studies also reveal that the glycine in gelatin heals and protects the gut via its anti-inflammatory, immune regulatory, and cell-protective activities.[3, 4, 5]

This last point—gut health—is so important that I want to talk more about it right now. Most people (and even most doctors) don't fully appreciate that to be slim and healthy, you need to have a rock-solid gut. Here's why.

You have about 25 feet of intestines, and about 1,500 different species of bacteria and other flora live in them. That's trillions of gut microbes. It's strange to think about these alien beings living inside you, but in reality, they're working hard for you. They make enzymes that help you digest food, they produce hormones and help synthesize vitamins, and they clean up toxins.

Unfortunately, the modern world isn't kind to your gut flora. A typical diet high in sugar, carbs, and artificial chemicals and low in critical nutrients can kill off huge swaths of beneficial flora, while allowing levels of bad bacteria to skyrocket. Infections, antibiotics, nonsteroidal anti-inflammatory drugs (NSAIDs), stress, diet, alcohol, and many medications can also unbalance your gut flora.

This is dangerous, because when bad flora take control in your intestines, they cause inflammation that damages your gut wall. The result is intestinal permeability, or "leaky gut." In this condition, your weakened gut barrier allows toxins and digestive debris that should stay trapped inside your gut to escape from it instead.

Your immune system quickly spots these intruders and goes on the attack—often violently. The result is systemic inflammation that packs on pounds, makes you feel miserable, and makes your skin look terrible.

In addition to the problems stemming from increased intestinal permeability, an unhealthy gut makes you prone to infections and disease. That's because 80 percent of your immune system is inside your gut—and when your gut is sick, this system can't work correctly. So you're easier prey for the flu, coronaviruses like the one that caused the 2020 pandemic, or even autoimmune diseases or cancer.

Gelatin helps restore the integrity of your intestines, healing a leaky gut and optimizing your immune function. This in turn makes extra pounds slide off more easily and sets off a cascade of other positive changes throughout your entire body. For instance, I've treated patients whose acne, arthritis, headaches, allergies, ADHD, dizziness, or fibromyalgia cleared up like magic when they cut out processed foods and added bone broth (and other healing foods I'll talk about in Chapter 4) to their diets.

By the way, adding powdered gelatin to your diet—not the sugary, artificially colored and flavored stuff in a box, but natural gelatin—can also help heal your gut. In addition, it can give you strong hair and nails. You'll find some great gelatin recipes in Chapter 8.

"POWER UP" YOUR RESULTS BY COMBINING BONE BROTH AND HYDROLYZED COLLAGEN!

In addition to getting the building blocks of collagen from bone broth, you can use *hydrolyzed collagen* in your shakes for a double dose of fat-melting, anti-aging power.

What's the difference between the two? Bone broth contains the building blocks of collagen in the form of gelatin, which is cooked collagen. Hydrolyzed collagen (which is collagen broken down into short pieces called peptides) gives you a big dose of collagen in a highly assimilable powder form.

Both hydrolyzed collagen and bone broth will give you the gut-healing, skin-smoothing, nail-strengthening, hair-beautifying collagen you want. But bone broth is also rich in other nutrients including glucosamine, chondroitin, hyaluronic acid, and minerals like magnesium. That's why I'm big on including *both* collagen and bone broth in your daily regimen.

Vitamins, minerals, fats, and alkylglycerols

One surprising thing about bone broth is that it's not high in the one nutrient you'd expect: calcium. However, the calcium that's present in bone broth is highly bioavailable (that is, easy for your body to absorb) because broth is an optimal vehicle for transporting it—along with other minerals that bone broth contains in larger amounts, like phosphorus, magnesium, and iodine (in fish broth). This bioavailability means that these nutrients can have powerful effects.

■ The iodine in fish broth helps regulate your thyroid hormones, while the calcium in all types of bone broths helps keep your endocrine hormones in balance—and balanced hormones are crucial to efficient metabolism and weight loss.

- The phosphorus in bone broth plays a critical role in energizing your cells.
- The magnesium in bone broth enhances your digestion and repairs your skin.

Bone marrow—the jellylike substance at the heart of the bone—is also a nutritional treasure trove. For instance, it's an outstanding source of healthy fats, and it contains iron and vitamin A. In addition, it contains compounds called alkylglycerols that can help protect you against cancer by boosting your immune system function. In fact, marrow is so nutritionally dense that wild animals will actually break the bones of their prey and eat the marrow first, before even touching the meat!

Joint-protecting nutrients

Joints are the spots where the bones in your body meet. These joints contain cartilage, which is like a slippery Teflon coating that allows your joints to slide over each other without grinding.

Animal bones contain cartilage, too. (The stuff on the end of a chicken drumstick, for instance, is cartilage.) In addition to being rich in the collagen building blocks I talked about earlier, cartilage is packed with glucosamine and chondroitin sulfate—the very same nutrients many doctors prescribe as supplements to keep joints young and healthy.

Some arthritis experts are skeptical about the effects of oral glucosamine and chondroitin on joint pain. However, a randomized, double-blind clinical trial[6] found that oral chondroitin and glucosamine are as effective as the arthritis drug Celebrex in reducing pain, swelling, and functional limitation caused by knee osteoarthritis. (Notably, glucosamine and chondroitin also have a perfect safety profile, while Celebrex [celecoxib] significantly increases the risk of heart attack and stroke.)

That's not all that these two nutrients do. In another study,[7] researchers noted that long-term use of glucosamine and chondroitin supplements "is associated with lower incidence of colorectal and lung cancers and with lower mortality." To find out why, the researchers asked overweight people to take these nutrients or a placebo for about a month. At the end of the month, the people taking glucosamine and chondroitin had far lower levels of C-reactive protein, a marker for inflammation. The researchers conclude, "Glucosamine and chondroitin supplementation may lower systemic inflammation and alter other pathways in healthy, overweight individuals." It's like I keep saying: *Everything circles back to inflammation.*

By the way, glucosamine and chondroitin aren't the only joint-healing nutrients in bone broth. It also contains hyaluronic acid, which lubricates your joints and muscles. One study[8] found that oral hyaluronic acid caused "statistically significant improvements in pain and function" in obese people with knee osteoarthritis. In addition, hyaluronic acid hydrates your skin,[9] erasing fine wrinkles. So along with happier joints, it'll give you smoother skin.

Glycine and other key amino acids

Bone broth is brimming with amino acids that are classified as "conditional" rather than "essential" because under ideal conditions, the body can make enough of these amino acids without getting them from food. But in today's stressed-out, toxified world, it's a good bet that you're not getting enough of some or all of them. Luckily, you can obtain an ample supply of four key conditional amino acids—glycine, proline, arginine, and glutamine—from bone broth. Here's a quick look at each one.

I mentioned earlier that glycine plays a key role in fighting inflammation. It's also one of the key building blocks of collagen. But that's just one of this amino acid's many roles. Here are still more.

- It's a key part of a liver detoxification pathway, helping to ferry toxins out of your body.

- It reduces oxidative damage (damage to cells that is caused by unstable molecules).[10]

- It enhances insulin sensitivity, making it easier for your body to burn fat and reducing your risk of metabolic syndrome and diabetes.[11]

- It helps regulate the secretion of human growth hormone, powering up fat-burning.[12]

- It helps you sleep well[13] (and, as I'll discuss in Chapter 12, sleeping soundly helps you take off pounds even faster).

Your body needs a good supply of proline, arginine, and glutamine to keep your muscles, joints, gut, and skin healthy. Proline helps your body synthesize proteins, metabolize food well, heal wounds, and protect itself against oxidative stress. Arginine has wound-healing properties,[14] may help prevent erectile dysfunction,[15] and may protect against Alzheimer's disease.[16] Glutamine is a powerful gut healer and may even protect against ulcers.[17]

For Dr. Kellyann's Bone Broth Diet–approved supplements, visit the Resources page on my website, drkellyann.com/resources.

A VICTORIAN CURE-ALL?

As a kid, did you read old-fashioned novels in which spunky heroines like Pollyanna went around delivering calf's foot jelly to invalids? I used to shudder whenever I read that.

Now, however, I know that these do-gooders really were doing a good deed. That's because in an age when antibiotics and fever reducers didn't exist, calf's foot jelly (basically, a bone broth made from calves' hooves and then chilled until it jelled) was one of the most powerful immune system enhancers and anti-inflammatories around. In fact, in the early 1900s, calf's foot jelly was one of the primary treatments hospitals offered to soothe patients' inflammation and help them heal.

However, if it's all the same to you, I'll take my bone broth steamy hot in a mug instead!

As you can see, bone broth isn't simply a fun and trendy food—it's a systemic healer, revitalizer, and metabolism optimizer. When you add up all of bone broth's nutritional benefits, it's easy to understand why every culture around the world believes in its healing power. Jewish grandmothers who treat colds with chicken broth, Caribbean parents who give their kids "cow foot soup" when they're sick, and Korean healers who prescribe fish bone broth to enhance immune function and promote weight loss all prove that the famed Middle Ages physician Maimonides was right when he said that soup is "an excellent food as well as medication."

BONE BROTH + FASTING = DYNAMITE WEIGHT LOSS

Bone broth fills you up and satisfies you deep down, and it makes it easy for you to stick to a fast. That's critical, because fasting is one of the biggest keys to turning your body into a fat-burning machine.

Back in Chapter 1, I outlined some keys ways in which fasting revs up weight loss. Now I want to talk more about how it dramatically changes your biochemistry and your metabolism.

Here's the primary thing to understand about fasting: It works because it stresses your body. (This is similar to making your muscles stronger by stressing them during a workout.) Now, you may think of stress as a bad thing—and that's true for chronic stress. (In fact, I talk in Chapters 13 and 14 about why you need to lower your stress levels if you want to stay slim for life.) But a quick dose of

FALSE FEARS ABOUT LEAD

In 2013, researchers in Britain alarmed bone broth fans everywhere when they reported finding high levels of lead in bone broth made from organic chickens.[18] Since I prescribe bone broth and drink it myself every day, you can believe that I was worried.

Fortunately, people following up on this study found no evidence to support its findings. For example, the National Food Lab tested and retested bone broth from grass-fed beef and pastured chicken and found no lead in either one.[19] These findings are very reassuring. So is an earlier study[20] in *Food Additives and Contaminants,* which found only very small traces of lead in a beef bone broth—less than in a beef casserole containing red wine. The levels were far below those considered to be concerning, and the researchers actually determined the primary source of lead in food was tap water.

After doing my own research, I've concluded that this is basically a nonissue. If you're following the 3-week diet, you can use either organic or nonorganic meat without concern (although I strongly recommend organic if you can afford it). If you plan to stay on the diet longer or make bone broth a regular part of any diet, just make sure you purchase pastured or organic meat. Also, consider using distilled or filtered water in your broth to eliminate any traces of lead from this source.

stress is like Mother Nature's energy drink. It revs up your cells' defenses and healing mechanisms, and it sends your body's fat-burning machinery into overdrive.

Here's what happens when you do a fast:

■ **Your insulin levels plummet.** As I said earlier, insulin puts on pounds. In fact, insulin is the biggest driver of excess weight. The bottom line is, excess insulin lays down fat.

When your insulin levels are chronically high, your cells react by becoming insulin resistant. This means that when insulin knocks on the door of a cell and asks to escort glucose in, the cell is likely to slam the door in its face. This forces your body to reroute that glucose to your liver, where it gets transformed into fat.

When your insulin levels drop on your intermittent fasting days, your cells will rapidly start becoming more sensitive to insulin. Rather than barring the door to it, they'll welcome it in, along with its package of glucose—so that glucose will get burned as fuel rather than wind up on your waistline.

■ **You burn more existing body fat.** To get rid of fat, you need to break fatty acids out of your fat stores and get them into your bloodstream. This is called lipolysis, and it depends on glucagon—a hormone whose job is the opposite of insulin's. While insulin escorts glucose out of the bloodstream, glucagon ushers it back in.

When you fast, here's what happens: Within hours, your glucose levels start to drop, and your body realizes that it needs to mobilize its fuel reserves. In response, it churns out large amounts of glucagon. Rising levels of glucagon cause your body to start releasing fatty acids into your bloodstream so they can be transported to your cells for burning. The result: Fat, and in particular belly fat (which is easily mobilized), melts away.

In addition, fasting causes your levels of adrenaline and norepinephrine to rise. These hormones rev up the amount of energy you burn at rest, making your body pull even more fat from your stores.

■ **You clean up your cells.** When you fast, your body has a chance to "take out the trash." You can't do this efficiently if you're always eating.

■ **You lower inflammation.** I know I keep coming back to that word *inflammation*. But remember that anything that increases inflammation puts on weight and makes you look older, and anything that reduces inflammation takes off weight and makes you look younger. And fasting fights inflammation at its roots.

Recently, researchers at Yale reported that fasting makes your body release a compound called beta-hydroxybutyrate, or BHB.[21] BHB inhibits one part of a set of proteins called the inflammasome—and when you inhibit the inflammasome, you knock out inflammation. That translates into easier weight loss, as well as a healthier body and even healthier skin.

■ **You optimize your immune system.** In a 2019 study, researchers found that during fasting, memory T cells become better at protecting the body. When mice in the study were injected with a pathogen they had already encountered, the fasting mice cleared the infection in two days while it took well-fed mice a week.[22] A second study, also conducted in 2019, found that fasting reduces the inflammatory activity of cells called monocytes. In this study, fasting lowered inflammation in mice with multiple sclerosis–like symptoms[23]—an effect also seen in some human trials of fasting for people with MS.[24]

■ **You beef up your levels of BDNF.**[25] Intermittent fasting increases your levels of a protein called brain-derived neurotrophic factor (BDNF). This protein improves your insulin sensitivity, accelerating weight loss—and as a bonus, it helps you think more clearly and brightens your mood.

■ **Your levels of human growth hormone (HGH) surge.** During a 24-hour fast, HGH increases an average of 1,300 percent in women and nearly 2,000 percent in men.[26] As I mentioned earlier, this hormone helps you burn fat faster and sculpts lean muscle. It also promotes healthy skin, thus reducing wrinkles.

■ **You even increase your life span!** Studies show that fasting animals live longer. They're also less prone to cancer, heart disease, and other age-linked diseases.

Recently, researchers at the University of Florida asked 24 people to alternate 1 day of fasting with 1 day of overeating for 3 weeks. They found that

Bone Broth and Your Hormones

Tami Meraglia, MD, bestselling author of *The Hormone Secret*
drtami.com

Dr. Tami, as her patients call her, is one of my best friends and a renowned expert on anti-aging techniques and the role of hormones in health. Here's what she has to say about the anti-aging hormonal effects of bone broth.

"Let me introduce you to your adrenal glands, two very tiny glands the size of a walnut that sit on top of your kidneys. The adrenals are best known for releasing the hormone cortisol, which is often called the stress hormone. But in truth, the adrenals do so much more. They produce testosterone, estrogen, progesterone, and DHEA. Their job is especially important in women past childbearing age, when the ovaries have completed their work.

"Every athlete knows that muscular strength and endurance are affected by the adrenal hormones known as steroids. And did you know that the adrenals also affect skin, blood pressure, blood sugar, sleep, the immune system, muscle building, and electrolyte balance? If you've noticed your waist expanding as you get older, you can blame the adrenals' impact on the distribution of fat. Even cardiovascular and gastrointestinal functioning is affected by these glands. Your entire health state suffers when the adrenals perform poorly.

"Why am I telling you all this? Because in the last 10 years, a condition called adrenal fatigue has become one of the most common threats to our well-being. Yet adrenal fatigue is frequently misdiagnosed or, worse, missed as a diagnosis, this feast-and-famine cycle caused an up-regulation of a gene that produces a protein called SIRT3. SIRT3 triggers protective responses in cells exposed to stress.

The researchers believe that fasting slightly increases oxidative stress—damage to cells caused by unstable molecules—causing protective responses to kick in. While prolonged oxidative stress is very bad for your body, the researchers hypothesize that "if the body is intermittently exposed to low levels of oxidative stress, it can build a better response to it."

How powerful an antiaging effect can fasting have? In one study,[27] researchers tested the effects of a "fast-mimicking diet" designed to create the same changes as fasting (for instance, low glucose levels and high levels of ketone bodies—which also occur on my diet). They asked their study subjects to follow the diet for 5 days a month for 3 months. The result: Compared with

despite being present in the medical literature since the 1800s.

"Adrenal fatigue is a general collection of symptoms that affects multiple body systems and can literally hijack your quality of life. Do you feel tired when you wake in the morning and fatigued throughout the day? Do you experience the 3:00 p.m. crash? Are you grumpy or depressed? Are you gaining weight even though you're not eating more or exercising less? If you answered yes to one or more of these questions, you may be battling this condition. Adrenal fatigue drains your hormones, causing deficiencies that can turn your life upside down. Even a mild case stops you from looking and feeling your best.

"The great news is that adrenal fatigue can be healed by what and when you eat, supplements, and lifestyle changes. An amazing and powerful form of food to heal the adrenal glands is bone broth. There are many aspects of bone broth that are beneficial to health, but the amino acid component is the part that is especially protective against adrenal fatigue. When you are ill or run-down, your body cannot produce conditional amino acids effectively. This is exactly what eating bone broth replaces. These conditional amino acids are also known as arginine, proline, glycine, and glutamine, and together they possess a large number of beneficial properties. These are essential for the proper functioning of the adrenals and for your adrenals to give you the energy and vitality to enjoy your life."

people who ate a standard diet, the people on the fast-mimicking diet showed reductions in risk factors linked to diabetes, cancer, cardiovascular disease, and aging. Improvements included weight loss, reduced markers of inflammation, and lower blood glucose. That's pretty amazing for just a few days of fasting each month!

Why is fasting so healthy for you? Because you're genetically designed to do it. These days, we're conditioned to think that "normal" is three square meals a day plus a couple of snacks. But to our ancestors, that would seem really weird.

Think about it. Our ancestors didn't have grocery stores and mini-marts, so finding food took work and luck. Some days they scored big. Other days they came back empty-handed. In that feast-or-famine lifestyle, going a day or two without eating was par for the course. And over the millennia, our bodies learned to take advantage of that "downtime" to refresh, restore, and rejuvenate cells.

In short, intermittent fasting is a natural healing process. So don't think of it as something abnormal. Think of it as getting back to normal, because it's exactly what your body is engineered to do.

See more facts about intermittent fasting on the Resources page on my website, drkellyann.com/resources.

THE BIGGEST REASON INTERMITTENT FASTING WORKS

So far, I've talked about how both bone broth and intermittent fasting rev up your cells and make you burn fat faster. But there's an even bigger reason a bone broth mini-fast strips weight off your body: It creates a huge calorie deficit.

Now, I don't belong to the "a calorie is a calorie" school. Trust me when I say that calories from carbs will put weight on you faster than the same number of calories from fat or protein because carbs affect your metabolism adversely. But the fact is that cutting way down on your overall calories—no matter where they come from—forces your body to burn your fat stores like crazy. (Don't believe the myth that fasting will cause your metabolism to slow down to a crawl, because it's just that: a myth. In fact, one recent study found that when volunteers fasted for 84 hours, their basal metabolic rates went up.[28])

On a typical day, you probably eat about 2,000 calories if you're a woman and around 2,500 calories if you're a man. On your bone broth fast days, you'll hover around 300 to 500. That's a big difference your body has to make up by releasing

BONE BROTH DIET DEVOTEES

Stephanie Miley

I initially started this diet because I was having frequent breakouts of shingles. I'm not big on meds, so I tried to find other alternatives to resolve the issue. And this worked for me. Within the first 21 days, I didn't have any breakouts, and I also lost the weight. The other day I actually paid attention—I'm like "Oh, my skin. I really kind of have a glow," like I did when I was pregnant. I lost 14 pounds, and I think it was 6 inches around my waist.

BEFORE   AFTER

fat—especially from your belly. As a result, your spare tire will start to vanish before your eyes . . . and thanks to the filling, satisfying properties of bone broth, you'll lose that fat without having to suffer.

CALCULATING YOUR PAYOFF

I know that weight loss and wrinkle reduction are at the top of your mind right now. And I hope I've convinced you that bone broth intermittent fasts can accomplish both of these goals—*fast.*

But as you can see, the benefits of bone broth intermittent fasting go far beyond getting you back into your favorite skinny jeans and making you look 10 years younger. They include rejuvenating your cells, reducing inflammation, healing your joints, and even helping to protect you from cancer, diabetes, and heart disease. That's a huge payoff for an occasional day of enjoying liquid gold, isn't it?

And remember this, too: Once you're done with each fast, you can look forward to eating like royalty. In Chapters 7 and 8, I'll introduce you to the scrumptious, fat-blasting foods you'll get to enjoy 5 days a week.

BONE BROTH DIET DEVOTEES

Dolores Griffin

My mood has been amazing, I'm happy, I feel good, and I have so much more energy than I did. I feel it in my gut. When I look at the measurements, I have lost about 4 inches around there, which is amazing. It's awesome. You've got to try it yourself. You've got to feel the amazement of it after 21 days.

BEFORE   AFTER

CHAPTER 4

Metabolic Magic for Your Nonfasting Days

Foods That Melt Off Fat and Erase Wrinkles

HAVE I CONVINCED YOU that you can survive and even enjoy two intermittent fasts a week? Then let's talk about the other 5 days of the week—because I know you're going to love these.

On the Bone Broth Diet, you'll spend 5 days a week for the next 3 weeks eating like a gourmet. Yes, you'll still be on a diet . . . but trust me when I say that it won't feel like a diet.

To make sure you're dining in style on your 5 nonfasting days, I've created 3 weeks' worth of mouthwatering recipes for you. Whether you're a gourmet cook, a busy person who likes to cook but wants quick-and-simple recipes, or an I-just-want-to-lose-weight-fast dieter, you'll find recipes that suit your desires.

However, while these are star-quality meals, that isn't the most important thing about them. The real story here is that the foods you'll be eating are high-octane fat blasters and wrinkle erasers. These are the same foods I use to take hundreds of pounds off my patients and take years off their faces as well. And they're the same foods I use to help Hollywood celebrities achieve the sculpted figures and flawless skin you see on-screen.

In this chapter, I'll tell you what these foods are and why they're so effective. I think you'll be excited about all the amazing things you can eat while your pounds melt away—especially if you're a veteran of dreadful low-fat and low-cal diets. I promise you this: You have a treat in store. (Here are some hints: Think fajitas. Pot roast. Spicy chorizo sausage. Creamy roasted sweet potatoes. Are you getting hungry yet?)

However . . .

Before we get to the green-light foods on the Bone Broth Diet, let's get the hard part out of the way. Yep—it's time to talk about temporarily clearing your pantry of the red-light foods that put those extra pounds and wrinkles on you in the first place.

TAKING THE PLUNGE: GIVING FAT-PROMOTING FOODS THE (TEMPORARY) KISS-OFF

There are a number of food groups I need you to slash from your diet for the next 3 weeks. And I admit it: It's a long list, and it's going to hurt a little. But trust me—you'll thank me 3 weeks from now, when your skin is gorgeous and you can slide right into those jeans or that party dress. And with all the good food you *can* eat, you won't feel too deprived.

Remember, too, that you don't need to give these foods up forever. Just kiss them good-bye for 3 weeks, and then you can invite them back in . . . if you still want to.

However, for the next 21 days, my job is to turn you into a natural fat burner. And to transform yourself into a fat-burning machine, you need to do three things.

1. You need to "flip the switch" from glucose-burning (sugar-burning) to fat-burning.

    For years, you've supplied your body with a constant flood of glucose (sugar) from foods like bread, pasta, and potatoes. When you turn off that spigot, your body will initially freak out a little. (I think of this as "good confusion.") Then it will respond by flipping the switch and starting to burn ketone bodies— basically, a type of fatty acid—for fuel. This is called ketosis, and it's the biggest secret to ramping up your weight loss to incredible levels. That's because ketosis pulls your fat out of storage and burns it up.

2. You need to drive your inflammation levels way down.

    Increasingly, research is revealing that obesity is an inflammatory disease.[1] To prevent or treat this disease—or even to get a minor weight problem under control—you need to reduce that inflammation.

    When you lower inflammation, you'll also see astonishing changes in your skin texture and your energy levels. If you're battling digestive problems, acne, or autoimmune issues, I predict that your symptoms will take a dramatic turn for the better.

3. You need to heal your gut.

    If you want to lose weight and have radiant skin, you must have your gut on your side—and that means cutting out any foods that damage your intestinal wall or kill off good bacteria. Remember that there's one of you and trillions of those gut flora. You need those trillions of players on your weight-loss team!

To achieve all three of these goals, you must be absolutely ruthless about cutting out foods that stand in your way. And I mean no-holds-barred, take-no-prisoners ruthless. This isn't about compromise. It's about transformation—and that takes determination. That's why you're going to cut out any food that's standing between you and the body you want.

Are you ready to be ruthless? Good. Then here are the foods I need you to say no to for the next 21 days. First I'm going to tell you what they are, and then I'm going to tell you why you need to give them the boot.

FOODS YOU'LL ELIMINATE FOR THE NEXT 3 WEEKS

Grains and Grain-Containing Foods
Barley

Breads

Cereal

Chips

Cookies

Cornstarch and other food starches

Crackers

Granola

Oats

Pasta

Quinoa

Rice

Rye

Spelt

Waffles

Wheat

Corn-Based Products
Corn

Popcorn

Products that contain corn oil (for instance, mayonnaise and salad dressings)

Refined Processed Fats
Canola oil

Corn oil

Grapeseed oil

Margarine and vegetable shortening

Peanut oil

Safflower oil

Soybean oil

Sunflower oil

Vegetable oil

Any foods containing these fats

Artificial Sweeteners
Acesulfame K

Aspartame

Erythritol

Saccharin

Sucralose

Truvia

Soy
Hoisin sauce

Soy hot dogs and other soy "meats"

Soy milk

Soy sauce

Teriyaki sauce

Tofu

Dairy Products

Butter (except clarified butter and ghee; see page 119)

Cheese

Cream

Flavored creamers

Frozen yogurt

Half-and-half

Ice cream

Milk

Yogurt

Commercial Condiments with Added Sugar or Artificial Ingredients

Barbecue sauce

Bottled salad dressings and marinades

Ketchup

Sweet-and-sour sauces

Sugars

All sugars including honey, maple syrup, molasses, and jams and jellies

Packaged Processed Foods

Including "healthy" processed foods in boxes or freezer containers, which often contain wheat, soy, sugars, or dairy

Commercial Sauces, Soups, and Stews

These typically contain flour and artificial colors or flavors

Canned Foods with Sugar, Soy, or Additives

Canned fruits packed in syrup

Canned tuna packed in soybean oil

Any other canned food with artificial ingredients or "mystery" ingredients

Sodas, Fruit Juices, Sweetened Coffee/Tea, and Alcohol

Sugar-sweetened and artificially sweetened drinks

Wine, beer, and hard liquor

Ice Pops and Frozen Fruit Bars with Sugar and/or Artificial Ingredients

Processed Meats

Lunch meats, bacon, and sausage containing gluten, nitrites, soy, or sweeteners

Note: Lunch meats, sausage, and bacon that don't contain these ingredients are fine.

Beans/Legumes

Beans

Lentils

Peanut butter

Peanuts

Peas

Note: Green beans and sugar snap peas are fine.

Did that list make your heart stop for a few seconds? I know I'm asking a lot of you here. It's a big deal to give up pasta, bread, pizza, cereal, sugary treats, milk, cheese, quick-fix processed foods, and wine for 3 weeks. And I totally get that.

But remember these four things.

- It's only for 3 weeks.
- The payoff is huge.

- You'll replace these foods with fabulous fat-burning foods you'll love.

- To turn yourself into a fat-burning machine, you need to be ruthless.

Now, I'm guessing that some of the foods on my "no" list surprise you, while others don't. Here are my reasons for excluding all of them.

Sugar and sugary foods

I'm sure you're already aware that sugar isn't a health food, but it's bad for you in ways you may not know about. Here are some of them.

- **Sugar drives your insulin levels sky-high.** This causes the insulin resistance I've talked about, leading to belly fat, metabolic syndrome, and even diabetes.

- **Sugar is inflammatory.** When you eat sugar, your body reacts by activating proinflammatory molecules called cytokines.[2]

- **Sugar ages you.** As you get older, your body accumulates destructive molecules called advanced glycation end products (AGEs). These aptly named molecules turn protein fibers dry and brittle, making your skin dull and saggy and increasing your risks of diabetes, cataracts, and even Alzheimer's disease. While we all accumulate AGEs over time, sugar sends the "AGEing" process into hyperdrive.

- **Sugar causes digestive problems.** Fructose is a particular culprit here. Research shows that an extraordinarily high percentage of both children and adults suffer from bloating, gas, digestive pain, or belching after ingesting fructose. For instance, one study found that more than 50 percent of children with unexplained abdominal pain had fructose intolerance.[3]

And here's another reason to cut your sugar intake way down. I know you're focused on quick weight-loss results right now, but I also know that you care about your long-term health—and especially about protecting yourself from cancer. One of the best ways to do that, according to researchers, is to stay away from sugar. Studies link a diet high in sugary foods to pancreatic cancer,[4] show that a high-sugar diet raises your risk of getting breast cancer,[5] and reveal that ingestion of fructose in particular is associated with more aggressive cancers.[6] If you ask me, that's very scary stuff. So if you need an extra incentive to give up sugary junk food, there it is.

Now, you may need that extra incentive—because of all the foods I'm asking you to give up for 3 weeks, sugar may be the hardest one for you to let go. As I've mentioned, sugar is actually addictive. So be prepared for sugar cravings, and recognize them for what they are: the siren song of a food that's bad for you in every way.

Be aware, too, that sugar goes by many names. When you cut it out, don't let it tiptoe back into your diet in a different form. Here are some of sugar's sneaky aliases.

Agave nectar	Invert sugar
Barley malt syrup	Lactose
Cane crystals	Maltodextrin
Corn sweetener	Maltose
Corn syrup	Malt syrup
Crystalline fructose	Monosaccharide
Dehydrated cane juice	Polysaccharide
Dextrin	Ribose
Dextrose	Rice syrup
Disaccharide	Saccharose
Evaporated cane juice	Sorghum
Fructose	Sorghum syrup
Fruit juice concentrate	Sucrose
Galactose	Treacle
Glucose	Turbinado sugar
High-fructose corn syrup	Xylose

Artificial sweeteners

It may surprise you that in addition to asking you to swear off sugar for 3 weeks, I'm asking you to say no to diet sodas and other artificially sweetened foods. Why am I doing this? Because there's strong evidence that artificial sweeteners affect your metabolism in ways that make you gain weight.

For instance, in a recent study,[7, 8] researchers fed three artificial sweeteners—saccharin, aspartame, and sucralose—to mice. To the researchers' shock, the mice developed glucose intolerance, which is the first step on the road to obesity and diabetes.

The researchers wondered if this applied to humans as well as mice. To find out, they looked at data collected from about 400 people and found that those who drank lots of diet soda had slightly higher HbA1C numbers than those who

Breaking Free from Sugar

**JJ Virgin, CNS, CHFS, celebrity nutrition and fitness expert and author of the
New York Times bestsellers *The Virgin Diet* and *Sugar Impact Diet***
jjvirgin.com

Here's what my good friend JJ Virgin has to say about sugar.

"Sugar holds your health, tastebuds, and waistline hostage. When you eliminate sugar, which experts argue can become eight times more addictive than cocaine, you finally untether from the vicious bind that high-sugar impact foods create, so you don't get those midafternoon brownie cravings after you eat a healthy lunch. You're not hungry every 2 or 3 hours and constantly resisting the hot cinnamon buns your coworker brought in.

"There are so many amazing benefits to eliminating high-sugar impact foods. For most people, losing fat quickly becomes the big motivator. You'll also break free of cravings; regain control of your appetite; and enjoy high, steady energy and laser-sharp focus. You'll ditch gas, bloating, and 'running to the bathroom' after meals. You'll look and feel younger as well as nix those nagging symptoms that make you constantly feel crummy. More important, losing the high-sugar impact foods means you'll begin to reverse chronic diseases like obesity, diabetes, and heart disease.

"Seeing becomes believing: Take this challenge (you can do anything for 3 weeks!) and you'll immediately begin reaping its glorious benefits."

didn't touch it. (The HbA1C test measures blood sugar over time, and even a slightly elevated number is an indication of glucose intolerance.)

Pursuing this trail further, the researchers then asked seven lean, healthy people who weren't diet soda drinkers to consume the maximum acceptable daily dose of artificial sweeteners every day for a week. Four of the volunteers developed blood sugar problems—and in some cases, their blood glucose soared to levels considered prediabetic!

What caused this to happen? The researchers discovered that artificial sweeteners alter the balance of gut bacteria in a way that can lead to glucose intolerance.

This means that diet soft drinks are doing the opposite of what they should do. Instead of helping you get thin, they're making you glucose intolerant, which in turn will make you fat. So I need you to give up diet soda for the next 3 weeks at a minimum—and if you can, cut way down on diet drinks after that.

Grains

The most important thing to realize about grains is that from your body's point of view, these foods are just sugar in another form—and that includes those whole grains your doctors probably tell you to eat all the time. In fact, two slices of "healthy" whole wheat bread raise your blood sugar more than a candy bar does.

But grains don't just jack up your insulin levels, leading to insulin resistance and metabolic syndrome. In addition, they cause your body to become resistant to leptin.

Leptin is a hormone that your fat cells use to tell your brain how much energy they need. High levels of leptin make you feel full, while low levels make you feel hungry. That's why I call leptin your hunger trigger.

A constant diet of high-carb grains leads to chronically high levels of leptin. That's bad, because eventually your brain becomes resistant to leptin's cues. (This is similar to insulin resistance.) When this happens, you don't get the mes-

---

Are You Heading for "Diabesity"?

Mark Hyman, MD, author of *The Blood Sugar Solution*

drhyman.com

Here's what Dr. Hyman, the internationally renowned medical director of the UltraWellness Center in Massachusetts, has to say about America's biggest health problem today.

"Right now, we're experiencing an epidemic of *diabesity*—a combination of diabetes or prediabetes and obesity. And if you're eating a standard American diet, you're at high risk.

"But here's the good news: Diabesity is almost 100 percent curable and preventable. The simple answer to preventing or reversing diabesity is to balance your blood sugar. To do this, you need to stop eating sugar, flour, and artificial Frankenfoods and start eating the real foods your

body needs. It's all about working with your body instead of against it.

"Doctors may prescribe drugs for you to take for the rest of your life to prevent diabesity. But that's like mopping up the floor around an overflowing sink instead of turning off the faucet. You need to turn off the faucet—the chronic supply of sugar, flour, and chemicals that's making you overweight and sick.

"Here's what Kellyann and I know from decades of transforming people's lives: What you put on your fork is more powerful than anything you'll find in a prescription bottle. So if you don't want to become another diabesity statistic, change what you eat—starting now."

sage that you're full. So even when you don't physically need to eat, you experience deep cravings that are nearly impossible to resist.

There are other reasons to give up grains. For one thing, they're high in "antinutrients" called lectins. Lectins make it harder for your body to use insulin efficiently and can damage the lining of your intestines. Grains are also high in phytic acid, which blocks the uptake of important nutrients.

Finally, most grains contain gluten. That's bad news, because up to a third of people are gluten sensitive or gluten intolerant. If you're one of them, grains that contain gluten can cause intestinal permeability—that leaky gut I talked about back in Chapter 3—and trigger wildfire inflammation throughout your body, leading to digestive problems, joint pain, blotchy skin, and a host of other ailments.

In short, grains strike out on all of my three criteria: They boost your insulin, cause inflammation, and damage your gut. And that means they've got to go for now.

In particular, you need to make sure that no gluten sneaks into your diet. To ensure that you clean it out of your pantry, watch out for these sneaky ingredients that indicate that a product possibly or definitely contains gluten.

Artificial flavoring	Natural flavoring
Bleached flour	Seasonings
Dextrin	Vegetable protein
Hydrolyzed plant protein (HPP)	Vegetable starch
Hydrolyzed wheat protein	What germ oil
Hydrolyzed wheat starch	Wheat grass
Malt	Wheat protein
Maltodextrin	Wheat starch
Modified food starch	

Another grain that often slinks in through a side door is corn. When you read labels, avoid any products that contain these ingredients:

Artificial flavoring	Dextrin
Caramel color	Dextrose
Corn alcohol	Food starch
Corn flour	High-fructose corn syrup
Cornmeal	Maltodextrin
Corn oil	Mazena
Cornstarch	Modified gum starch
Corn sweetener	MSG
Corn syrup solids	Natural flavorings

Sorbitol	Vegetable starch
Vegetable gum	Xanthan gum
Vegetable protein	Xylitol

Dairy

Some people tolerate dairy just fine, while others don't. So normally, my advice is: Do what works for you.

However, it takes time for most people to figure out if dairy causes them any problems. In my experience, about 80 percent of people don't handle dairy

---

The Inflammation Connection

Thaddeus Gala, DC, author and speaker

drthadgala.com

As a health coach, Thad transforms patients by removing inflammatory foods like sugar and grains from their diets. Here's his take on the role of inflammation in disease.

"In your life, you've experienced overt or clinical inflammation. Classic examples include when you get sunburned, cut yourself, or sprain your ankle. This immediate clinical inflammation differs from the more serious and less obvious and deleterious subclinical inflammation. Because the cause and effect of subclinical inflammation are much more delayed, we often miss the health connection as the damage often manifests slowly as chronic pain, being overweight, elevated blood pressure, high cholesterol, sleep apnea, Alzheimer's, heart disease, cancer, fibromyalgia, and diabetes, to name a few.

"When you focus on lifestyle habits and foods that reduce this low-grade inflammation, often within days or weeks you can begin to experience an improvement or reversal of chronic symptoms. You will begin to lose weight, have more energy, and feel refreshed, so you make strides toward breaking free from fatigue and prescription medications and ultimately looking and feeling great.

"Eliminating the guesswork about which foods to include and avoid is necessary for a win. The Bone Broth Diet has hit the nail on the head in defining the core elements necessary for success. Whether it's losing weight or reversing chronic disease, reducing inflammation is paramount in feeling and looking great, no matter your age. Recent research has shown that reducing subclinical inflammation may hold the key to living to 150 quality and fulfilling years."

BONE BROTH DIET DEVOTEES

Sara Katzman

BEFORE AFTER

I feel like I've really changed my life. I was very sick before I started this, and I knew I needed to do something that drastically would change me.

Today I went to the endocrinologist, and he completely took me off insulin and one of my diabetes meds. This diet healed me so much, and it's given me so much energy that I'm having trouble sleeping, I'm so wired! I would recommend that anyone at least give it a try. I've tried all kinds of things, and this is what works for me. I don't go around hungry, and that's the most amazing thing. And I can actually go without eating some meals—that's how full I feel.

well, and many of them don't even realize that they have a problem. These people's symptoms—which range from weight gain and bloating to acne and allergies—often clear up when they drop milk and other dairy products from their diets.

So consider these 3 weeks as a test. When you're done with your Bone Broth Diet, try adding high-quality, full-fat dairy back in (cautiously) and see if any symptoms that cleared up during your diet return. If not, add dairy back to your "yes" list. But for now—can I say it again?—be ruthless.

Soy

Okay, this one may shock you. I know you've heard over and over again that soy is a health food—but in reality, that's one of the biggest lies in history. In fact, I strongly suggest that even after you finish your diet, you reduce the amount of soy you eat to a bare minimum. (It's hard to eliminate soy altogether, because it's so pervasive in processed foods—which is another good reason to eat natural, unprocessed foods.)

Why am I so down on soy? Well, here's the truth about this "healthy" food.

■ Eating soy puts you at risk for hypothyroidism, and an underactive thyroid packs weight on your body. Research shows that soy harms your thyroid by suppressing your uptake of the crucial nutrient iodine and by promoting autoimmunity.[9]

■ Soy contains phytoestrogens, and women consuming the equivalent of 2 cups of soy milk per day get the estrogenic equivalent of one birth control pill.[10] Soy phytoestrogens disrupt other hormones and have the potential to cause breast cancer[11] and breast cancer metastasis[12] in women. Soy affects men's

---

Food and Your Thyroid

**Alan Christianson, NMD, naturopathic medical doctor
and *New York Times* bestselling author**

drchristianson.com

If you have thyroid issues, here's important information from an expert.

"Being on a healthy diet is necessary in managing Hashimoto's thyroiditis. Since thyroid disease is primarily an autoimmune disease, it's important to recognize that the wrong foods can stress the immune system and worsen its attack against the thyroid.

"How does this work? The more your immune system is attacking things from your intestinal tract, the greater the chances are that it will attack proteins within your thyroid. Some of the most common food culprits include dairy, eggs, gluten, almonds, bananas, and sugar. Although many foods can be triggers, people do not react to the same ones. It is best to learn through testing or elimination diets which foods are the culprit for you. Some people take the approach of cutting out all possible reactive foods just to be safe. Although this might make sense, it can cause the digestive system to become less able to digest a variety of foods.

"Foods with soy protein like soy protein isolate, tofu, and soy milk should be avoided by anyone with early disease. There has been a great deal of misinformation about goitrogens. Many healthy foods like kale, broccoli, or Brussels sprouts have been unnecessarily avoided by those with Hashimoto's. Not only did these foods not worsen Hashimoto's, but they improved gene abnormalities that are common with those who have the disease."

reproductive systems negatively, too; for instance, research involving male partners in couples having difficulty conceiving shows that men with a high soy intake have lower sperm counts than men who don't eat soy.[13]

- Soy, like grains, contains phytic acid, which reduces your absorption of several key nutrients.

- The processing of soy proteins such as soy burgers, hot dogs, and sausage results in the formation of lysinoalanine and nitrosamines. These toxins damage your cells and make them sluggish, causing you to put on weight. Processed soy foods are also high in MSG, an excitotoxin that excessively stimulates and can damage your cells.

Now, I'm guessing you've heard that soy must be healthy because people in Asia—who are extremely healthy overall—eat large amounts of it. However, they don't consume anywhere near as much soy as you may think. The average consumption of soy foods in China is 10 grams (about 2 teaspoons per day); in Japan, it's about 30 to 60 grams. Basically, people in Asian countries tend to use soy as a condiment—not as a meal or a replacement for animal foods as we do in the United States and other Western countries.

Moreover, the soy we eat is highly processed for the most part, while the soy products in Asian countries are usually fermented and unprocessed. This fermentation makes a big difference, because it partially neutralizes the toxins in the soybean—toxins that you're otherwise getting in full strength.

Frankly, I'm hoping that after reading my list of soy's negative effects, you'll toss out your soy Frankenfoods and soy milk and replace them permanently with real foods. But at a minimum, I need you to give soy the boot for the next 3 weeks so you optimize your hormones and clear your body of toxins.

To make sure you're eliminating soy from your diet, cut out these foods as well. All of them contain soy.

Hydrolyzed plant protein (HPP)	Stabilizer
Hydrolyzed soy protein	Tamari
Hydrolyzed vegetable protein (HVP)	Tempeh
Miso natural flavoring	Textured soy flour (TSF)
Soy albumin	Textured soy protein (TSP)
Soy fiber	Textured vegetable protein (TVP)
Soy flour	Tofu vegetable broth
Soy lecithin	Vegetable gum
Soy protein	Vegetable starch
Soy sauce	

Industrial seed oils

If you think that seed oils like corn, soybean, sunflower, safflower, and vegetable oil are good for you, think again. Even canola oil—billed as a health food—belongs in a landfill, in my opinion.

Never Settle for Bland!

Mark Sisson, fitness expert and bestselling author of *The Primal Blueprint*

thrv.me/primalmayo

Mark, one of the biggest superstars in the world of primal nutrition and fitness, is living proof that healthy food can keep you strong, fit, and young . . . even into your sixties and beyond. Here's his advice on eating well and loving what you eat.

"One of the primary sacrifices of almost any weight-loss plan or healthy-living program is taste. We trade in taste for bland in the name of health and weight management, ditching condiments like mayo and ketchup in order to cut calories and health-leaching ingredients from our diets. The effort is commendable but not necessary, at least not in this day and age.

"Yes, the majority of commercial condiments should be avoided. They are made with industrial seed oils and vegetable oils such as soybean and canola oil. Let's take a more in-depth look at canola oil, which is a genetically modified oil. It comes from rapeseed oil, which is high in eruic acid, a poisonous toxin. In order to strip rapeseed oil of eruic acid and make canola oil, it needs to be processed at temperatures higher than 500°F, which means a good portion of the omega-3s in canola oil are rancid and toxic before they hit your tongue. Not only are partially hydrogenated oils like canola oil in most of the condiments you eat, but they also hang out in virtually every processed and packaged food you buy . . . if you don't source the right products, that is.

"I personally live a primal-inspired life and eat a diet made of only real food ingredients, but my meats and salads got pretty boring pretty fast without sauces and condiments. So I set out to create a line of paleo-friendly condiments made of only healthful natural fats, superfoods, and antioxidant-rich herbs. Primal Kitchen Mayo, for example, is made of nutrient-dense avocado oil, organic and cage-free eggs, organic vinegar from non-GMO beets, a dash of sea salt, and some rosemary extract. No canola or soy, no sugar or high-fructose corn syrup, no dairy, and no artificial colors, flavors, or fillers. Quite simply, these are condiments you can trust, so you no longer have to sacrifice taste to meet your health goals."

Why? First of all, seed oils (even canola) contain high ratios of omega-6 to omega-3 fatty acids. In fact, because our Western diet is heavy in seed oils, we now consume 10 to 25 times more omega-6 fatty acids than our early ancestors did. That's bad, because omega-3 fatty acids fight inflammation, while omega-6 fatty acids are proinflammatory. So it's no surprise that we're seeing an epidemic of "aging" diseases linked to inflammation, including obesity, diabetes, cardiovascular disease, autoimmune disease, and cancer.

Second, seed oils are heavily processed. They undergo caustic refining, bleaching, and degumming processes, and the end result is hardly food at all. They also go rancid quickly, making them even more toxic to your cells. Ick. Out they go.

Beans

The primary reason to say no to these foods for the next 3 weeks is that they're high in carbs. And by now, you know what carbs do to your insulin levels.

Another downside of beans is that they're hard for our bodies to digest, which is why legumes so often leave us feeling worse after we eat them. You want your gut to glow during your diet, and beans can make it ache instead. Beans are also high in those lectins I talked about earlier, so they can damage your gut.

That said, it's true that many people handle legumes just fine. If you're one of them, they can be a healthy part of your maintenance diet after you finish your 3-week diet. But for now . . . yeah, you got it. Be ruthless.

Artificial ingredients

The number of artificial chemicals added to our food these days is astonishing: fake colors, fake flavors, fake thickeners, you name it. Unfortunately, the more we learn about these additives, the worse they sound.

For instance, research shows that chemical emulsifiers used to thicken foods like soup and ice cream break down your protective gut barrier and increase your risks of inflammatory bowel disease and metabolic syndrome.[14] MSG, which is ubiquitous in processed foods, is linked to obesity.[15] And that fake caramel coloring in your soda may increase your risk of cancer.[16]

Basically, if you eat foods containing additives, you're rolling the dice. We don't know what most of these additives do to us, but we do know that our bodies aren't designed to handle them because they're not food. Right now we want to fine-tune your metabolism rather than slow it down with fake foods it can't handle, so I need you to cut these chemicals out for the next 3 weeks—and you'll do your body a favor if you limit them after that.

Alcohol

Ouch! I know—that's a burn. But don't quit on me now. When I tell people they need to give up drinking for 21 days, I frequently see a look of sheer panic on their faces. This is by far the hardest thing for most people to forgo on this diet. I look forward to a glass of wine or a shot of potato vodka after a hard day myself, and I confess that it's one thing I miss when I'm following this plan.

But if you really want to melt off fat for the next 21 days, I need you to white-knuckle this one. Alcohol can damage your digestive system, giving you that leaky gut I've talked about—and right now we need your gut functioning at the highest possible level. Also, alcohol doesn't do your skin any favors at all. And it can lower your willpower, making carbs and junk food look a lot more tempting.

Fast-Food Diet = Fast-Food Brain

Daniel G. Amen, MD, founder, Amen Clinics and author of *Change Your Brain, Change Your Life*

danielamenmd.amenclinics.com

Daniel Amen is one of the world's most influential psychiatrists and experts on optimizing brain function. If you need added incentive to kick artificial colorings and flavors and other junk-food ingredients out of your life, here's what he has to say.

"Your brain is the CEO that runs your life. When your brain works right, you work right; and when it is troubled, you are much more likely to have trouble in your life.

"With a healthy brain, you feel happier and physically healthier because you make better decisions; you're likely to be wealthier, also because you make better decisions; and you're more successful in everything you do. When your brain is unhealthy for whatever reason, from a concussion to drinking too much alcohol to being diabetic or having sleep apnea, you are more likely to be sadder, sicker, poorer, and less successful.

"Your brain uses 20 to 30 percent of the calories you consume, so if you consume a fast-food diet, you will have a fast-food mind. Great nutrition is the cornerstone of a healthy mind and body. Get your food right and nearly everything else will follow."

So please, *please* bear with me on this one. It's only for 3 weeks. I know you can do it.

You can add alcohol right back into your diet as soon as you move to the maintenance phase after 21 days. So if you find yourself pining for a nip of the

---

Good Fat, Bad Fat

Jonny Bowden, PhD, CNS, coauthor of *Smart Fat: Eat More Fat. Lose More Weight. Get Healthy Now.*

jonnybowden.com

Jonny Bowden, a national expert on weight loss, nutrition, and health, knows absolutely everything there is to know about fats. So if you're skeptical when I tell you to toss your canola oil and switch to coconut oil, here's what he has to say about it.

"For years we thought we knew the definition of *good fat* and *bad fat*. 'Bad' fats were saturated and trans fats while 'good' fats were everything else, specifically vegetable oils and omega-3s.

"We were wrong.

"Two major meta-analyses—which is where researchers pool the very best and most rigorous data from dozens of published studies, put them all together, and see what the science really shows—have found saturated fat not guilty of any role whatsoever in heart disease. In fact, some of the fats we thought were so good for us— namely, vegetable and seed oils like canola, soybean, corn, and safflower— are actually very high in proinflammatory omega-6s while being vanishingly low in omega-3s. That's precisely the wrong balance for human health. In fact, the soybean oil we consume in virtually every processed food product and the vegetable oils used to cook in just about every restaurant in America may be having a much more diabolical effect on our health than saturated fat ever did.

"Tropical oils—like coconut oil and palm oil from Malaysia (where it is sustainable)—are fantastic oils with many healthy compounds in them, and both are mostly saturated fat. And we have nothing to fear from saturated fat when it's sourced from grass-fed, pastured animals raised organically.

"Higher-fat diets—especially when accompanied by less sugar and carbs— will help you lose weight. Carbs raise your levels of insulin, also known as the fat-storage hormone. Protein can also raise insulin, though not nearly as much as carbs. But the one class of food that has absolutely *no* effect on insulin is fat. And as a bonus, fat from healthy, nontoxic sources has a balancing effect on both hormones and the brain."

bubbly or a sip of scotch, make a plan to treat yourself to an expensive, high-quality bottle of your favorite alcoholic beverage when your diet ends. It'll be a nice reward for your willpower!

A few tips for later: If you do drink during your maintenance phase, choose champagne, gin, scotch, whiskey, potato vodka (my favorite by a long shot), or wine. All of these are just fine in moderation. Avoid liqueurs, sweet specialty drinks, premixed cocktails, and beer containing gluten.

If you like mixed drinks, good mixers in the maintenance phase include blended or juiced vegetables, blended or muddled fruits, club soda (my favorite), lime/lemon/orange juice, coconut milk, and coconut water.

Do keep in mind that booze lowers your willpower and can lead you to overeat—and you don't want to put those pounds right back on! I recommend eating a high-protein, low-carb meal before you have anything to drink and having healthy snacks on hand so you won't be tempted by junk food. Also, decide ahead of time how many drinks you'll have, and stop when you hit that number.

Finally, practice the "every other" rule. Try to have a glass of water or a nonalcoholic "mocktail" in between drinks. This will keep you hydrated and cut down on the amount of alcohol you consume.

If you're struggling with how to handle the Bone Broth Diet when you're out with friends or family, see my "Dinner Party Pitch" on the Resources page of my website, drkellyann.com/resources.

NOW . . . ON TO THE GOOD NEWS!

Are you still with me? If so, I know you're truly serious about getting slim and healthy. Now that you know which foods you'll need to give up, it's time for us to talk about the fantastic foods you'll get to enjoy for the next 3 weeks.

Here's why I've carefully selected these foods.

■ **They're low in carbohydrates.** This means they shut off the flood of glucose to your cells, likely putting your body into ketosis—that rapid fat-burning state that strips weight right off you. Lower glucose also translates into less insulin resistance, so you'll start reversing any symptoms of metabolic syndrome. And it means less leptin resistance, so you won't crave food when you're not hungry.

What's more, you'll feel great. When you balance your blood sugar by cutting down on carbs, you'll enter what I call the zone. Most people don't realize how many issues they have that trace back to blood sugar problems.

When they balance their blood sugar, my patients often say, "I forgot what it was like to feel this great."

- **Many of them are lipotropic.** As I mentioned earlier, lipotropic nutrients carry fat away from your liver and help you break it down and metabolize it. In particular, many of the foods you'll be eating are loaded with choline, the body's primary lipotropic substance. (By the way, banned diet drugs like ephedra worked because they were lipotropic—but in contrast to these unhealthy drugs, lipotropic foods work in a healthy way.)

- **They provide healthy fats that nourish your body and skin.** I know you've heard for years that fat is bad. However, this is yet another destructive myth. It's true that those heavily processed seed oils I talked about earlier are horrible for you. But healthy fats optimize your metabolism, and they're essential components of your skin and hair. (You know those skin-smoothing ceramides that wrinkle creams boast about having? Healthy fats feed your skin ceramides from the *inside*.) When you eat the right amount of these fats, you lose weight, your hair gets glossier, your skin gets its glow back, and those fine wrinkles disappear. Add these fats to your diet every day, and you'll be amazed at the results.

- **They sweep your cells clean of toxins.** Right now, if you've been eating a standard high-carb, high-sugar diet, your cellular matrix—the "sea" your cells swim in—is clogged and acidic. The clean, nutrient-dense foods I'm asking you to eat are brimming with antioxidants and other detoxifying nutrients that will clear the sludge out of your cellular matrix, making your cells vibrant and young and rejuvenating your skin and hair.

- **They regulate your hormones.** These real foods will help bring all of your hormones—not just insulin—into balance. As a result, you may experience relief from such problems as wide-ranging as acne, oily or dry skin, PMS, excess facial hair, fatigue, headaches, low sex drive, and depression.

- **They lower inflammation.** The healthy proteins, fats, vegetables, and fruits you'll eat on the Bone Broth Diet are loaded with anti-inflammatory nutrients. In addition to erasing wrinkles and making your pounds fall off, these foods will help heal you from head to toe. In fact, the results my patients see when they cut out proinflammatory foods and start eating these anti-inflammatory foods often are nothing short of stunning.

Okay. Now that I've told you why these foods will melt fat off you, erase wrinkles from your face, and make you feel younger and more energetic, it's time to meet them! Are you ready? Here are the foods you can eat 5 days a week for the next 3 weeks.

continued on page 66

Julie and Merris

When Julie attended one of my talks, she said she knew "there was something there." As she heard me speak about how inflammation can make you fat, she realized that this was true for her because she was always puffy and her weight simply wouldn't budge, no matter what she did.

Julie began an earlier variation of the Bone Broth Diet, and what happened to her was amazing. She says, "I literally shrank." She lost 30 pounds and, as she puts it, "the inches just melted away."

Julie says, "People keep asking me, 'How do you keep looking younger, when I'm getting older?' "

Before she started her diet, Julie had, as she called it, the heartbreak of psoriasis. She never wanted to be in photos or draw any attention to herself, even though she's very pretty and has a bubbly personality. She was one of those "invisible" women I talk about.

When Julie made all the lifestyle changes I recommended, her psoriasis cleared up 70 to 80 percent. In addition, she has more energy than ever. She's lost her bloat and her saddlebags and sleeps like a baby, waking up refreshed instead of groggy.

Julie's family was so impressed that all of them jumped on the bandwagon. Her husband lost 45 pounds, his achy joints cleared up, and he's athletic once again. Her daughter lost 20 pounds, and her allergies and eczema are completely gone. And Julie's 21-year-old son lost 20 pounds and got rid of his acne.

Unlike Julie, Merris didn't need to lose weight when she came to see me. Instead, she needed to save her life.

Merris has celiac disease, an autoimmune condition that affects the intestines. When people with celiac disease eat any food containing gluten, their immune system attacks the villi, tiny structures in the intestines. The result: diarrhea, constipation, abdominal pain, nausea, and absolute misery.

The standard treatment for the disease is a strict avoidance of gluten. Merris had tried that for a year and a half, but it didn't work. Her doctor suspected that she had refractory celiac disease—a severe and potentially fatal condition that's treated with powerful immune-suppressing steroids and other dangerous drugs.

Merris wanted a better solution. And when she saw me on TV one day talking about treating inflammation with food, she decided to give me a chance.

After she followed my protocol for only 4 days, Merris's severe diarrhea completely stopped. Within a month, her pain and cramps vanished. After being unable to sleep for more than an hour or two at a stretch, she could sleep soundly through the night.

Now, at 66, Merris says, "I feel like a teenager." She's living proof that when it comes to autoimmune disease, the wrong foods can hurt or even kill you—and the right foods can heal you.

You can see Julie's and Merris's stories at drkellyann.com/resources.

YOUR FAT-BURNING BONE BROTH DIET "YES" FOODS

Meats
  Beef
  Bison
  Chicken
  Lamb
  Pork
  Turkey
  Wild game

Note: Buy pastured meat and free-range poultry if you can afford them. Avoid pork unless you can find pastured pork.

Fish
  Fresh or canned. Buy wild-caught fish if possible, and make sure canned fish is packed in water or olive oil.

Eggs
  Buy organic/free-range if possible.

Organ Meats
  Look for organic liver.

Nitrite- and Gluten-Free Deli Meats, Bacon, and Sausages
Note: Read labels carefully and make sure you're not getting any sugars or artificial additives.

Vegetables
  Acorn squash*
  Artichokes
  Arugula
  Asparagus
  Bamboo shoots
  Beets*
  Bell peppers
  Bok choy
  Broccoli

Broccoli rabe
Brussels sprouts
Butternut squash*
Carrots*
Cauliflower
Celery
Celery root*
Chile peppers
Cilantro
Cucumber
Daikon
Eggplant
Fennel
Garlic
Ginger
Green beans
Green cabbage
Green onions
Greens (beet, collard, mustard, turnip, etc.)
Horseradish
Jalapeños
Jicama*
Kale
Kohlrabi*
Konjac root (shirataki)
Leeks
Lettuce
Mushrooms
Napa cabbage
Okra
Onions
Parsnips*
Plantains*
Pumpkin
Radicchio
Radishes
Red cabbage
Rutabaga*

Seaweed

Snap peas

Snow peas

Spaghetti squash*

Spinach

Sprouts

Summer squash

Sweet potatoes and yams*

Swiss chard

Tomatillos

Tomatoes (including canned or sun-dried tomatoes)

Turnips*

Watercress

White Potatoes*

Yucca*

Zucchini

Etc.

These are starchy vegetables and fruits. Add them to a meal only if you need extra fuel after a workout or you're feeling weak and tired and you know it isn't the carb flu (see my troubleshooting notes at the end of this chapter).

For more info on which starchy vegetables have the fewest carbs—some, like turnips and kohlrabi, are surprisingly low—check the carb counter on page 371.

Buy organic veggies if possible.

Corn is not on this list and is not Bone Broth Diet approved.

___

Fruits

Apples

Applesauce, unsweetened

Apricots

Bananas

Bitter melon

Blackberries

Blueberries

Cantaloupe

Cherries

Cranberries

Dragonfruit

Durian

Elderberries

Figs

Grapefruit

Grapes

Guava

Honeydew melon

Kiwifruit

Kumquat

Lemons

Limes

Lingonberries

Loquat

Lychee

Mandarin oranges

Mangoes

Nectarines

Oranges

Papayas

Peaches

Pears

Persimmons

Pineapple

Plums

Pomegranates

Raspberries

Rhubarb

Strawberries

Tangerines

Ugli fruit

Watermelon

Notes: Buy organic if possible; also, emphasize berries, which are lower in sugar than most fruits. Avoid dried fruits, fruit

(continued)

juices, and smoothies—other than smoothies that contain only foods allowed on the diet.

Healthy Fats

Avocado mayonnaise

Avocado oil

Avocados

Coconut/coconut chips

Coconut butter

Coconut flour

Coconut milk

Coconut oil

Ghee or clarified butter

MCT oil

Nut butters (unsweetened)

Nuts

Olive oil

Olives

Seeds

Sesame oil

Tallow

Healthy Meal-Replacement Shakes

These shakes must have protein only from one of the Dr. Kellyann–approved sources.

Collagen protein

Egg protein

Hydro beef protein

Whey protein isolate

Pea protein (approved if doing a vegan or vegetarian version of the diet)

Natural Sweeteners

Stevia

Monk fruit

Fermented Foods

Coconut kefir

Kimchi

Pickles (unpasteurized, refrigerated)

Sauerkraut

Condiments

Cocoa powder, unsweetened/cacao

Coconut aminos (to replace soy sauce)

Fish sauce

Herbs

Hot sauce, gluten-free

Mustard, gluten-free

Nutritional yeast

Pepper

Pickles, unsweetened and sulfite-free

Salsa

Salt, Celtic or pink Himalayan (instead of regular table salt)

Spices

Vinegar (except rice vinegar)

Note: While regular table salt contains iodine, it also contains additives you don't want. To get a good supply of iodine, be sure to include sea vegetables (like SeaSnax) and fish in your diet.

Flours and Thickeners

Almond flour

Arrowroot powder

Coconut flour

Beverages

Coffee

Mineral water

Sparkling water

Tea

Note: Try not to overdo caffeinated coffee or tea if you're experiencing the carb flu— instead, add a little extra fat to your diet to ease your symptoms.

For shopping guides, specific brands, and recommendations, go to my Resources page on drkellyann.com/resources.

When you eat these foods, you're going to rediscover a remarkable truth that people have forgotten in an age of "bling" food: Real, nutrient-dense food is powerful. Real food trims your weight, wipes out your wrinkles, and heals your body because it transforms you at the cellular level. It has curative powers stronger than any powders, pills, or drops.

Each of the foods on your "yes" list will contribute in its own way to revving up your fat-burning, as well as smoothing and beautifying your skin and de-aging your body. Here are just some examples.

- Pastured beef contains conjugated linoleic acid (CLA), which reduces body-fat mass.[17]

- Eggs are loaded with lipotropic choline as well as other fat-burning nutrients.

- Citrus fruits, garlic, onions, and cruciferous vegetables such as broccoli, cauliflower, and kale aid the liver's detoxification pathways, helping to cleanse your body.

- The omega-3 fatty acids in fish do double duty, lowering inflammation while they "inflate" your skin cells and make them bouncy.

- Bacon (yes, bacon!) is high in fat-blasting choline.

- Coconut fat and avocados are incredible wrinkle blasters because their fatty acids strengthen your cell membranes. The lauric acid in coconut oil fights weight gain.

- Fermented foods like kimchi, sauerkraut, coconut kefir, and unpasteurized pickles are *probiotics* that feed your gut beneficial bacteria, helping you digest foods more easily and protecting against leaky gut.

- Foods like asparagus, onions, garlic, and jicama are *prebiotics*. This means that they provide soluble fiber that creates a healthy "soil" for the microbes in your gut.

- Fish and seaweed are rich in iodine, which helps optimize your thyroid function.

- The nutrients in blueberries promote collagen formation, erasing wrinkles and skin flaws.

- The minerals in mineral salt pull water into your skin cells, minimizing eye bags.

- The fiber in veggies helps you take off pounds. One study, for instance, found that increasing the fiber intake of adults significantly increased their

WANT A SHORTCUT?

If you're feeling a little overwhelmed by my "no" and "yes" lists, here's an easy way to approach your nonfasting days: Simply eat three meals a day chosen *only* from the recipes in Chapters 7 and 8, and eat nothing else except for two snacks of bone broth (with the two exceptions I outline in the "Troubleshooting Tips" section at the end of this chapter). Or, if you don't want to cook at all, check out my section in Chapter 7 on no-cook foods like rotisserie chicken or turkey lunch meat. Just make sure you follow my guidelines later in this chapter for controlling your portions.

If you love to be creative in the kitchen, however, feel free to range beyond the recipes in this book and invent your own breakfasts, lunches, and dinners. Just stick religiously to the list of "yes" foods I've outlined in this chapter and you can happily get your culinary freak on.

populations of *Bacteroidetes* bacteria and decreased the population of *Firmicutes*. A higher ratio of *Bacteroidetes* to *Firmicutes* is associated with a lower body mass index.[18]

Like these foods, all of the other foods on my "yes" list have fat-burning and anti-aging superpowers. Better yet, they work synergistically, boosting one another's effects. So when you load your diet with them—and especially when you add them to the healing power of bone broth—you'll see pounds and wrinkles vanish, and you'll feel younger and more vibrant than you've felt in years.

For quick-tip shopping guides, go to the Resources page on my website, drkellyann.com/resources.

Now, I do have one caution about a specific group of foods on the "good guy" list. Some people have problems with nightshade fruits and vegetables, which include bell peppers, hot peppers, potatoes, eggplant, paprika, and tomatoes. If you're still experiencing digestive problems and inflammation after a week or two on the Bone Broth Diet, try cutting out these foods and see if it helps. (You can easily alter most of my recipes to remove the nightshades.)

ONE MORE IMPORTANT ELEMENT OF YOUR DIET: WATER

On your bone broth days, you'll be getting plenty of water (especially if you add in coffee or tea). On your other days, make a conscious effort to drink lots of

Are You Getting Enough MCTs and Other Healthy Fats?

Dave Asprey, author of *The Bulletproof Diet* and creator of Bulletproof Coffee
bulletproofexec.com

Here's what my good friend Dave Asprey has to say about the importance of eating fats—and why it's so critical to pick the *right* fats.

"Millions of people are overweight, sick, and tired right now because they're not getting enough healthy fat. Our hormones are made of saturated fat, our brains are made of fat, and the membranes of all of our cells are made of fat. When you eat a low-fat diet, you limit the performance of so many key systems in your body that it's no wonder you have cravings and feel fatigued.

"So take Kellyann's advice: Eat fats. The key, however, is to make sure you're eating high-quality fats—not vegetable oils or peanut butter. Saturated fats like coconut oil and grass-fed butter or ghee will not cause hardened arteries; instead, they will help your body perform and look better. Eating a diet rich in healthy fats teaches your body to burn fat instead of sugar, keeping you lean. It balances your blood sugar. It gives you insane energy. And it keeps you satisfied, preventing cravings.

"In particular, your body needs a steady supply of MCTs (medium-chain triglycerides) like those found in coconut oil. These are the cleanest, most direct sources of energy for your body. These fats will take weight off your body—not put it on. In addition, MCTs promote the formation of lean muscle. That's why so many high-level athletes take MCT oil supplements.

"Butter or ghee from grass-fed cows is also an essential. A 14-gram serving of grass-fed butter or ghee contains 500 IU of vitamin A, more carotenes than carrots, and large amounts of vitamins K_2, D, and E. Butter or ghee also contains a short-chain saturated fatty acid called butyrate, a powerful inflammation fighter. In animal studies, butyrate has been shown to protect against mental illness, increase energy expenditure, improve body composition, and decrease intestinal permeability ('leaky gut').

"In short, healthy fats like those in coconut and butter or ghee are one of the biggest keys to keeping your body strong, slim, and young and keeping your brain healthy. My advice? When in doubt—eat more healthy fat, not less!"

water. Water flushes toxins out of your body and helps prevent you from feeling hungry. Often when people are thirsty, they experience "signal confusion" and think they're hungry instead.

Here's a low-tech way to make sure you're drinking enough water: Simply check your pee. You should be urinating at least six times a day, and your urine should have a slightly yellow color. If you aren't urinating that often or your urine is a deeper yellow, that's a sign that you need more water.

One quick tip: You'll enhance the results of your diet if you start off each morning with a big glass of water with a little lemon squeezed in it. Oddly, while lemons are acidic, lemon water helps make your body more alkaline (which is very good).

IMPORTANT! LET'S TALK ABOUT PORTIONS

There's one more crucial thing we need to talk about before you start your diet, and that's "portion control."

In Chapter 2, I told you that I don't want you counting calories, carbs, or fat grams. Measuring your meals like this is unnatural, plus it takes the fun out of eating (and I firmly believe that eating should be fun!). Besides, virtually everyone who tries to lose weight that way fails.

Instead, I want you to be able to eat naturally—now and for the rest of your life. I want you to be wise about what your body needs and choose your portions instinctively, just like people did for millions of years.

To do this, however, you need to know what a natural portion size is. This is something you're actually born knowing, which is why babies and kids hardly ever overeat when they're eating real, natural foods. Unfortunately, if you're used to restaurant portions—which typically are double or triple what you need—you may have trouble instinctively knowing just how much food your body really requires.

Luckily, there's an easy way to "mentally measure" your portions. You don't need a scale or a calculator. On the following pages, you'll find a handy chart for measuring portions, as well as an At-a-Glance Meal Plan that makes it supereasy to calculate how many servings of each "yes" food group you'll include in each meal.

To see the big picture, check out my "Bone Broth Diet Quick Plate" on the Resources page of my website, drkellyann.com/resources.

Easy Tips for Portion Control
A PERFECT PLATE

PROTEIN PORTIONS

A serving of meat, fish, or poultry should be about the size and thickness of your palm. A serving of eggs is as many as you can hold in your hand (that's about 2 or 3 for women and 3 or 4 for men). A serving of egg whites alone is double the serving for whole eggs. Each meal should include a serving of protein.

NONSTARCHY VEGETABLE PORTIONS

A serving of these vegetables should be at least the size of a softball. You can't eat too many of them, so fill your plate with at least 2 or 3 softballs' worth.

STARCHY VEGETABLE PORTIONS

A serving of starchy vegetables (such as sweet potato, jicama, kohlrabi, or winter squash) should be about the size of a baseball for women and the size of a softball for men. *Note:* Eat starchy vegetables only if you're recovering from a workout or you're feeling weak and tired and you know it's not due to the carb flu (see "Troubleshooting Tips" later in this chapter).

FRUIT PORTIONS

A serving of fruit is half an individual piece (half an apple, half an orange) or a tennis-ball-size serving of berries, grapes, or tropical fruits (about ½ cup). That's a closed fistful, or about ½ cup if they're diced. Eat only 1 portion of fruit per day, preferably at breakfast.

FAT PORTIONS

A serving of liquid fat should be about the size of a Ping Pong ball, a typical bouncy ball, or 1 to 2 thumb-size portions (that's about 1 tablespoon).

A serving of nuts, seeds, coconut flakes, or olives is about 1 closed handful.

A serving of avocado is one-quarter to one-half an avocado.

A serving of coconut milk Is one-third of a cup.

Each meal should include 1 or 2 servings of fat.

At-a-Glance
WEEKLY PLAN

	BREAKFAST	LUNCH	DINNER	SNACK
Day 1	1 portion protein 2 portions non-starchy vegetables 1 to 2 portion fats 1 portion fruit	1 portion protein 2 portions non-starchy vegetables 1 to 2 portion fats	1 portion protein 2 portions non-starchy vegetables 1 to 2 portions fat	Bone broth*
Day 2	Sip on bone broth. May also drink: • Coffee (black only)/tea • Water	Sip on bone broth. May also drink: • Coffee (black only)/tea • Water	Sip on bone broth. May also drink: • Coffee (black only)/tea • Water	Bone broth if you're doing Plan 1, or 7:00 p.m. snack or approved shake if you're doing Plan 2
Day 3	1 portion protein 2 portions non-starchy vegetables 1 to 2 portions fat 1 portion fruit	1 portion protein 2 portions non-starchy vegetables 1 to 2 portions fat	1 portion protein 2 portions non-starchy vegetables 1 to 2 portions fat	Bone broth*
Day 4	1 portion protein 2 portions non-starchy vegetables 1 to 2 portions fat 1 portion fruit	1 portion protein 2 portions non-starchy vegetables 1 to 2 portions fat	1 portion protein 2 portions non-starchy vegetables 1 to 2 portions fat	Bone broth*
Day 5	Sip on bone broth. May also drink: • Coffee (black only)/tea • Water	Sip on bone broth. May also drink: • Coffee (black only)/tea • Water	Sip on bone broth. May also drink: • Coffee (black only)/tea • Water	Bone broth if you're doing Plan 1, or 7:00 p.m. snack or approved shake if you're doing Plan 2
Day 6	1 portion protein 2 portions non-starchy vegetables 1 to 2 portions fat 1 portion fruit	1 portion protein 2 portions non-starchy vegetables 1 to 2 portions fat	1 portion protein 2 portions non-starchy vegetables 1 to 2 portions fat	Bone broth*
Day 7	1 portion protein 2 portions non-starchy vegetables 1 to 2 portions fat 1 portion fruit	1 portion protein 2 portions non-starchy vegetables 1 to 2 portions fat	1 portion protein 2 portions non-starchy vegetables 1 to 2 portions fat	Bone broth*

*When you feel tired or weak or need more energy, up to 2 mugs of bone broth are allowed per day for a snack.

TROUBLESHOOTING TIPS

The Bone Broth Diet is easy to follow, and you should see quick results, but occasionally problems crop up. Here's how to handle them easily.

Problem 1: "I'm hungry!"

On this diet, you'll be getting all the calories and food energy you require. However, there are two reasons you may find yourself craving extra food.

The first is that carb flu I talked about in Chapter 2. (Make sure you've read that section, because it's really important. If you didn't read it yet, check it out now.) You can tell if you have the carb flu based on the timing and your symptoms. It typically starts 2 to 7 days into your diet and lasts for 3 to 7 days. As I said earlier, it'll make you feel tired, cranky, wired, and weird.

If the carb flu is making you feel hungry, the solution is to add a tiny bit of extra fat to your diet. So eat a handful of unsweetened coconut chips, some olives (rinse off the salty brine), or half an avocado. Remember that you just need to ride out this stage. It won't last long.

If you're past the carb flu stage and you occasionally feel famished, it may be because you really do need a tiny extra shot of energy. If that's the case, simply add a bit of starchy vegetables (I call them "energy veggies") to your next meal. For instance, have half a sweet potato or some jicama. Jicama is one of my favorites because it's rich in that soluble fiber that feeds your gut flora and keeps your microbiome—or your bag of bugs—superhealthy.

Problem 2: "I'm not losing weight!"

After a few days on the Bone Broth Diet, you should start burning fat like crazy.

Occasionally, however, I get a call from a patient who says, "The magic isn't happening, Kellyann." When I hear this, I do a little troubleshooting. Nearly 100 percent of the time, I narrow the problem down to one of seven issues.

If you're not seeing the fat melt off your own body, here's my seven-step troubleshooting drill. Just ask yourself: Are you . . .

■ **Eating too much fruit?** Fruit is high in fructose, and although a little fruit is good for you, too much can create havoc. Remember: A good serving size is a closed handful of berries or chopped fruit, or half of a larger piece of fruit like a grapefruit or a large apple.

- **Eating too many nuts?** Nuts are on the "yes" list, but it's important to eat them in moderation. Stick to a closed handful.

- **Keeping foods on the "no" list in your kitchen?** Don't keep chips and cookies and other high-carb stuff in your pantry or fridge, where they can tempt you to cheat. Donate or, better yet, toss them.

- **Skipping the fat?** I can't say this often enough: Adding the right quantities of fat to your diet actually helps you lose fat. Try it and you'll see.

- **Eating too much healthy fat?** Use the measuring system I taught you earlier and you won't go wrong.

- **Not measuring your other foods properly?** Keep that "plate picture" in mind. Don't overdo your proteins, and don't short yourself on nonstarchy veggies.

- **Not completely letting go?** Clutching on to that one food or drink you struggle to let go of can thwart your weight-loss efforts. Remember: Be ruthless.

GETTING ENOUGH . . .

You will be shocked at how satisfied you feel eating this food. This is the healthiest and most satisfying kind of cleanse you can get. The trick here, though, is to make absolutely sure you are sticking to the key fundamentals of the diet—getting protein, veggies, and a healthy fat with every meal. You can't short-cut, or you will not feel totally satisfied and in the zone. Getting the fat is truly your safeguard. When you don't, you'll feel the difference.

Once you've spotted your issues, correct them—and then be patient and trust that your body will do what it needs to do. When you fine-tune your diet, the magic will happen!

Eating clean doesn't mean you need to turn into a hermit! There is a way to communicate with others and keep your relationships strong while starting a healthy lifestyle. Check out my "Dinner Party Pitch" on the Resources page of my website, drkellyann.com/resources.

A GENTLE WORD ABOUT "CHEATS"

As I said back in Chapter 2, I don't want you to feel like a failure if you cheat. If you say "Screw it, Kellyann, I'm having a bowl of oatmeal"—or you give in to a plate of spaghetti, a bowl of ice cream, or a scotch and soda—that's perfectly okay. I'm not the diet police . . . and like I said before, sometimes I'm beautifully imperfect myself.

However, here's the reality. I've made a promise to turn you into a natural fat burner and help you lose weight and wrinkles in 21 days. To keep that promise, I have to keep you constantly low carb.

If you cheat at any point during your 3-week diet—even once—you're going to be back to square one. Your body will revert to burning glucose for fuel, and it'll take time for it to get back to mega-fat-burning. But there's more. You will not stop the inflammation cycle, heal your gut, or balance your blood sugar. And I truly want this for you.

So remember what I said earlier: If you fall off the wagon, don't kick yourself. Simply reset your 3-week calendar and start over again. Some of my patients have two or three "oopsies" before they make it through 3 weeks without a cheat. They're surprised when I say, "Hey, no problem"—but I know from experience that they'll get there!

CHAPTER 5

My Bone Broth Lifestyle Plan—or How to Keep Those Pounds Off FOREVER

OKAY, WE'VE TALKED ABOUT what my Bone Broth Diet is going to do for you. It's going to slim you down, take years off your face, and give you the energy of a teenager.

Now, let's talk about what's going to happen AFTER your diet . . . starting on Day 22.

I'm not psychic, but here's something I think I know about you. I'm pretty sure you've lost weight before, and then, within months, you gained it back. What's more, there's a good chance you gained back more pounds than you lost.

In fact, I'm betting you've ridden this roller coaster again and again. It's frustrating, upsetting, and even a little heartbreaking.

Well, right now, I want to make you a promise: If you do what I'm about to tell you to do, *that's not going to happen this time*. That's because this time I have your back, and I'm not going to let you down.

That's a bold promise, I know. But remember: I've personally guided thousands of people through this diet, and hundreds of thousands more through my books. I'm not an expert on everything in life, but I can guarantee you that I'm an expert on this.

Here's my promise to you. If you follow the rules of the Bone Broth Lifestyle that I spell out here, you're going to keep those pounds (and those wrinkles) off for life. And you're going to do it without starving, and without saying goodbye forever to your favorite foods. You have my word.

Ready? Here's how the magic works.

STEP 1: REACH YOUR GOAL WEIGHT.

If you still want to lose some pounds after you finish your 21 days, simply continue on the Bone Broth Diet. This is a healthy, gentle plan you can follow as long as you like. I've had hundreds of patients lose 100, 200, or even 300 pounds on this plan.

Alternately, if you're just a few pounds shy of your goal, and you have a big event coming up—for instance, a wedding or a class reunion—you can switch over to my five-day Cleanse and Reset or my 10-Day Belly Slimdown. You're running the show, so choose the plan that works for you and your lifestyle.

Once you reach your goal, it's time for the next step.

STEP 2: FOCUS ON THE FOODS THAT KEEP YOU SLENDER—BUT LET YOURSELF CHEAT!

After 21 days on my diet, you've witnessed first-hand the incredible power of cutting the carbs and focusing on lean proteins, bone broth, healthy fats, and nonstarchy veggies (along with a touch of fruit and starchy vegetables). You've seen the magic at work, so you know these are the foods that will keep you slim, healthy, and youthful for life.

So if life were simple, you'd be all set. You'd choose all your meals from these foods and stay away from junk food and carb overloads.

Simple, right? But there's just one catch: Like me, *you're human*. That means that like me, you're "perfectly imperfect"—and sometimes you're going to want to indulge in pancakes and syrup, macaroni and cheese, or your mom's to-die-for lasagna. I know . . . because I do, too.

Well, guess what: That's not a problem. In fact, you'll get to have regular cheats on this plan. That's what I do, and I know it works.

Being able to cheat a little is a powerful thing, because you never need to say "never" to any food you love. The trick, as I like to say, is to put enough credits in your good-food bank that you can sin without paying a price. Here's how to do it.

MY TWO BONE BROTH LIFESTYLE OPTIONS— PICK YOUR FAVORITE!

There are two ways to do my Bone Broth Lifestyle plan; one is to follow the 80/20 rule, and the other is to count carbs. You can pick whichever method is easiest for you—you know I'm all about personal play!

Here's how each approach works. Check out both of them carefully before you make up your mind.

METHOD #1: THE 80/20 SYSTEM

If you pick this approach, here's what you'll do:

- For 80% of your meals, you'll stick to slimming, wrinkle-blasting, inflammation-fighting, blood-sugar-lowering foods (I'll give you the list shortly). And you'll fill your plate full at every meal.

- For the other 20% of your meals, you'll get to splurge. As long as you keep your proportions reasonable, nothing is off limits.

- If you go too far off the rails and wind up putting a few pounds back on, you'll be able to erase the damage like it never even happened (more on this later as well).

Now let's take a closer look at each stage.

YOUR 80% MEALS

For 80% of your meals, you're going to stick to the Bone Broth Diet "yes" foods on pages 66–68. These include:

- **Proteins.** fish, poultry, beef, lamb, eggs, organ meats, bone broth, and collagen powder. Look for meats that are free from nitrates, nitrites, and sugar, and choose pastured meats and eggs if they fit into your budget. (If not, remove the skin from your chicken and take the skin off your beef, because that's where most of the toxins collect.)

COCKTAILS? YES, YOU CAN!

Just make alcoholic drinks an *occasional* treat and be smart about the type of liquor and mixers you choose. Beer is carb-heavy and contains gluten (unless it's specifically labeled as gluten-free), which can cause inflammation. And commercial mixers are sugar bombs. Choose wine or distilled spirits, and mix drinks with sparkling water, muddled berries, or even bone broth. (Really. Check out "A Healthier Way to Mix: Collagen and Bone Broth Cocktail Recipes," on the Resources page of my website at drkellyann.com/resources. Cheers!)

- **Healthy fats.** Clarified butter or ghee, avocados and avocado oil, olives and olive oil, coconut and coconut oil, nuts, and seeds. Remember: This is where you'll get those skin-plumping ceramides I talked about on page 63.

- **Nonstarchy vegetables.** Don't skimp on these, because they're rich in slimming nutrients and they give you the fiber you need to stay regular and battle the bloat.

- **Small "accents" of starchy veggies and fruits.** Add these to your plate if you need an extra boost of energy.

If you focus on these foods for 80% of your meals, and you watch your portion sizes (see "Your 80% Template" below), you're going to maintain your goal weight with no effort at all. It really is that simple.

YOUR 80% TEMPLATE

Protein Portions

A serving of meat, fish, or poultry should be about the size and thickness of your palm. A serving of eggs is as many as you can hold in your hand (that's about two or three for women, three or four for men). A serving of egg whites alone is double the serving for whole eggs. Each meal should include a serving of protein. Note: See "A Word About Protein," page 121.

Fruit Portions

A serving of fruit is half an individual piece (half an apple, half an orange, half a banana) or a tennis ball–size serving of berries, grapes, or tropical fruits (about half a cup). That's a closed fistful if they're diced. Eat no more than two servings of fruit per day and break them up across meals and snacks to distribute your sugar intake.

NonStarchy Vegetable Portions

A serving of nonstarchy vegetables should be at least the size of a softball. These are fabulous for you, so if possible, fill your plate with at least two or three softballs' worth!

Starchy Vegetable Portions

A serving of starchy vegetables (such as sweet potato, jicama, kohlrabi, or winter squash) should be about the size of a baseball for women and the size of a softball for men. Eat these veggies only when you need an extra burst of energy—for instance, on days when you do strenuous workouts.

Fat Portions

A serving of oil or clarified butter is 1 tablespoon.

A serving of nuts, seeds, coconut flakes, or olives is about one closed handful.

A serving of nut butter is 1 tablespoon.

A serving of avocado is ¼ to ½ an avocado.

A serving of canned coconut milk is ⅓ cup.

A serving of chia seeds is 4 teaspoons.

A serving of flaxseed is 2 tablespoons.

A serving of hemp seeds is 2 tablespoons.

To help make your gut glow, I also want you to work *probiotic* and *prebiotic* foods into your meals as often as you can. Probiotics are fermented foods that contain healthy bacteria to reseed your gut; they include kimchi, sauerkraut, and pickles. (Be sure to buy these in the refrigerated case, because the versions on the store shelf are pasteurized, which kills off the bacteria.) Prebiotics are foods that act as fertilizer for your gut bacteria; they include asparagus, onions, jicama, garlic, leeks, Jerusalem artichokes, and unripe bananas.

For your 80% meals, I want you to continue to avoid grains, dairy (unless you know you don't have problems with it), soy, and seed oils. If you want a quick refresher on why these foods aren't good for you, check out pages 52–59.

In addition to avoiding these foods, I want you to steer clear of foods with artificial sweeteners or additives. When you shop for your 80% meals, be sure to read labels. If a product's label lists ingredients you can't pronounce, put it back on the shelf. Buy fresh food as often as you can; the fewer bar codes you wind up with in your cart, the better. When you can't go fresh, choose a brand you can trust; see my list of recommended brands on the Resources page of my website at drkellyann.com/resources.

Now, a word about beans and lentils. This one comes down to doing what's right for your own body. Beans and lentils contain large amounts of substances called phytates and lectins, and some people can handle these well, while others can't. (Personally, I enjoy black beans and lentils, but I need to steer clear of the others.) If you do fine with them, you can add them in small amounts to your 80% list; otherwise, make them a 20% food or eliminate them entirely.

Now that you know all about the foods you'll eat for 80% of your meals, put all those good food credits in your food bank. So let's talk about the other 20%—or as I call them, your "splurge" meals.

YOUR 20% MEALS

Think for a minute about your favorite foods—the ones that you consider taboo. Now imagine getting to enjoy them—guilt-free!—on a regular basis.

Well, that's what you're going to do now. For 20% of your meals, you can indulge in a favorite food that's not on the yes list. That works out, roughly, to four "splurge" meals each week. And I'm talking about eating whatever you want (within reason) for these meals. There are *no taboo foods*.

I'm serious. Cookies for breakfast. Pizza for lunch. Pad Thai and rice on date night. As long as you stick to reasonable servings, you're good.

Now, this is where a little bit of what I call "personal play" enters the picture.

You can stick to 20% or tweak that number a little bit. To decide, ask yourself these questions:

- Do you still want to lose more weight? If so, try sticking to a 90/10 plan until you reach your goal weight.

- Do you have an autoimmune condition or any other serious health problem? Consider keeping your splurges to a minimum.

- Is your blood sugar higher than you'd like? If so, take your blood sugar measurements regularly so you can determine just how many carbs your body can handle. (For more on this, see my article "How to Measure Your Blood Sugar" on the Resources page of my website at drkellyann.com/resources.)

By the way, when you're getting a feel for how many carbs your body can handle, remember that it's the *net* carbs on the label that count. (For more on this, see page 85.)

Once you decide how many "splurge" meals are right for you, *enjoy them*. There's no guilt, no shame, no I-wish-I-didn't-eat-that. Because you have my blessing.

YOUR 80/20 MEALS AT A GLANCE

To make it easier for you to see how my 80/20 system works, here are samples from two different patients. Sarah still wants to lose a few pounds, so she sticks to three splurge meals each week—and she saves them for the weekend, so she can enjoy them with her kids. David is at his goal weight, so he enjoys four splurge meals that he spreads out over the week.

Sarah's 80/20 Week

	MONDAY	TUESDAY	WEDNESDAY	THURSDAY	FRIDAY	SATURDAY	SUNDAY
BREAKFAST	80% Meal	80% Meal	80% Meal	80% Meal	80% Meal	20% Meal: Bagels and cream cheese	20% Meal: Home-made waffles with the kids
LUNCH	80% Meal	80% Meal	80% Meal	80% Meal	80% Meal	80% Meal	80% Meal
DINNER	80% Meal	80% Meal	80% Meal	80% Meal	80% Meal	20% Meal: Girls' night out— Linguini with Clam Sauce	80% Meal

David's 80/20 Week

	MONDAY	TUESDAY	WEDNESDAY	THURSDAY	FRIDAY	SATURDAY	SUNDAY
BREAKFAST	80% Meal	80% Meal	80% Meal	20% Meal: Oatmeal with sliced banana	80% Meal	80% Meal	80% Meal
LUNCH	20% Meal: Restaurant meal with friends—cheeseburger and fries	80% Meal	80% Meal	80% Meal	80% Meal	20% Meal: Game-day pizza, wings, and beer	80% Meal
DINNER	80% Meal	80% Meal	20% Meal: Tacos and refried beans with the kids	80% Meal	80% Meal	80% Meal	80% Meal

To make it easier for you to keep track of your "splurge" meals, I suggest either writing them down on your calendar or creating a routine so you know which meals they'll be. That way, it's easy to make sure you're sticking to the plan.

METHOD #2: CARB CONTROL

You don't have to count carbs on my lifestyle plan—but you can if you prefer this method. First, do some up-front work to determine what your ideal carb range is. Stick to this range nearly every day, and you'll be in total control of your weight.

On average, here's the range that works for most people:

- Lose weight: 50 to 75 net carbs (you may need to go lower)
- Maintain weight: 75 to 150 net carbs
- Gain weight: 150 to 200 net carbs

However, each one of us is unique. Your age, your metabolism, and your activity level will all help to determine the carb range that's right for you.

To track your carb intake, use an online carb counter like MyFitnessPal, Senza, or Carb Manager: Keto Diet Tracker & Macros Counter by Wombat Apps LLC. The carb counter beginning on page 371 of this book can also help.

To find out what your limit is, start at 50 carbs per day. If you hold your weight steady there, you can try adding in more starchy veggies, fruits, and other carbs very gradually, keeping a careful eye on how they affect your health and waistline. If you get lots of heavy-duty exercise every day, you may find that you need more than 50 carbs per day. If you want to lose weight, you may find that you do better dropping below 50.

For the rest of your diet, aim for about 100 grams of protein each day (see my box on protein on page 121) and round out your meals with leafy greens and healthy fats.

Stick as much as possible to healthy foods—the "yes" foods on pages 66–68 will work for this option as well as the 80/20 option—and avoid foods that contain soy, seed oils, dairy (unless you know you can handle it), sugar, and artificial sweeteners. If you eat grains, keep them to a minimum and pay close attention to how they affect you.

Keep track of your carb intake over several months, and you'll discover how many carbs you can eat on an average day while maintaining your ideal weight. (For extra points, track your blood sugar using a glucose monitor and see how many carbs you can eat without it spiking too high. You want your fasting blood sugar to stay in the low 90s at a maximum.)

Now let's talk about counting carbs—because there's a right way and a wrong way to do it. When you're counting carbs, you don't want to look at the *total* carbs in a food. Instead, you want to look at the *net* carbs.

The carbohydrates in food fall into four categories:

- Fiber
- Starch
- Sugar alcohols
- Sugars

Not all of these types of carbs affect your blood sugar the same way. Starches and sugars get absorbed rapidly and converted to glucose, causing your blood sugar and insulin levels to spike. This packs pounds on you quickly. Fiber and sugar alcohols like erythritol, however, are absorbed slowly (or not at all) and metabolized differently. As a result, they don't cause your blood sugar and insulin levels to rise. The net carbs consist of the carbs that will raise your blood sugar and insulin, so that's the number you want to count.

Here's the formula for calculating net carbs: Total Carbohydrates - Dietary Fiber - Sugar Alcohols = Net Carbs. The following are a few examples:

- **Raspberries.** A half-cup serving contains about 7 grams of carbs, but 4 grams of this comes from dietary fiber. So you only need to count the 3 net carbs.

- **Almonds.** A quarter cup of almonds has 11 total carbs, but 6.5 of those carbs are fiber. So in this case, you only need to count the 4.5 net carbs.

- **Avocados.** A half-cup serving of avocado has 6.4 total carbs, but 5 grams of that is fiber—so your net carb total is a mere 1.4 grams.

- **Baked potato.** A baked potato has about 27.4 total carbs, and only about 2.4 grams are fiber, so your net carb count is a whopping 25 grams.

Now let's talk a little bit about those "cheats" I mentioned earlier. Once you determine what your ideal carb range is, you'll be able to exceed it on occasion without doing any harm. So enjoy that piece of birthday cake or that plate of pasta . . . just make sure you get right back on track the next day.

And if you don't, well, that's what I'll talk about next.

Interested in knowing more about calculating and measuring your protein and fat intake, too? If you want even more control over your diet, go to my Resources page at drkellyann.com/resources for more information on calculating and measuring your personal protein and fat requirements.

WHEN YOU STRAY TOO FAR . . .

Now that you're totally up to speed on how to live the Bone Broth Lifestyle, I want to talk about one more thing: what to do when you fall off the wagon. And you'll notice that I said *when*, not *if*.

Let's be honest. Sooner or later, it's going to happen to you: You're going to drown your sorrows in a family-size bucket of macaroni and cheese or celebrate your joys with waaaay too much cake and champagne. That's because, as I said before, you're only human, and that means you're perfectly imperfect.

Since I'm in confession mode, I'll tell you the last time it happened to me. It was back in March 2020, during the early days of the COVID-19 pandemic. While I was safe in my home, I was terrified for my friends and medical colleagues a few miles away on the front lines. I worried myself sick about how my patients would cope when I couldn't get together with them face-to-face. And I wept to see my most beloved city in the world—New York City—in agony.

I'll tell you . . . for a few days, it broke me. I just wanted to crawl into bed and make it go away. Eventually, I picked myself up and got back into action, because I knew I had to stay strong. But by then I'd eaten way more ice cream than one very short Italian girl can pack away without starting to look like a Weeble.

I'm not going to judge you when you stray, because I do, too. And I know it's a cliché, but it's not how many times you fall down; it's how many times you get up.

Tips for Staying Gluten-Free in Your Maintenance Phase

Jennifer Fugo, gluten-free expert and founder of Gluten Free School

glutenfreeschool.com

Going gluten-free may sound overwhelming at first. But follow my friend Jennifer's ABCs and you'll discover that it's far easier than you think.

"If you're like many people, you may discover during your maintenance phase that you're sensitive to gluten and should eliminate it completely from your diet forever. While going gluten-free can seem daunting, knowing where to start and understanding a few key initial steps can take you from confusion to confidence.

"First, get to know exactly where gluten hides. This spongy protein occurs in certain grains such as wheat. An easy way to remember gluten-containing grains is to think of the acronym BROWS, which stands for *barley, rye, oats* (which are contaminated and must be purchased clearly labeled "gluten-free"), *wheat,* and *spelt*. While there are other grains that contain gluten, such as farro and einkorn, they are less frequently found in the North American diet.

"Many amazingly delicious and nutrient-dense foods are naturally gluten-free, such as fresh vegetables and fruit, nuts, seeds, meat, seafood, fish, poultry, and dairy (but see Dr. Kellyann's caution about dairy). It doesn't matter how big (or small) your local store's "gluten-free" aisle is, because you can still shop through a huge portion of the store. And there are many companies that now clearly label their food products with the words *gluten-free*. Before buying anything (or taking the time to scan the ingredients on the label), look for the words *gluten-free* and then double-check that you don't see any questionable ingredients. Contact companies if you think that their products might be gluten-free if they aren't labeled as such.

"Remember, the best food to make and serve is that which is naturally gluten-free so that no one (not even you) misses the gluten that's not supposed to be on your plate! Plus it's a healthier, more nutritious path to take that will help you feel better sooner."

So don't worry about falling down. Just pick yourself up.

How? You're going to love this, because it's ridiculously simple. Just do two bone broth fasts per week, having nothing but bone broth for twenty-four hours each time. (You can drink bone broth at any time, day or night.) If you only

I TRAVEL EVERY MONTH. HOW CAN I STICK TO THE BONE BROTH LIFESTYLE WHEN I'M ON THE ROAD?

I work coast to coast, so I've come up with lots of tricks for staying on the plan even when I'm in hotels. Here are my best tips:

Keep some dried bone broth or collagen powder in your suitcase. When you get to your hotel, just heat some water and you have a healthy snack.

Pack low-carb treats like nuts, coconut chips, protein bars, and keto granola (there are some great brands online).

If you'll be eating out with clients or friends, go online ahead of time and check out menus. If you can't find healthy options, most restaurants will allow you to make substitutions. (Or you can always go with a salad with vinegar-and-olive-oil dressing). You can also schedule a few splurge meals to enjoy on your travels.

sinned a little bit, you'll undo the damage in a week. If you hit the ice cream harder, like I did, it might take a little longer than that. But eventually, you'll undo the damage like it never even happened.

MY SEVEN BEST TIPS FOR LIFELONG SUCCESS

When you follow my Bone Broth Lifestyle plan, you'll be set for life—no yo-yo dieting, no starving, and no cravings for "forbidden" foods. To make sure you're set up for a long-term win, here are seven final tips:

1. Watch those portion sizes. If you see a pound or two creep back on, it's probably due to "portion creep"—especially when it comes to starchy veggies, nuts, or your "cheat" meals. Stick to the 80/20 template (page 83) or your ideal carb range as closely as you can, because small cheats will add up over time.

2. Be proactive. Don't wait until you've gained five, ten, or fifteen pounds. Instead, the instant you feel that waistband getting tight or you spot a little "pooch" reappearing, do a couple of 24-hour bone broth fasts.

3. Remember those healthy fats every day! They'll balance your hormones and conquer cravings—and they're loaded with ceramides (see page 63) to keep your skin moist and young-looking.

4. Make bone broth and collagen a daily habit. Mix bone broth into soups and stews, drink it straight, or add it to cocktails. Stir collagen into soups, and blend it into shakes and smoothies.

5. Fill up on fiber. High-fiber foods slim you down and blast the bloat, so fill your plate with them at every meal.

6. Bust your stress. When you're stressed, you crave sugar and fat—and over time, excess levels of the stress hormone cortisol will give you a "cortisol tire" around your waist. Make it a habit every day to do at least one stress-relieving activity (see Chapter 13).

7. Move every day. Exercise is one of the most powerful ways to keep your body young, slim, healthy, and beautiful (see Chapters 11, 12, and 15).

PART II

RECIPES, MEAL PLANS, and BATCH-COOKING TIPS

CHAPTER 6

Fabulous Recipes
for Beautiful Bone Broth

(Plus Intermittent-Fasting-Day Snacks)

To prepare for your Bone Broth Diet, you're obviously going to need a good supply of one essential: bone broth! These days, you can order bone broth online or find it in health food stores. But it's so easy to make bone broth that you can simply simmer it up yourself.

In this chapter, I offer up basic bone broth recipes as well as gourmet recipes that rival anything you can buy. There's even a no-bones vegetarian broth. In addition to being nutritionally dense, all of these broths taste absolutely amazing—and you can make them for just a few dollars.

On your fasting days, you can pick any version of bone broth you prefer. But here's a word of advice: Try several different recipes. That way, you'll keep your palate intrigued and treat your body to a wider range of nutrients.

And speaking of taste and nutrition, let's take a minute to talk about the starring ingredient of bone broth: the bones. To make the most delicious and nutritious broth, you need to start with the right bones. Here's my advice on which bones make the best broth, along with some tips on where to find them.

But . . . before you read on, do me a favor: Don't get too obsessive about this! There's really no wrong way to make bone broth. I'm going to give you tips for making the very *best* broth, but don't worry about perfection. If you can toss a half-dozen ingredients into a stockpot and turn on the stove burner, you're set. Remember: Cave people used to cook broth in animal skins over a fire. It's not rocket science.

If the gourmet recipes intimidate you, simply make the basic chicken or beef recipes. It doesn't get any easier than that. And even if you make the gourmet recipes, feel free to leave out any ingredients you don't want. Basically, you only need bones and water—that's probably the original cave person recipe!

MEET YOUR NEW BEST FRIEND: THE BUTCHER

Everyone always asks me, "How do I select the best bones for bone broth?" It's really very simple, and these guidelines should help.

The biggest key is to make friends with your butcher. My team is always cooking and testing new recipes, and my butcher is a fabulous resource for getting the bones I want. He's more than happy to order something special if he doesn't have it available.

In selecting bones, strive to get bones from organic, grass-fed, pasture-raised animals if at all possible. These bones are more nutrient-dense, and they come from healthier animals raised in an environment with as few toxins as possible. Select bones with a lot of cartilage, because the collagen in that cartilage breaks down into gelatin when slowly heated—and gelatin, as you've seen, is a powerful healing and antiaging nutrient. (It's that "natural Botox" I keep talking about, so don't short yourself.)

The best beef bones to use are knuckles, joints, feet, and marrow bones. If your butcher doesn't stock knuckle and joint bones, he or she should be able to easily order them for you. A calf's or beef's foot is rich in cartilage. Neck bones are good, too, and you can often find them in the beef case. I also throw in some meaty bones when I make broth, because they add a lot of flavor. Oxtail, shank, and short ribs are perfect in broth.

For chicken or turkey broth, you can use the full carcass, necks, backs, and feet. Again, your butcher should be able to provide you with these inexpensive cuts. I always add a whole chicken and extra legs, thighs, or wings to further enrich the flavor. If you're using pastured chicken, leave the skin on; it's rich in collagen.

For fish, ask your butcher for the carcasses of any nonoily fish. That means no salmon or tuna. You're better off with a low-fat whitefish such as halibut, turbot, tilapia, cod, or rockfish. Better fish markets often buy the entire fish, cut the fillets themselves, and throw away the carcasses, and they may be willing to save some bones for you.

Fish heads work really well in broth, too. I know they're not exactly pretty to look at, but they're rich in gelatin. Also, you can toss in shrimp shells to add more flavor to your fish stock. Fish bones are much softer and finer than beef or poultry bones and they break down quickly when you cook them, so be sure not to overcook your broth.

You can save yourself some money by keeping all the leftover bones from your day-to-day cooking and storing them in the freezer so you can use them whenever you make broth. However, it takes a while to get a big enough stash of "good" bones, so plan on initially buying some.

A FEW COOKING TIPS

Bone broth is about as simple as a recipe gets. But if you're new to making bone broth, there are a few things you should know.

First, your cooked broth should become bouncy, just like gelatin, when you chill it. Now, if it doesn't, *don't fret*—it's still rich in the nutrients you need. (Remember what I said about not getting too obsessive here!) To get more bounce in your broth next time around, check out these troubleshooting tips:

- **Did you select the right bones?** The bones need to be cartilage rich, because it's the collagen in the cartilage that "melts" into gelatin when cooked. If you aren't using the bones I mentioned above, you won't get the best results.

- **Did you use too much water?** Adding excess water can dilute your broth too much. When you make broth, you only need to cover the ingredients in the pot.

- **Did you boil the broth?** When you make your stock, keep it at a low simmer, barely bubbling. Also, use the right-size burner for your pot. Even though I use a huge stockpot when I make broth, I keep it on the smallest burner on low. If your stove cooks too hot for the size of your pot, use a slow cooker, buy a bigger pot (so you can make a larger batch), get a pot with a heavier bottom, or keep the lid off or askew.

- **Did you overcook or undercook the broth?** Follow the timing guidelines in each of the bone broth recipes. Beef will take the longest time to cook and fish the shortest.

Also, be aware that the vinegar in these recipes has an important job: It helps dissolve the bones so you'll get the maximum amount of nutrients out of them. You won't taste it at all when your broth is done, so don't skimp on it.

Once you have the basics of bone broth down, it's fine (and fun) to experiment! Try different herbs and spices; let your creativity loose. Thyme is particularly nice with chicken or turkey broth, and garlic works well. You can always test a new spice combination in a cup of broth before stirring it into your whole pot.

Now, here's a really important tip: Since you might use the broth in a variety of recipes, don't salt your entire batch. Instead, salt just the broth you plan to drink.

If your slow cooker is small (2 quarts or less), you can cut back on the quantities in the recipe. (Your measurements don't need to be specific when you're making broth.) However, it'll be easier if you use a large saucepan or stockpot on the stovetop.

Now, let's talk a little about bones.

The number of pounds of bones needed will vary based on the size of your slow cooker or stockpot. You want the bones to fill the vessel so you can barely cover them with water. If you have bones from any leftovers, also add those.

If it's difficult to get chicken or turkey bones from your butcher, you may be able to get backs and necks. These make excellent bone broth.

Meaty bones add great flavor to beef broth—don't skimp on these. If you choose, you can roast the meaty bones in a 350°F oven before placing them in the pot, but roasting is not necessary.

HOW TO MAKE YOUR BROTH IN AN INSTANT POT

If you're busy and don't have time to watch over a pot of bone broth, I have an easy solution for you: Make your broth in an Instant Pot! Here are some tips for creating Instant Pot broth.

Cooking on both high and low pressure can result in a rich, gelatinous broth. However, if you have the extra time, low-pressure cooking may give you better and more consistent results.

The length of time required for making bone broth in an Instant Pot depends on several factors, including which pressure setting you select as well as the type and quantity of bones you're using. However, for a six-quart Instant Pot on high pressure, chicken bone broth typically takes ninety minutes while beef bone broth usually requires two hours. For low pressure cooking, chicken bone broth takes two hours and beef requires approximately three hours.

These times refer only to the actual pressure-cooking time. Allow for additional time:

- if you choose to first roast your beef bones (to enhance the flavor)
- for presoaking in apple cider vinegar
- for the Instant Pot to reach the appropriate pressure
- to naturally release the pressure at the end (this can take up to ninety minutes)

The whole process from start to finish typically takes four to six hours—which is still much faster than making broth in a slow cooker or on the stovetop. And if you're like me, every extra minute you can save in a day counts!

	POULTRY	BEEF	FISH
Stove/Slow Cooker	6 to 8 hours	12 to 24 hours	1 hour 15 minutes
Instant Pot	1.5 to 2 hours on high; 2 to 3 hours on low	2 to 3 hours on high; 3 to 4 hours on low	do not use

CHICKEN BONE BROTH

PREP TIME: 15 MINUTES • COOK TIME: 6–8 HOURS

*Yield: Varies depending on pot size; these ingredients are sufficient
for 1 gallon of broth*

- 3 or more pounds raw chicken bones/carcasses (from 3–4 chickens)
- 1 whole chicken and 4–6 additional legs, thighs, or wings
- ¼ –½ cup apple cider vinegar, depending on the size of the pot
- Purified water to just cover the bones and meat in the pot
- 2–4 carrots, scrubbed and roughly chopped
- 3–4 ribs organic celery, including leafy part, roughly chopped
- 1 onion, cut into large chunks
- 1 tomato, cut into wedges (optional)
- 1–2 garlic cloves
- 2 teaspoons peppercorns
- 1 bunch parsley

Place all the bones and meat in a large stockpot or slow cooker. Add the vinegar and enough purified water to cover everything by 1". Cover the pot.

Bring the water to a simmer over medium heat. Use a shallow spoon to carefully skim the film off the top of the broth. If you're cooking in a slow cooker, wait for about 2 hours until the water gets warm before skimming, but continue with the next step.

Add the carrots, celery, onion, tomato (if using), garlic, and peppercorns and reduce the heat to low. You want the broth to barely simmer. Skim occasionally during the first 2 hours. Cook for at least 6 hours or up to 8, adding water as needed to ensure the bones are always covered with water and adding the parsley in the last hour. (You will have to add water during the cooking process.)

When the broth is done, remove the pot from the heat or turn off the cooker. Using tongs and/or a large slotted spoon, remove all the bones and meat. Save the chicken for another recipe. Pour the broth through a fine-mesh strainer and discard the solids.

Let cool on the counter and refrigerate within 1 hour. You can skim off the fat easily after the broth is chilled, if desired. When chilled, the broth should be very gelatinous. The broth will keep for 5 days in the refrigerator and 3 or more months in your freezer.

NOTE:

In a pressure cooker or Instant Pot, using your cooker's instructions, bring up to full pressure. Reduce the heat to low, maintaining full pressure, and cook for 1.5 to 2 hours or 2 to 3 hours on low. Allow the pressure to naturally release.

TURKEY BONE BROTH

PREP TIME: 15 MINUTES • COOK TIME: 6–8 HOURS

*Yield: Varies depending on pot size; these ingredients are sufficient
for 1 gallon of broth*

- 3 or more pounds raw turkey bones (backs and necks are usually available)
- 4–5 pounds turkey thighs or drumsticks
- ¼–½ cup apple cider vinegar, depending on the size of the pot
- Purified water to just cover the bones and meat in the pot
- 2–4 carrots, scrubbed and roughly chopped
- 3–4 ribs organic celery, including leafy part, roughly chopped
- 1 onion, cut into large chunks
- 1 tomato, cut into wedges (optional)
- 1–2 garlic cloves
- 2 teaspoons peppercorns

Place all the bones and meat in a large stockpot or slow cooker. Add the vinegar and enough purified water to cover everything by 1". Cover the pot.

Bring the water to a simmer over medium heat. Use a shallow spoon to carefully skim the film off the top of the broth. If you're cooking in a slow cooker, wait for about 2 hours until the water gets warm before skimming, but continue with the next step.

Add the carrots, celery, onion, tomato (if using), garlic, and peppercorns and reduce the heat to low. You want the broth to barely simmer. Skim occasionally during the first 2 hours. Cook for at least 6 hours or up to 8, adding water as needed to ensure the bones are always covered with water. (You will have to add water during the cooking process.)

When the broth is done, remove the pot from the heat or turn off the cooker. Using tongs and/or a large slotted spoon, remove all the bones and meat. Save the turkey for use in another recipe. Pour the broth through a fine-mesh strainer and discard the solids.

Let cool on the counter and refrigerate within 1 hour. You can skim off the fat easily after the broth is chilled, if desired. When chilled, the broth should be very gelatinous. The broth will keep for 5 days in the refrigerator and 3 or more months in your freezer.

NOTE:

In a pressure cooker or Instant Pot, using your cooker's instructions, bring up to full pressure. Reduce the heat to low, maintaining full pressure, and cook for 1.5 to 2 hours or 2 to 3 hours on low. Allow the pressure to naturally release.

BEEF BONE BROTH

PREP TIME: 15 MINUTES • COOK TIME: 12–24 HOURS

*Yield: Varies depending on pot size; these ingredients are sufficient
for 1 gallon of broth*

4–5 pounds grass-fed beef bones, preferably marrow, joints, and knuckle bones

3 pounds meaty bones such as oxtail, shank, or short ribs

¼–½ cup apple cider vinegar, depending on the size of the pot

Purified water to just cover the bones and meat in the pot

2–4 carrots, scrubbed and roughly chopped

2 ribs organic celery, including leafy part, roughly chopped

1 onion, cut into large chunks

2 dried bay leaves

1–2 garlic cloves

1 tablespoon peppercorns

Place all the bones in a large stockpot or slow cooker. Add the vinegar and enough purified water to cover everything by 1". Cover the pot.

Bring the water to a simmer over medium heat. Use a shallow spoon to carefully skim the film off the top of the broth. If you are cooking in a slow cooker, wait for about 2 hours until the water gets warm before skimming, but continue with the next step.

Add the carrots, celery, onion, bay leaves, garlic, and peppercorns and reduce the heat to low and cover the pot. You want the broth to barely simmer. Skim occasionally during the first 2 hours. Cook for at least 12 hours or up to 24, adding water as needed to ensure the bones are always covered with water. (You will likely have to add water during the cooking process.)

When the broth is done, remove the pot from the heat or turn off the cooker. Using tongs and/or a large slotted spoon, remove all the bones and meat. Save the beef for another recipe. Pour the broth through a fine-mesh strainer and discard the solids.

Let cool on the counter and refrigerate within 1 hour. You can skim off the fat easily after the broth is chilled, if desired. When chilled, the broth should be very gelatinous. The broth will keep for 5 days in the refrigerator and 3 or more months in your freezer.

NOTE:

In a pressure cooker or Instant Pot, using your cooker's instructions, bring up to full pressure. Reduce the heat to low, maintaining full pressure, and cook for 2 to 3 hours or 3 to 4 hours on low. Allow the pressure to naturally release.

ROTISSERIE CHICKEN BONE BROTH

PREP TIME: 15 MINUTES • COOK TIME: 6–8 HOURS
DEPENDING ON COOKING MODE

Yield: 1 gallon of broth

3 or more carcasses from rotisserie chickens

Drumsticks, thighs and wings from a rotisserie chicken or 2 or more pounds chicken thighs, legs, and/or wings

¼ cup apple cider vinegar

Purified water

2–4 carrots, scrubbed and roughly chopped

3–4 celery stalks, including leafy part, roughly chopped

1 medium onion, cut into large chunks

1–2 garlic cloves

1 bay leaf

2 teaspoons Celtic or pink Himalayan salt

1 teaspoon peppercorns

FAT-BURNING SPICES YOU CAN ADD FOR MORE FAT-BURNING POWER:

1" piece fresh ginger, sliced

Handful of parsley or cilantro

1 teaspoon fresh or ground turmeric

1/16–1/8 teaspoon cayenne

1–2 teaspoons ground cumin

Place all the bones into a large stockpot or slow cooker. Add the vinegar and enough purified water to cover everything by 1". Add all the vegetables, herbs, and spices. Add more water, if necessary.

On the stovetop on medium heat, bring the water to a simmer and reduce the heat to low. Cover and let simmer for at least 6 hours and up to 8. Add water as needed so the bones are always covered.

In a slow cooker, set to low, cover, and let cook for 6 to 8 hours.

When the broth is done, remove all the bones and the meat and pour the broth through a fine-mesh strainer into a large bowl. Discard the solids and reserve the meat for another use. (You can also refrigerate or freeze the bones and reuse them to make more broth.)

Let the broth cool completely before covering and placing into the refrigerator. When chilled the broth should be very gelatinous.

The broth will keep for 5 days in the refrigerator and 3 or more months in your freezer.

NOTE:

In a pressure cooker or Instant Pot, using your cooker's instructions, bring up to full pressure. Reduce the heat to low, maintaining full pressure, and cook for 2 to 3 hours or 3 to 4 hours on low. Allow the pressure to naturally release.

TRY BONE MARROW, TOO!

Like bone broth, bone marrow is packed with healing nutrients—and it's delicious. Bone marrow is considered a delicacy in many cultures, and more and more fancy restaurants are adding it to their menus in the United States.

Here's an interesting historical fact: Specially shaped marrow bone spoons were very popular in Europe and England in the 19th century because they made it easy to scoop out and enjoy this delicacy.

You can add these bones to any meal as a special treat on a nonfasting day. Enjoy!

ROASTED MARROW BONES

PREP TIME: 1 MINUTE • COOK TIME: 30 MINUTES

1 or more pounds beef marrow bones
Celtic or pink Himalayan salt
Ground black pepper

Preheat the oven to 425°F.

Place the marrow bones in a shallow roasting pan and bake for about 30 minutes. Season with salt and pepper. Save the bones for your next batch of bone broth.

FISH BONE BROTH

PREP TIME: 15 MINUTES • COOK TIME: 1 HOUR 15 MINUTES

Yield: *Varies depending on pot size; these ingredients are sufficient for 1 gallon of broth*

5–7 pounds fish carcasses or heads from large nonoily fish such as halibut, cod, sole, rockfish, turbot, or tilapia (see Notes)

2 tablespoons ghee (see page 119)

1–2 carrots, scrubbed and coarsely chopped

2 ribs organic celery, including leafy part, coarsely chopped

2 onions, coarsely chopped

Purified water to just cover the bones in the pot

1 bay leaf

1–2 garlic cloves

2 teaspoons peppercorns

1 tablespoon bouquet garni or a small handful of fresh parsley and 4–5 stems fresh thyme

Wash the fish and cut off the gills if present.

In a large stockpot, melt the ghee over medium-low to low heat. Add the carrots, celery, and onions and cook, stirring occasionally, for about 20 minutes.

Add the fish and enough water to cover everything by 1". Increase the heat to medium and bring the water to a bare simmer. Use a shallow spoon to carefully skim the film off the top of the broth. Add the bay leaf, garlic, peppercorns, and bouquet garni or parsley and thyme and reduce the heat to low. Cook at a bare simmer for about 50 minutes, uncovered or with the lid askew. Continue to skim the surface as needed.

When the broth is done, remove the pot from the heat. Using tongs and/or a large slotted spoon, remove all the bones. Pour the broth through a fine mesh strainer and discard the solids.

Let cool on the counter before refrigerating. You can skim off the fat easily after the broth is chilled, if desired. When chilled, the broth should be very gelatinous. The broth will keep for 5 days in the refrigerator and 3 or more months in your freezer.

NOTES:

Nonoily fish is necessary because the fish oils in fatty fish such as salmon become rancid in cooking.

The cartilage in fish bones breaks down to gelatin very quickly, so it's best to cook this broth on the stovetop.

Because of the short cooking time, a pressure cooker is not recommended.

BONE BROTH DIET DEVOTEES

Rosita and Rohit Lobo

Rosita: Being able to do the diet as a couple makes it so much easier. . . . It has brought us closer as a family. . . . We're eating dinner together, and that to me is priceless.

Rohit: This is not a diet. More so, it's a detoxification. But more importantly, it's a way of how you want to live your life. I feel much healthier. . . . I wanted to prove to myself that I had no dependency on alcohol, and I didn't even have a craving. March 31 was my birthday. We go out to a party, and this guy's got single malt, he's got everything we like, and I said, "I'll just have a fresh lime soda."

It was around 14 pounds [of weight loss] for me.

Rosita: Nine for me.

BEFORE   AFTER

VEGETARIAN POTASSIUM-RICH BROTH

IF YOU'RE A VEGETARIAN, YOU CAN SUBSTITUTE THIS BROTH FOR BONE BROTH.

1
VEGETARIAN
BROTH
Recipe

PREP TIME: 20 MINUTES • COOK TIME: 2 HOURS

Yield: Makes 12 cups • *Portions: no fat, protein, or vegetables*

- 2 medium or 1 large sweet potato or yam, scrubbed and cut into 2" pieces
- 1 bunch Swiss chard, cut into 2" pieces, including the stems (about 6 leaves)
- 2–3 big handfuls spinach, about ½–¾ of one 5-ounce box/bag
- 3 medium zucchini, cubed into 2" pieces
- 2 stalks celery, cut into 2" pieces
- 2–3 plum tomatoes, quartered (optional)
- 1 medium onion or 1 leek; cut the onion into wedges; slice the white part of the leek in 2" pieces
- ½ bunch parsley
- 2 garlic cloves, smashed
- 2–3 teaspoons salt
- 1 teaspoon ground black pepper or 8 whole peppercorns
- 2 bay leaves
- 1 or more tablespoons of coconut aminos (optional)

Wash all the vegetables well and put all ingredients except for the coconut aminos into a large pot. Cover with 1 gallon of filtered or bottled water. Bring to a boil over high heat, then immediately reduce the heat to low, cover, and simmer for about 2 hours. When done, let cool, strain, and add the coconut aminos (if using), one tablespoon at a time, to taste. Store broth in glass jars or covered containers in the refrigerator in glass jars for up to 5 days. If you are not using immediately, freeze for up to 1 month.

NOTE:

You can also make this broth in a slow cooker. Cook it on low for about 2 hours.

To make a smaller amount of broth, halve the recipe.

Because of the short cooking time, a pressure cooker is not recommended.

THANKSGIVING TURKEY BONE BROTH

PREP TIME: 5 MINUTES • COOK TIME: 5–10 MINUTES

Yield: Makes 4 cups (1 quart)

4 cups (1 quart) Turkey Bone Broth (page 99)

2 ribs celery, diced

1 carrot, diced

1 small clove garlic, crushed

¼–½ teaspoon ground sage or Bell's Seasoning (see Note)

1 clove

Celtic or pink Himalayan salt

Ground black pepper

Heat the broth in a saucepan over medium heat. Add the celery, carrot, garlic, sage or Bell's Seasoning, and clove. Reduce the heat to medium-low or low so the broth barely simmers for 5 to 10 minutes, or just until the carrots and celery are tender.

Remove and discard the garlic and clove. Season with salt and pepper and serve.

NOTE:

Bell's Seasoning is a salt-free blend of herbs and spices containing rosemary, oregano, sage, ginger, and marjoram.

SPICE UP YOUR BROTH!

The herbs and spices in bone broth will tickle your tastebuds—and at the same time, they'll boost your metabolism, burn fat, and promote good digestive health. Here's a look at what some of these herbs and spices do for you.

Ginger: This warming spice has anti-inflammatory properties. It also soothes your intestinal tract. Ginger may have thermogenic properties that help boost your metabolism.

Garlic: A nutrient-dense food, garlic is rich in antioxidants. Allicin, a powerful antioxidant, is released when you smash, cut, or chew garlic. Garlic also reduces LDL cholesterol, which may lower your risk of heart disease. Garlic reduces oxidative damage from free radicals, slowing the aging process. It's been used medicinally for thousands of years. The ancient Greek physician Hippocrates, often called the father of Western medicine, prescribed garlic to treat a variety of medical conditions.

Turmeric: Curcumin is the active ingredient in turmeric. It slows the formation of fatty tissue and may contribute to lower body fat and enhanced weight control. It's also an anti-inflammatory agent and reduces insulin resistance.

Black pepper: Piperine is the compound that gives pepper its pungent flavor. Piperine enhances the serum concentration, absorption, and bioavailability of curcumin, the active ingredient in turmeric.

Cayenne pepper (ground red pepper): Capsaicin, the compound that gives chile peppers their heat, may help shrink fatty tissue and lower blood fat levels. Because capsaicin creates heat in the body, it may temporarily increase fat-burning.

Cumin: This herb aids digestion and is active in energy production in the body.

Cardamom: This is another warming, thermogenic spice that may help boost your metabolism and your body's ability to burn fat.

ASIAN CHICKEN BONE BROTH

PREP TIME: 5 MINUTES • COOK TIME: 5–10 MINUTES

Yield: Makes 4 cups (1 quart)

- 4 cups (1 quart) Chicken Bone Broth (page 98)
- 3" length of lemongrass, cut into 1" pieces
- 1 small clove garlic, smashed
  One handful of shiitake mushrooms, sliced
- 2 scallions, white and green parts, cut into ½" pieces
  Celtic or pink Himalayan salt
  Ground black pepper
- 2 tablespoons coarsely chopped cilantro leaves

Heat the broth in a saucepan over medium heat. Add the lemongrass, garlic, mushrooms, and scallions. Reduce the heat to medium-low or low so the broth barely simmers for 5 to 10 minutes.

Remove and discard the lemongrass and garlic. Season with salt and pepper. Top with the cilantro.

EASTERN EUROPEAN BEEF BONE BROTH

PREP TIME: 5 MINUTES • COOK TIME: 5–10 MINUTES

Yield: Makes 4 cups (1 quart)

- 4 cups (1 quart) Beef Bone Broth (page 100)
- 1 small clove garlic, smashed
  Large handful of shredded cabbage
- 1 rib celery, diced
- 1 bay leaf
- 1 teaspoon dried dill
- 1 peppercorn
  Celtic or pink Himalayan salt

Heat the broth in a saucepan over medium heat. Add the garlic, cabbage, celery, bay leaf, dill, and peppercorn. Reduce the heat to medium-low or low so the broth barely simmers for 5 to 10 minutes, just until the vegetables are tender.

Remove and discard the bay leaf, garlic, and peppercorn. Season with salt and serve.

FRENCH ONION BEEF BONE BROTH

PREP TIME: 5 MINUTES • COOK TIME: 5–10 MINUTES

Yield: Makes 4 cups (1 quart)

4 cups (1 quart) Beef Bone Broth (page 100)

1 small clove garlic, smashed

   About 1 cup Roasted Sweet Onions (page 229)

¼ teaspoon herbs de Provence

1 peppercorn

   Celtic or pink Himalayan salt

Heat the broth in a saucepan over medium heat. Add the garlic, onions, herbs, and peppercorn. Reduce the heat to medium-low or low so the broth barely simmers for 5 to 10 minutes.

Remove and discard the garlic and peppercorn. Season with salt.

ITALIAN BEEF BONE BROTH

PREP TIME: 5 MINUTES • COOK TIME: 5–10 MINUTES

Yield: Makes 4 cups (1 quart)

4 cups (1 quart) Beef Bone Broth (page 100)

1 small clove garlic, smashed

¼ cup tomato sauce, sugar-free

¼ teaspoon Italian seasoning

   Celtic or pink Himalayan salt

   Ground black pepper

6 fresh basil leaves, cut into fine chiffonade (see Notes, page 162) ribbons

Heat the broth in a saucepan over medium heat. Add the garlic, tomato sauce, and Italian seasoning. Reduce the heat to medium-low or low so the broth barely simmers for 5 to 10 minutes.

Remove and discard the garlic. Season with salt and pepper and serve topped with the basil.

NEED BONE BROTH ON THE RUN? HERE'S THE SOLUTION!

Homemade stocks and broths tend to be much healthier than store-bought versions, which often contain MSG and other additives. However, on days when life is crazy, you may not have time to cook up a batch of bone broth. Luckily, it's now possible to buy dehydrated bone broth that's nutrition-packed and free of toxins and additives.

One big benefit of dehydrated bone broth is that it's portable. If you travel, you can carry on a lightweight packet of dehydrated broth when you fly and not have to worry about checking in a liquid. You can almost always get hot water in hotels or airports, and an emergency "meal" of a cup of broth can hold you over until you are able to get a full meal. You just add hot water, mix, and sip!

Also, if you or someone in your household has a sudden illness and you don't have any bone broth handy in the refrigerator, the dehydrated version can save the day.

If you buy dehydrated bone broth, make sure the broth is organic and the salt (if any) is mineralized salt or sea salt. If you can't find high-quality bone broth in a packet in your local stores, I offer a high-quality, powdered bone broth in easy-to-go packets at drkellyann.com.

7:00 P.M. SNACKS FOR YOUR INTERMITTENT-FASTING DAYS

In Chapter 2, I outlined two options for your intermittent-fasting days. If Plan 1 sounds best for you, simply drink bone broth all day. If you choose Plan 2 instead, you'll substitute a snack around 7:00 p.m. for your last cup of bone broth. This is a good choice if you find that you're very hungry or not sleeping well on mini-fast days.

If you choose Plan 2, keep your snacks simple and nourishing by including:

- An excellent protein source, about the size of your palm
- A serving of nonstarchy vegetables (see Chapter 4), the size of a softball or more
- 1 tablespoon olive oil or one serving of any of the Bone Broth Diet salad dressings or sauces (see Chapter 8). You can also enjoy any portion of the three salsas (pages 267, 269, and 272) or the Santa Fe Sauce (page 270).

LOOKING FOR OTHER SOURCES OF COLLAGEN?

Here's another way to add wrinkle-fighting power to your diet: grass-fed collagen protein. This is my absolute favorite protein outside of grass-fed meats and pastured eggs. If you're looking for a great protein in shakes and bars, this is it. If you have a hard time with food allergies or can't find a quick protein source that agrees with you, then you just hit the mother lode!

Grass-fed collagen protein is amazing. It has the same gut-healing, joint-healing, wrinkle-erasing benefits as the collagen building blocks in bone broth.

Collagen is lacking in our diets, so drink your bone broth—which is loaded with collagen building blocks—and get collagen in the form of protein powder and as the main protein in grab-and-go nutrition bars. Just make sure the label specifies that it's grass-fed, enzymatically hydrolyzed collagen. Quality matters, so don't skimp—you want the good stuff.

For more information on why collagen is considered "liquid gold," view the Resources page on my website, drkellyann.com/resources.

Here are 16 quick and easy snacks for fasting days. Each contains one protein, one vegetable, and one fat. None of them take more than a few minutes to prepare.

1. 3–4 ounces smoked salmon with sliced tomatoes and lettuce, drizzled with 1 tablespoon olive oil or 1 serving salad dressing*

2. 3–4 ounces cooked chicken breast, roast turkey breast, or whole roast chicken and steamed broccoli, drizzled with 1 tablespoon olive oil or ghee

3. 3–4-ounce turkey or chicken burger wrapped in large lettuce leaves with 1 tablespoon approved mayonnaise*

4. 3–4-ounce beef or bison burger topped with your choice of salsa, plus a small salad of lettuce and tomatoes with 1 tablespoon salad dressing* or 1 tablespoon olive oil and vinegar or lemon juice

5. 3–4 ounces sliced leftover Easy Pot Roast (page 179) with a sliced tomato drizzled with 1 tablespoon olive oil

*Whenever salad dressing or mayonnaise is included, it refers to one of the Bone Broth Diet salad dressing or mayonnaise recipes. Or you can use 1 tablespoon Primal Kitchen Mayo, which is available on Amazon.

6. 2 scrambled eggs with 1 tablespoon ghee and sautéed spinach

7. 1 Baked Scotch Egg (page 126) and sliced cucumbers or tomatoes drizzled with 1 tablespoon olive oil

8. 1 serving Bone Broth Egg Drop Soup (page 207) with 1 tablespoon olive oil or ghee added after you take the soup off the stove

9. 1 slice Turkey Meatloaf Loaded with Vegetables (page 169) with Ketchup (page 262), plus steamed cauliflower with 1 tablespoon ghee

10. 3–4 slices Applegate turkey breast, 1 tablespoon approved mayonnaise, and 3–4 asparagus spears to make roll-ups

11. 2–3 cups mixed salad greens and other vegetables from the Bone Broth Diet vegetables list (Chapter 4), topped with a small can of tuna or salmon with Lemon Vinaigrette (page 256) or 1 tablespoon olive oil and lemon juice

BONE BROTH DIET DEVOTEES

Don and Cindy Fuller

Don: I think Cindy lost 7 or 8 pounds, and I lost just over 14. One of the things I've noticed is that I have more breath. I don't know if the fat was pushing up or what, but I have more breath now. I noticed it almost right away. When we go to Florida, we walk the beaches a lot, and I had noticed that I was starting to get winded very easily. When we were walking down there recently, I didn't have that problem at all.

Cindy: What do you call it?

Don: Delicious bone broth!

Cindy: He's been walking around for 3 weeks saying, "Delicious bone broth!"

BEFORE   AFTER

12. 2–3 cups mixed salad greens and other vegetables from the Bone Broth Diet vegetables list, topped with a sliced hard-cooked egg and Creamy Avocado Salad Dressing (page 253)

13. 4–5 ounces baked or broiled whitefish such as cod drizzled with 1 tablespoon olive oil or ghee, plus Napa Slaw with Creamy Ginger Dressing (page 227)

14. 6 large boiled or steamed shrimp with ¼ cup Cocktail Sauce (page 258), plus steamed green beans with 1 tablespoon olive oil or ghee

15. 1 cup leftover Rich and Hearty Turkey Chili (page 168) with steamed spinach drizzled with 1 tablespoon olive oil or ghee

16. A Bone Broth Diet–approved shake (page 68). For more on everything you need to know about Dr. Kellyann's approved shakes, go to the Resources page on drkellyann.com/resources.

HOW TO MAKE YOUR BONE BROTH EXTRA TASTY

While a basic batch of bone broth is delicious, that doesn't mean you can't mix it up from time to time. There are endless ways to enhance the flavor of bone broth, and here are my most favorite.

Healing Your Heart

Joel Kahn, MD, author of *Dead Execs Don't Get Bonuses*

drjoelkahn.com

Joel Kahn, an interpreventional cardiologist and the director of wellness programs at Michigan Healthcare Professionals, knows that real food is powerful medicine for your heart. Here's what he has to say about it.

"I am a broken record in my heart clinic, preaching that food is medicine, food can heal, and food can reverse chronic diseases. I have seen so many powerful examples of patients turning around their lives by grasping the power of eliminating Western toxic processed foods and permitting their bodies to heal by nourishing heart and arteries with nutrient-dense whole foods.

"The Bone Broth Diet is a path to restore health and vitality while permitting healing to take place. Taking the challenge for 3 weeks can be your first step to living the life you always wanted.

"Too many patients have told me that Dr. Kellyann has improved their health and energy for me to have any doubts about her gifts. She is a gifted healer with an amazing bone broth program. If Dr. Kellyann teaches it, you can trust it has a proven record of helping so many."

When I want to keep it simple, I add a dash or two of some of the following:

- Salt
- White or black pepper
- Garlic powder
- Onion powder or dried minced onion
- Lemon juice
- Lemon zest
- Hot sauce
- Worcestershire sauce
- Vinegar (apple cider vinegar is my favorite)
- Truffle oil
- Smoked salt
- Coconut aminos
- Fish sauce

When I'm craving something reminiscent of my Italian roots, I'll add various combinations of the following:

- Parsley
- Oregano
- Basil
- Thyme
- Rosemary
- Marjoram
- Sugar-free tomato paste (½ to 1 teaspoon)
- Italian seasoning

When I want something mild but bursting with flavor, I'll go with one of these combinations:

- Salt, pepper, chives, and lemon juice
- Ginger, garlic powder, and lemon juice
- Truffle salt and ginger
- Garlic and onion powder, salt, and smoked paprika
- Garlic powder, ginger, cilantro, coconut aminos, and lime juice

When I really want to spice it up, I go for one of the following:

- Hot sauce (or cayenne pepper) and lemon juice
- Hot sauce or Sriracha, lime juice, salt, garlic powder, and coriander (or cilantro)

- Chili powder, cumin, cayenne pepper, garlic powder, onion powder, and paprika
- Turmeric, garlic powder, and black pepper

Don't Forget to Visit the Spice Aisle

There are so many interesting flavor combinations sitting on your local grocery store shelf! Every time I stock up on spices, I'm amazed at the new seasoning combinations I find. If you have a favorite ethnic food, I guarantee there is a seasoning for it. Try some out, but be sure to be mindful of added ingredients and skip ones with monosodium glutamate and added sugar.

Here are some of my go-to combination spices and pastes:

- Italian seasoning (of course)
- Herbs de Provence
- Taco seasoning
- Mexican adobo

- Curry powder or paste
- Garam masala
- Chinese five-spice
- Blackening seasoning

- Umami seasoning
- Za'atar
- Harissa

Make It Creamy

A little healthy fat, a tablespoon or two per eight ounces of bone broth, can turn any soup into a creamy soup. My favorite way to make a soup creamy is canned coconut milk, but pureed avocado works great, too. (Just remember to count the fat while you're on your Bone Broth Diet.)

Bottom Line . . . Make It Your Own

You know what you like. Play around with your favorite flavors and make it a daily adventure to try something new! If you do that, you'll never be bored with your bone broth.

CHAPTER 7

Fat-Blasting Entrées and Soups for Your Nonfasting Days

IF YOU'VE HAD IT up to here with doctors telling you that you can't eat anything good and still lose weight, guess what? Here's your chance to prove them all wrong!

In the next two chapters, I'm going to prove to you that dieting and fine dining can go hand in hand. It's time to reintroduce your tastebuds to formerly taboo foods like beef, eggs, avocados, bacon, and coconut oil—foods that will slash your insulin levels, reverse inflammation, heal your gut, burn off pounds, and take years off your skin.

First, in this chapter, I'll serve up dozens of no-sacrifice main courses and entrée/side soups that will make you drop weight while you indulge in foods you thought were sinful. In the next chapter, you'll get recipes for everything from veggie sides to shakes to desserts.

NOTE

I've included portion sizes for each recipe to make things easier for you. And in Chapter 9, you'll find 3 full weeks of meal plans, along with a convenient shopping list.

Because I know that some people love to cook and others don't, I'm providing something for everyone in these chapters, including:

- Gourmet recipes you'll enjoy if you love to cook
- Simple recipes that are perfect if you're short on time
- Easy entrée soups

- "Grab-and-go" meals you can make with leftovers
- Tips for no-cook meals you can buy at the grocery store

As a bonus in this chapter, I'm also serving up six "call-to-action" entrée soup recipes that will give you additional fat-melting, wrinkle-blasting, and energizing results. (Think of these as "power-ups.")

REMINDER
On your nonfasting days, you can have 2 cups of bone broth for snacks.

Of course, you can also come up with your own recipes, if you're feeling creative—just follow the guidelines in Chapter 4. Or if you don't want to cook at all, read on.

HATE TO COOK? NO PROBLEM!

I've designed these recipes to be fun and simple, even if you're a beginning cook. However, there's a chance that you're too busy to cook or that cooking isn't your thing. If so, don't worry! It's still easy to do this diet. Here are easy tips for eating well without cooking (or at least cooking only a little).

First, get precut veggies and lettuce at the salad bar in the supermarket. If possible, select a store that uses mostly fresh ingredients. Walk past the cottage cheese, canned fruit, and bottled dressings and select all fresh vegetables. If you plan on eating immediately, dress your salad with oil and vinegar or lemons. Keep the oil to 1 tablespoon.

You can also select the salad bar's cut-up vegetables such as broccoli, cauliflower, shredded carrots, mushrooms, and tomatoes, and then head to the produce area and buy prepared triple-washed lettuce, spinach, or cabbage. Mix them when you get home and voilà!—salad.

You may find vegetables precut and ready to pop in the microwave, bag and all. But don't microwave them in the bag if you can help it. (Who knows what chemicals may leach into the food?) Steam them on the stovetop if you possibly can.

While you're in the produce section, buy blueberries. They're the best fruit for you, and you can have a handful with your breakfast.

When it comes to veggies, your best choices are any fresh vegetables that you steam or roast. But if you know you won't have time to prepare them, frozen vegetables are an option. Just make sure you select veggies without butter sauces.

For protein, purchase lots of eggs, which are supereasy to cook—or even buy already hard-cooked eggs. Also get smoked salmon (make sure it's sugar-, dextrose-,

MAKING A MEMORABLE ENTRÉE SALAD

Entrée salads quickly solve the "I really don't feel like cooking" problem. The trick is making a delightfully delicious salad that feels like a meal, not like a diner's lifeless dinner salad. You want a salad that's satisfying and has enough of the right protein, vegetables, and fat to keep you energized, comfortably full, and burning fat. Here are my guidelines for a memorable entrée salad.

Choose a protein that you really like.
You don't have to eat tilapia when you want steak. Enjoy your meal! Protein will keep you satisfied for several hours because your body digests it more slowly than vegetables. And protein combined with vegetables and healthy fat will actually help you burn fat.

Select greens for their crispness.
Greens make a salad refreshing, invigorating, and energizing. Fresh greens are nutrient powerhouses, and there are so many to choose from: romaine, Bibb, green leaf, red leaf, oak leaf, spinach, kale, cabbage, frisée, arugula, dandelion greens, mesclun (spring mix), watercress, endive . . . the list goes on. Check out the Bone Broth Diet vegetables list on pages 66–67. Have two or three handfuls.

Add vegetables for the crunch factor.
Crunchify your salad. Use vegetables that you have to chew. Texture matters, and the action of crunching satisfies. People like to crunch—that's part of the reason the junk-food industry is huge. Walk down any snack aisle in the grocery store and you'll find that nearly everything fulfills the need to crunch. The good news is, vegetables crunch! Think radishes, cucumbers, snap peas, peppers, blanched broccoli or cauliflower, carrots, scallions . . . you get the picture. Take a look at the Bone Broth Diet vegetables list on pages 66–67. Enjoy about two softball-size servings.

Top with salad dressing for bold flavor and healthy fat.
All those vegetables are delicious, but a good salad dressing makes them sing. It also adds the smooth, almost creamy mouthfeel of fat. Just as crunch gives us a satisfying feeling, fat gives us a comforting feeling. It's smooth, creamy, silky, and very easy to swallow. I've included seven salad dressing recipes in Chapter 8, and most of them take less than 5 minutes to prepare.

and nitrite-free and preferably not farm raised). Canned tuna and salmon packed in water or olive oil are great choices, too.

Ask the folks at the deli if there are any additives in their rotisserie chicken. If not, it's a winner. If you shop at a store that caters to health-conscious consumers, you're more apt to find additive-free birds. While you're at the deli, also ask for sugar-, dextrose-, nitrite-, and gluten-free turkey. If the person behind the counter looks at you like you're crazy, simply ask for Applegate deli turkey (it usually comes prepacked, and many stores are familiar with it). If the store doesn't carry it, ask them to order it for you.

Buy a good extra-virgin olive oil and one or more vinegars that you enjoy. That way you can whip up a quick salad dressing. Just be sure there are no additives. Balsamic, white wine, and red wine vinegars are good choices.

Rest assured that it's easy to stay on your diet if you eat out. If possible, choose a restaurant that caters to health-conscious clients. Be very specific when you order. If the waitperson looks at you like you're from Mars, just smile pleasantly. Order plain grilled or roasted meat, chicken, or fish. Hold the sauces. Hold the rolls. Hold the bun for your burger. Order double veggies and skip the starch. Order a salad and ask for oil and vinegar or lemons. Simple!

See my shopping guide on the Resources page on my website, drkellyann .com/resources.

LOVE TO COOK? HERE ARE MY FAVORITE RECIPES

If you enjoy your time in the kitchen, this is the diet for you—because you can make delicious, satisfying *real* food. In this chapter, you'll find entrées ranging from hearty breakfasts to gourmet dinners you can serve to company. (And in

---

MAKING GHEE

When recipes call for butter, you'll use ghee (because it doesn't contain dairy solids). You can buy ghee in the grocery store these days, but it's easy to make your own.

To make ghee, gently melt a stick of butter over low heat. Once the solids begin to separate from the melted fat, raise the heat to medium and continue to simmer the butter. Skim off the froth that appears on the surface and simmer the butter until it turns golden. (The milk solids will sink to the bottom and turn brown.) Strain your ghee through cheesecloth to remove the last of the milk solids, and voilà! You have ghee.

Note: If you stop cooking when the milk solids have separated but your butter is still pale yellow, you'll have clarified butter, which is also just fine on the diet. You can use it in place of ghee if you like.

Chapter 8, you'll find great sides, condiments, desserts, and extras to pair with them.) From morning to night, I've got you covered.

Enjoy! Below, there's another look at the meal plan I showed you back in Chapter 4, just to refresh your memory now that you're ready to start choosing your recipes.

ASSEMBLING THE PERFECT PLATE

Each meal on the Bone Broth Diet should contain 1 portion protein, 2 portions of nonstarchy vegetables, and 1 to 2 portions of fat. If you need a little extra energy after exercising, you can include a serving of a starchy vegetable. Breakfast can also contain 1 portion of fruit.

PROTEIN PORTIONS

A portion of meat, fish, or poultry should be about the size and thickness of your palm (that's 4 to 6 ounces). A portion of eggs is as many as you can hold in your hand (that's 2 or 3 for women and 3 or 4 for men). All recipes contain 1 portion of protein per serving.

NONSTARCHY VEGETABLE PORTIONS

A portion of these vegetables should be at least the size of a softball. You can't eat too many of them, so fill your plate with at least 2 or 3 softballs' worth.

STARCHY VEGETABLE PORTIONS

A portion of starchy vegetables should be about the size of a baseball for women and the size of a softball for men. REMEMBER: Eat starchy vegetables only if you're recovering from a workout.

FRUIT PORTIONS

A portion of fruit is half an individual piece (half an apple, half an orange) or a closed fistful, about ½ cup, of diced fruit or berries. Consume only 1 portion of fruit per day, preferably at breakfast.

(continued)

A WORD ABOUT PROTEIN

I keep my eye on all the latest medical research, especially when it comes to fighting aging. And emerging science is showing that one of the best ways to stay youthful, gorgeous, and healthy as you age is *to eat more protein.*

For years, we've heard that eating lots of protein is a no-no, especially for women. But guess what: To keep your metabolism high, repair tissue damage, optimize your hormones, and prevent sarcopenia (that's the muscle wasting that happens with age), you need to eat lots of protein . . . and you need to eat *more* as you get older.

Follow the guidelines I outline while you're on your Bone Broth Diet. Then, when you're on your Bone Broth Lifestyle Plan, continue to follow the same guidelines if you're in your twenties or thirties, but consider adding even more protein if you're forty or older. In fact, if you're a woman, you can bump your protein intake up to 100 grams a day. If you're a man, you can shoot for 150 grams. That's double (or more) the serving size for younger men or women.

In short, don't fear the protein— embrace it!

MY NEW TAKE ON WHEY

You know that saying "It's a woman's prerogative to change her mind"? Well, guess what: That's exactly what I'm doing right now.

Why? Because I'm open-minded, and sometimes I discover that a food I've put on my "no list" deserves to move over to the "yes list." Recently, the food that I moved from the naughty to the nice list is whey protein—but *only* the right form of this protein. Here's the story.

As I said earlier, I'm not a fan of dairy. I can't tolerate most dairy foods, and neither can my patients. I estimate that

about 80 percent of people have issues with dairy—gas, bloating, blotchy skin— and most of them don't even know it. So why am I moving whey isolate to my yes list? After all, it's a dairy product: a combination of proteins isolated from whey—the liquid part of milk that separates during cheese production.

Here are my reasons. When it comes to dairy sensitivity or allergies, whey typically isn't the issue. Instead, it's lactose. Whey protein isolate is lactose-free, because unlike whey protein concentrate (another common form of whey protein), it undergoes extra purification to remove this troublemaker. Look for the word *isolate* on the label, and you're good to go.

What's more, whey protein isolate is a nutritional powerhouse. After an intense workout, the amino acids in this super-food can help you build muscle fast—and as you age, they can fight sarcopenia, or age-related muscle wasting. And that's just the beginning, because whey is packed with other health-promoting nutrients that can enhance immune function,[1] lower high blood pressure,[2] and lower fasting insulin levels in overweight people.[3] It's also filling and satisfying, so you're less tempted to cheat.

And here's a finding that may surprise you, if you're worried about experiencing gut problems if you use whey. It turns out whey protein can actually help heal a leaky gut and reduce gut inflammation,[4] which is the most important step you can take if you want to prevent weight gain.

After doing a deep dive into the latest research, my new take is that whey protein isolate gives you all the advantages of whey without the disadvantages—and that's why it's on my "yes list" now.

FAT PORTIONS

A portion of liquid fat and oils should be about the size of a Ping-Pong ball, a typical bouncy ball, or 1 to 2 thumb-size portions (that's about 1 tablespoon). A portion of nuts, seeds, coconut flakes, or olives is about 1 closed handful. A portion of avocado is ¼ to ½ an avocado. A portion of canned coconut milk is ⅓ to ½ a cup.

One portion of fat for mayonnaise or mayonnaise-based condiments and salad dressings would be 1 tablespoon. One portion of fat for vinegar and oil based salad dressing would be 2 tablespoons. Because the recipes for salad dressings and condiments each make quite a few servings, I've included portions at the top of each of these recipes to make it easy to calculate the amount of fat per serving.

Each meal should include 1 or 2 portions of fat. If using one portion of fat for cooking you can add an additional portion of fat to your meal. If your meal is a salad, use two portions of fat per serving in salads. A portion of fat is approximately 11 to 14 grams of fat. Note: You do not need to count the fat contained in your proteins (just trim off extra fat).

When following a recipe with less than 1 to 2 fat portions, here are a few ways you can get an additional fat portion into your meal.

- Slice a quarter of an avocado and use it as a side to any meal.
- Whip 1 to 2 teaspoons of ghee or coconut oil into your coffee or bone broth for a latte-style drink.
- Grab a closed handful of nuts or seeds and sprinkle them on top of a salad or other meal.
- Add a closed handful of olives to a salad or as a side to any meal.
- One-third of a cup of canned coconut milk or coconut cream can be used as a fat portion in a smoothie or soup.
- Sprinkle a closed handful of coconut flakes onto a salad or blend it into a smoothie.

For instance, you can add a quarter of an avocado on top of the Egg and Tomato Skillet on page 131, because the oil used in the recipe is less than one portion of fat per serving. For the Chicken Stir-Fry recipe on page 157, you could sprinkle a closed handful of sliced almonds per serving as well.

ASPARAGUS AND MUSHROOM CRUSTLESS QUICHE

PREP TIME: 15 MINUTES • COOK TIME: 25–30 MINUTES

Yield: Makes 4 servings • **Portions:** *1 protein, ½ fat*

- 2 tablespoons + 1 teaspoon coconut oil or ghee, melted
- 1½ pounds asparagus, sliced into 1" pieces (about 2 cups)
- 1 cup mushrooms, sliced
- ½ onion, finely chopped
- 8 eggs
- 1 tablespoon + 1 teaspoon ghee, melted
- 1 teaspoon Dijon mustard
- 1 teaspoon dried Italian seasoning, herbs de Provence, or your favorite herb mix
- ⅛ teaspoon garlic powder
- 1 teaspoon Celtic or pink Himalayan salt
- ⅛–¼ teaspoon ground black pepper

Preheat the oven to 375°F. Brush a 9" × 9" baking dish with 1 tablespoon of the oil or ghee.

Put the asparagus, mushrooms, and onion in the baking dish. In a medium bowl, whisk the eggs with the remaining ghee, the mustard, Italian seasoning or herbs, garlic powder, salt, and pepper. Pour over the vegetables. Use a fork to distribute the vegetables evenly in the egg mixture.

Bake for 25 to 30 minutes, or until a knife inserted near the center comes out clean. The quiche will puff up while baking and deflate when removed from the oven. Let cool for 5 to 10 minutes before cutting and serving.

NOTES:

Serve with salsa, Pico de Gallo (page 267), or hot sauce, if desired.
This can be made ahead and refrigerated.

BAKED EGG CUPS WITH SPINACH

PREP TIME: 5 MINUTES • COOK TIME: 20–25 MINUTES

Yield: Makes 4 servings • *Portions:* 1 protein, ½ fat

2 tablespoons coconut oil, melted

2 scallions, white and green parts, chopped

2 handfuls of fresh baby spinach, chopped (about 2 cups)

8 eggs

½ teaspoon Celtic or pink Himalayan salt

⅛ teaspoon ground black pepper

⅛ teaspoon ground nutmeg (optional)

Preheat the oven to 350°F. Brush 8 cups in a muffin pan with the oil.

Divide the scallions and spinach among the cups. The spinach will likely pop up over the top of the cups until you add the eggs. Crack 1 egg into each cup. Sprinkle with salt, pepper, and a dash of nutmeg (if using). Alternatively, if you want scrambled eggs, whisk the eggs together in a bowl along with the salt, pepper, and nutmeg (if using), before pouring into the cups.

Bake for about 20 minutes for scrambled eggs or for 23 to 25 minutes for eggs with soft yolks. Remove from the pan and serve.

> **NOTES:**
> *Nutmeg is a great accent for eggs and spinach.*
> *Serve with hot sauce or any of the Bone Broth Diet salsas (pages 267, 269, and 272).*
> *These cups can be made ahead and refrigerated.*

VARIATIONS:

Add a handful of sliced mushrooms.

Brown ½ pound lean ground beef, drain well, and divide among the egg cups before baking.

Sprinkle a dash of smoked paprika in each cup for a smoky flavor.

Add a pinch of your favorite herbs or garlic powder.

Stir in a dash of hot sauce or cayenne to add heat.

BAKED SCOTCH EGGS

PREP TIME: 20 MINUTES · COOK TIME: 25–30 MINUTES

Yield: Makes 4 servings • *Portions: 1 protein, negligible fat*

1½ teaspoons Bell's Seasoning, dried Italian seasoning, herbs de Provence, or your favorite herbs

1 teaspoon Celtic or pink Himalayan salt

⅛–¼ teaspoon ground black pepper

Dash of cayenne (optional)

1 pound ground turkey

4 eggs, hard-cooked and peeled

Preheat the oven to 375°F. Brush or spray 4 cups in a muffin pan with coconut oil.

In a large bowl, mix the herb seasoning, salt, black pepper, and cayenne (if using) into the turkey and divide into 4 equal portions.

Lay a large piece of plastic wrap on your work surface. Place 1 meat portion in the middle. Press the meat into a circle about ½" thick.

Place 1 egg in the center, then lift the egg and meat using the plastic wrap and shape the meat into a ball around the egg, making sure the egg is completely enclosed. Remove the plastic wrap and place the egg into a prepared muffin cup. Repeat with the remaining 3 eggs.

Bake for 25 to 30 minutes. Cool for 5 minutes before serving. Serve warm or cold.

NOTES:

The eggs are great served with hot sauce.

These can be made ahead and refrigerated.

HOW TO MAKE PERFECT HARD-COOKED EGGS

Place raw eggs in a medium saucepan and add enough cold water to cover eggs with 2" water.

Add 1 tablespoon of Celtic or pink Himalayan salt. Place the pan over high heat until it reaches a boil.

Turn off the heat, cover, and let stand for 13 minutes.

After exactly 13 minutes, remove the eggs from the pan and place them in a bowl of ice water until cooled.

Carefully crack the eggshells. Peel under cold running water.

BEEF, EGG, AND MUSHROOM BREAKFAST

PREP TIME: 15 MINUTES • COOK TIME: 15 MINUTES

Yield: Makes 4 servings • *Portions: 1 protein, negligible fat*

1 onion, finely chopped

1 package (8–10 ounces) mushrooms, sliced (about 2 cups)

1 pound lean ground beef, sirloin, or bison

Pinch of garlic salt

1 teaspoon fresh thyme or marjoram or ⅓–½ teaspoon dried

2 teaspoons coconut aminos

1 teaspoon Celtic or pink Himalayan salt

¼ teaspoon ground black pepper

4 eggs

Generously spray or brush a skillet with coconut oil.

Cook the onion and mushrooms over medium-high heat until they start to brown. Add the beef, garlic salt, thyme or marjoram, coconut aminos, salt, and pepper and cook for 8 to 10 minutes, or until the meat is no longer pink.

Serve with the eggs prepared as you choose, or whisk the eggs and pour into a greased skillet over medium heat, stirring with a spatula until they are cooked through.

> **NOTE:**
> *This can be made ahead and refrigerated; don't prepare or add the eggs until you are reheating the meat mixture.*

BREAKFAST EGG MUFFINS WITH ITALIAN SAUSAGE

PREP TIME: 10 MINUTES • COOK TIME: 20 MINUTES

Yield: Makes 4 servings • *Portions: 1 protein, ½ fat*

- 2 tablespoons coconut oil or ghee, melted
- ½ small onion, finely chopped
- ½ pound ground turkey or chicken
- 1 teaspoon dried Italian seasoning
- ½ teaspoon Celtic or pink Himalayan salt
- ⅛–¼ teaspoon ground black pepper
- 8 eggs
- 2 plum tomatoes, seeded and diced

Preheat the oven to 350°F. Brush a skillet and 8 cups in a muffin pan with the oil or ghee.

Warm the skillet over medium heat. Cook the onion for 3 to 5 minutes, or until softened. Add the turkey or chicken, Italian seasoning, salt, and pepper and cook for about 10 minutes, or until the meat is no longer pink.

Whisk the eggs in a medium bowl. Divide the turkey mixture and tomatoes evenly among the prepared muffin cups. Pour the eggs into the muffin cups. Bake for about 20 minutes, or until the eggs are firm.

NOTE:

These can be made ahead and refrigerated.

VARIATION:

Add a dash of hot sauce or cayenne to the turkey mixture for a bit of heat.

BREAKFAST MEATBALLS (WITH AIR FRYER AND OVEN COOKING METHODS)

PREP TIME: 10 MINUTES • COOK TIME: 8–15 MINUTES
BASED ON COOKING METHOD

Yield: 4 servings • *Portions:* 1 protein; ½ fruit

1¼   pounds ground turkey or pork, or a combination of the two

1   medium apple, grated

½   teaspoon ground or rubbed sage

½   teaspoon fennel seed (optional, but it's really a complement to the apple and sage)

⅛–¼   teaspoon garlic powder

1   teaspoon Celtic or pink Himalayan salt

½   teaspoon ground black pepper

⅛   crushed red-pepper flakes (optional)

   Avocado, coconut, or olive oil pan spray

Place meat in a medium bowl. Use the large holes on a box grater or a food processor with the shredding disk to grate the apple. Squeeze as much juice as possible from the grated apple. Add sage, fennel seeds, garlic powder, salt, pepper, and red-pepper flakes (if using) and combine all ingredients. Wet your hands and roll into 1" balls. Try to keep them the same size so they will cook evenly. You should get 16 small meatballs, about 1½ ounces each.

AIR FRYER METHOD:

Preheat the air fryer to 350°F. Place half the meatballs into the basket in one layer and lightly spray with pan spray. Cook for about 8 minutes, shaking the basket halfway through. Remove and keep warm while cooking the second batch. Test for doneness with an instant-read thermometer. Turkey should be cooked to an internal temperature of 165°F and pork to 160°F.

OVEN METHOD:

Preheat the oven to 400°F, center the rack in the top half of the oven, and line a baking sheet with parchment. Place the meatballs in one layer, leaving a bit of room between each meatball. Lightly spray each meatball with pan spray and bake for 15 minutes, or until they are cooked through. Test for doneness with an instant-read thermometer. Turkey should be cooked to an internal temperature of 165°F and pork to 160°F.

NOTE:

If you make the meatballs larger or smaller, or if you make patties, you will need to adjust the cooking time.

CHILI OMELET

PREP TIME: 5 MINUTES • COOK TIME: 10 MINUTES

Yield: Makes 4 servings • **Portions:** *1 protein, ½ fat*

- 8 eggs
- ½ teaspoon Celtic or pink Himalayan salt
- ⅛ teaspoon ground black pepper
- 2 cups Rich and Hearty Turkey Chili (page 168), warmed
- 1 avocado, pitted and sliced or cubed
- 1 cup salsa or Pico de Gallo (page 267)

Whisk the eggs in a medium bowl and add the salt and pepper.

Spray or brush a 10" nonstick skillet with coconut oil. Heat the skillet over medium heat. When the pan is hot, pour in one-quarter of the egg mixture (2 eggs whisked together) and swirl the pan so the eggs spread evenly. Cook for 3 to 5 minutes, or until the eggs are cooked. Slide out onto a plate. Repeat with the remaining egg mixture. Top with the chili and avocado. Serve with the salsa or Pico de Gallo.

VARIATIONS:

Top with fresh lime wedges, chopped onions, and coarsely chopped cilantro.

Add hot sauce for a bit of heat.

EGG AND TOMATO SKILLET

PREP TIME: 10 MINUTES • COOK TIME: 15 MINUTES

Yield: Makes 4 servings • Portions: 1 protein, ½ fat

2 tablespoons coconut oil or ghee

1 onion, finely chopped

1 green or red bell pepper, finely chopped

1 can (28 ounces) diced tomatoes

2 tablespoons tomato paste

¼ teaspoon balsamic vinegar

1 teaspoon dried Italian seasoning, herbs de Provence,
  or your favorite herbs

Dash of garlic powder

¾ teaspoon Celtic or pink Himalayan salt

⅛–¼ teaspoon ground black pepper

8 eggs

Warm the oil or ghee in a 10" skillet* over medium heat. When the oil is hot, add the onion and bell pepper. Cook for about 5 minutes, or until the vegetables soften.

Add the tomatoes, tomato paste, vinegar, herb seasoning, garlic powder, salt, and black pepper and cook until the mixture is bubbling. It must be hot enough to poach the eggs. Crack the eggs into the tomato mixture, leaving some of the yellow yolk exposed. Partially cover the skillet with a lid. Let the mixture bubble for about 5 minutes, or until the whites are set and the yolks are still runny. If you don't like a soft yolk, continue to cook.

Serve immediately.

NOTES:

Serve with red-pepper flakes or hot sauce, if desired.

The tomato mixture can be made ahead and refrigerated. Add the eggs when you reheat the skillet, just before serving.

*If the skillet is much larger than 10", the liquid might be too dispersed to poach the eggs.

MEDITERRANEAN SCRAMBLE

PREP TIME: 10 MINUTES • COOK TIME: 15–20 MINUTES

Yield: Makes 4 servings • Portions: 1 protein, ½ fat

2 tablespoons ghee or coconut oil

8 ounces mushrooms, sliced (1½–2 cups)

1 cup cherry or grape tomatoes, cut in half

1 shallot, minced, or ½ small onion, finely chopped

4 kalamata olives, chopped

2 cups fresh baby spinach

8 eggs

1 teaspoon dried Italian seasoning

Dash of garlic powder (optional)

1 teaspoon Celtic or pink Himalayan salt

Melt the ghee or oil in a skillet over medium-high heat. Add the mushrooms and cook for 3 to 5 minutes, until softened. Add the tomatoes, shallot or onion, and olives and heat through, about 3 minutes. Reduce the heat to medium. Toss in the spinach.

In a medium bowl, whisk the eggs with the Italian seasoning, garlic powder (if using), and salt. Pour over the vegetables in the skillet. Mix with a spatula until the eggs are done to your liking.

NOTE:

This can be made ahead and refrigerated.

PORK AND EGGS

PREP TIME: 10 MINUTES · COOK TIME: 10 MINUTES

Yield: Makes 4 servings • **Portions:** *1 protein, negligible fat, 1 fruit*

1 onion, finely chopped

1 red bell pepper, finely chopped

2 small apples, finely chopped

1 pound cooked pork loin, cubed (leftovers from Balsamic Roast Pork Loin, page 184)

Dash of garlic powder

½ teaspoon Celtic or pink Himalayan salt

⅛ teaspoon ground cinnamon (optional)

4 eggs

Spray or brush a skillet with coconut oil. Cook the onion, pepper, and apples over medium-high heat for about 5 minutes, or until softened. Add the pork, garlic powder, salt, and cinnamon (if using) and heat through, about 5 minutes.

Meanwhile, poach or fry the eggs. Plate the pork and top each serving with an egg.

NOTES:

Serve with hot sauce, if desired.

If you like smoky flavors, you can add smoked paprika.

The meat-and-vegetable mixture can be made ahead and refrigerated. Cook the eggs right before serving.

QUICK AND EASY LOX FOR BREAKFAST OR LUNCH

PREP TIME: 5 MINUTES

Yield: 1 serving • *Portions:* 1 protein

3–4 ounces of lox

1 ripe tomato, sliced

Several thin slices red onion

1–2 teaspoons capers, drained and rinsed (optional)

Bibb lettuce leaves (optional)

Serve lox with tomato, red onion, and capers. Serve on a Bibb lettuce leaf or as a lettuce roll-up, if desired.

NOTE:

A dab of horseradish adds a nice zing! Or combine 1 teaspoon horseradish, 1 tablespoon avocado oil mayonnaise, and a turn of freshly ground black pepper and use it as a condiment. This adds 1 fat portion to the meal and is quite delicious.

ROASTED RED PEPPER AND BASIL EGG BITES

PREP TIME: 15 MINUTES • COOK TIME: 10–13 MINUTES DEPENDING ON METHOD

Yield: 14 egg bites, 4 servings • Portions: ½ protein

5 **eggs**
½ **cup + 2 tablespoons almond milk or coconut milk (not canned)**
½ **teaspoon salt**
¼ **teaspoon ground black pepper**
½ **cup roasted red peppers, diced**
10–12 **fresh basil leaves, cut into chiffonade (see Notes, page 162) ribbons**
   Avocado, coconut, or olive oil pan spray

Blend the eggs, milk, salt, and pepper in a blender for about 30 seconds. You can also whisk them, but be sure they are thoroughly blended. Spray a silicone egg bite mold with pan spray, add the roasted red peppers and basil, and fill each cup a little over halfway full with the egg mixture.

INSTANT POT METHOD:

Pour a cup of water into the pot. Place the filled egg bite mold onto the trivet and gently lower it into the pot. Close the top and set the release valve to the sealed position. Set the Instant Pot to steam for 10 minutes. When done, manually release the pressure, remove the top, and let the eggs rest in the pot for about 5 minutes. Lift the trivet out of the pot and allow the eggs to cool. Pop out of the mold and serve.

STOVETOP METHOD:

Place a stock pot or Dutch oven on the burner and add 1 to 2 cups of water. You don't want the water to come over the mold. Place the filled egg bite mold onto the trivet and gently lower it into the pot. Turn the heat on high and wait for the water to come to a boil. Cover the pot, reduce the heat to medium-low, and steam the eggs for 12 to 13 minutes. When done, uncover the pot and lift the trivet out of the pot and allow the eggs to cool. Pop out of the mold and serve.

NOTES:

Egg bite molds are available online and anywhere kitchen tools are sold.

If you have two egg bite molds, it's best not to stack them. Make them in two batches.

There are countless fillings you can use to make egg bites. If you are using any meat, bacon, sausage, etc., it must be fully cooked before you place it in the mold. You should also precook any raw vegetables such as broccoli, mushrooms, asparagus, onions, bell peppers, etc., to soften them.

Store egg bites in a covered container in the refrigerator for up to 4 days. Reheat for about 30 seconds in the microwave.

SAUSAGE AND APPLE FRITTATA

PREP TIME: 10 MINUTES • COOK TIME: 30 MINUTES

Yield: *Makes 4 servings* • ***Portions***: *1 protein, ½ fat, 1 fruit*

2 tablespoons coconut oil or ghee

½ onion, finely chopped

1 pound ground turkey

1½ teaspoons Bell's Seasoning, dried Italian seasoning,
herbs de Provence, or your favorite herbs

2 apples, cut into small cubes

8 eggs

Dash of garlic powder

1–1½ teaspoons Celtic or pink Himalayan salt

¼ teaspoon ground black pepper

⅛–¼ teaspoon ground cinnamon

Move an oven rack to the center of the oven. Preheat the oven to 350°F.

Melt the oil or ghee in an ovenproof skillet, such as cast iron, over medium-high heat. Cook the onion for 3 to 5 minutes, or until softened. Add the turkey and seasoning and cook for about 10 minutes, or until no longer pink. Add the apples.

In a large bowl, whisk the eggs with the garlic powder, salt, pepper, and cinnamon. Pour the egg mixture into the skillet and use a fork to distribute the ingredients evenly in the egg mixture. Cook for 1 to 2 minutes, or until the eggs begin to firm.

Transfer the pan to the oven and bake uncovered for 20 to 30 minutes, or until the center is puffed, the frittata is set, and a knife inserted in the center comes out clean. Slice and serve.

NOTES:

If you don't have an ovenproof skillet, put all the ingredients into a baking dish and bake in the oven, uncovered, for 20 to 30 minutes.

This recipe can be made ahead and refrigerated.

SAVORY VEGETABLE WAFFLES

PREP TIME: 30 MINUTES • COOK TIME: 5 MINUTES/WAFFLE

Yield: 4 *servings* • *Portions*: ½ *protein*, ½ *fat*

- 2 large zucchini
- 1 large carrot
- 3 green onions, green and white parts, thinly sliced (⅓ cup)
- ½ cup almond flour
- 2 tablespoons arrowroot
- 3 eggs, lightly beaten
- 2 tablespoons avocado or olive oil
- ¼ teaspoon dried dill or ¾ teaspoon fresh
- ¾ teaspoon Celtic or pink Himalayan salt
- ¼ teaspoon ground black pepper
- ¼ teaspoon garlic powder
- ⅛ to ¼ teaspoon cayenne
- ⅛ teaspoon nutmeg (optional)
- Avocado, coconut, or olive pan spray (for waffle irons that are not nonstick)

Shred the zucchini and carrot separately on a box grater using the large holes or in a food processor using the shredding disk. Using both hands squeeze out as much liquid as you can. Place zucchini in a clean kitchen towel or several layers of paper towels and very thoroughly wring out/press out any remaining water. Repeat 3 or more times with a clean towel or paper towels. Then place carrots in a clean dish towel or several layers of paper towels and very thoroughly wring out any water. You should have 1½ cups zucchini and ½ cup carrot. Place zucchini, carrot, and green onions in a large bowl. Add the almond flour and arrowroot.

In a small bowl, beat the eggs, then add the oil, whisking to combine. Pour into the bowl with vegetables and add the dill, salt, pepper, garlic powder, cayenne, and nutmeg (if using).

Preheat waffle iron to medium-high. When the waffle iron is hot, spray with pan spray if you are not using a nonstick waffle iron. Scoop ½ cup of the vegetable mixture and pour onto the center of the preheated waffle iron. Cook for about 5 minutes until golden brown. Repeat with remaining vegetable mixture.

NOTE:

Since every waffle iron is a different, you may need to adjust the temperature. For variety, try adding 2 tablespoons nutritional yeast for a cheesy flavor.

SMOKED SALMON AND EGGS

PREP TIME: 5 MINUTES

Yield: Makes 4 servings • *Portions: 1 protein*

12 ounces smoked salmon (sugar-, dextrose-, nitrite-, and gluten-free, if possible)

4 hard-cooked eggs, sliced

2 large tomatoes, sliced

½ English cucumber, sliced

1 red onion, sliced

1 lemon, sliced (optional)

Slice the salmon into thin pieces. Arrange the eggs, tomatoes, cucumbers, and onions on a plate and serve with the lemon (if using).

VARIATION:

You can use baked salmon, canned salmon in water, or canned tuna in water.

SOUTHWEST BREAKFAST SCRAMBLE

PREP TIME: 10 MINUTES • COOK TIME: 15 MINUTES

Yield: Makes 4 servings • *Portions: 1 protein, ½ fat*

2 tablespoons ghee or coconut oil

2 small or 1 large bell pepper, any color, finely chopped

½ onion, finely chopped

2 Roma tomatoes, seeded and finely chopped

8 eggs

2 tablespoons cilantro, coarsely chopped

1 teaspoon Celtic or pink Himalayan salt

⅛ teaspoon ground black pepper

Pinch of cayenne

⅛ teaspoon ground cumin (optional)

Pinch of garlic powder (optional)

Melt the ghee or oil in a skillet over medium-high heat. Add the bell peppers and onion and cook for 4 to 5 minutes, or until the vegetables are softened. Add the tomatoes and heat through, about 2 minutes.

In a medium bowl, whisk the eggs, cilantro, salt, black pepper, cayenne, and cumin and garlic powder (if using). Pour over the vegetables in the skillet. Mix with a spatula until the eggs are done to your liking.

NOTES:

Serve with Santa Fe Sauce (page 270) or any of the Bone Broth Diet salsas (pages 267, 269, and 272).

This can be made ahead and refrigerated.

SWEET AND SAVORY BREAKFAST HASH

PREP TIME: 15 MINUTES • COOK TIME: 25 MINUTES

Yield: 4 *servings* • *Portions*: 1 *protein*, ½ *fat*, 1 *fruit*

2 tablespoons avocado oil, coconut oil, olive oil, or ghee, divided

1 pound ground turkey

½ teaspoon ground or rubbed sage

¼ teaspoon ground cinnamon

½ teaspoon salt

⅛ teaspoon ground black pepper

1 medium onion, diced (about 1 cup)

1 small jicama, peeled and diced (1 cup)

2 medium red bell peppers, diced (1½–2 cups)

2 small to medium apples, diced (1–1½ cups)

Heat 1 tablespoon oil in a large skillet over medium-high heat. Add the ground turkey, sage, cinnamon, salt, and pepper and sauté for about 15 minutes, until fully cooked. The turkey should be 165°F on an instant-read thermometer. Transfer the turkey to a plate and cover to keep warm.

Return the skillet to medium-high heat, add the remaining 1 tablespoon oil, onion, jicama, and red pepper and sauté for about 4 minutes. Add the apples to the same pan and sauté for 2 to 3 minutes more. Add the turkey, reduce the heat to medium, cover, and cook for another 2 to 3 minutes to warm through.

VEGETABLE FRITTATA

PREP TIME: 15 MINUTES • COOK TIME: 30 MINUTES

Yield: Makes 4 servings • *Portions:* 1 protein, ½ fat

- 2 **tablespoons coconut oil or ghee**
- 4 **Roma tomatoes, seeded and finely chopped**
- 2 **cups broccoli florets, broken into small florets or coarsely chopped**
- 4 **scallions, white and green parts, sliced**
- 12 **eggs**
- 1–2 **teaspoons dried Italian seasoning, herbs de Provence, or your favorite herbs**
  - **Dash of garlic powder**
- 1–1½ **teaspoons Celtic or pink Himalayan salt**
- ¼ **teaspoon ground black pepper**

Move an oven rack to the center of the oven. Preheat the oven to 350°F.

Melt the oil or ghee in a 12" or larger ovenproof skillet, such as cast iron, over medium-high heat. Add the tomatoes, broccoli, and scallions and cook for 5 to 10 minutes, or until the vegetables are softened.

In a large bowl, whisk the eggs with the herb seasoning, garlic powder, salt, and pepper. Pour into the skillet and use a fork to distribute the vegetables evenly within the egg mixture. Cook for 1 to 2 minutes, or until the eggs begin to firm.

Transfer the pan to the oven and bake, uncovered, for 20 to 30 minutes, or until the center is puffed, the frittata is set, and a knife inserted in the center comes out clean. Slice and serve.

NOTES:

If you don't have an ovenproof skillet, put all the ingredients into a baking dish and bake in the oven as you would a crustless quiche.

You can use any combination of vegetables to make this frittata, but this version is one of my favorites.

This recipe can be made ahead and refrigerated.

ZUCCHINI BREAKFAST CAKES

PREP TIME: 10 MINUTES • COOK TIME: 6 MINUTES

Yield: Makes 4 servings • ***Portions:*** *1 protein, ½ fat*

- 2 tablespoons coconut oil or ghee
- 8 eggs
- 1 zucchini, grated and strained well
- 2 large carrots, shredded
- ½ onion, shredded
- 1 clove garlic, minced, or a dash of garlic powder
- 1 teaspoon dried thyme
- 1 teaspoon Celtic or pink Himalayan salt
- ⅛ teaspoon ground black pepper to taste
- ⅛ teaspoon ground nutmeg (optional)

Melt the oil or ghee in a nonstick skillet over medium-high heat.

Whisk the eggs in a large bowl. Add the zucchini, carrots, onion, garlic, thyme, salt, pepper, and nutmeg (if using). When the skillet is hot, ladle batter into the pan to form 4" pancakes. Flatten slightly with the back of a spatula. Reduce the heat to medium and cook for 2 to 3 minutes. Turn the pancakes and cook for 2 to 3 minutes.

Remove the cakes from the heat and blot on paper towels. Serve hot or cold.

NOTES:

Zucchini contains a lot of water, so straining it well will yield a much better pancake. Put shredded zucchini in a fine mesh strainer and press the zucchini with a clean kitchen towel or paper towels until no more water is released. You can also put it in a clean kitchen towel or cheesecloth and squeeze it.

These are great served with Creamy Avocado Sauce (page 253).

They can be made ahead and refrigerated.

DISPELLING TWO MYTHS

When I describe the Bone Broth Diet to people, I often hear two questions—so let's tackle them right now.

1. Isn't it unhealthy to eat as many eggs as you have on this diet?

Not at all! In fact, one of the worst pieces of advice "experts" ever gave us was to limit ourselves to one or two eggs a week. That misguided advice stemmed from the idea that eggs significantly raised cholesterol levels, which proved to be a myth—a very destructive myth that deprived generations of people of one of the most amazing superfoods on the planet.

Fortunately, government authorities recently changed their minds after reviewing all the evidence, and the egg scare officially came to an end. According to the newest draft of the Dietary Guidelines for America, "Cholesterol is not a nutrient of concern for overconsumption."[5] Translation: Eggs are just fine.

2. How about the saturated fat in red meat? Isn't that bad for my cardiovascular system?

This is another myth that science is disproving. Here's a look at the most current evidence.

In a research review published in 2014,[6] scientists analyzed the results from more than 70 studies and found no support for a link between saturated fat and cardiovascular disease. They concluded, "Current evidence does not clearly support cardiovascular guidelines that encourage high consumption of polyunsaturated fatty acids and low consumption of total saturated fats."

In a separate study of 148 men and women in 2014,[7] researchers compared low-carb and low-fat diets. The low-carb dieters averaged about 13 percent of their daily calories from saturated fat, which is more than double the amount recommended by the American Heart Association. Here's what the scientists found: "The low-carbohydrate diet was more effective for weight loss *and cardiovascular risk factor reduction* [emphasis added] than the low-fat diet."

Now, I'm not saying to load up on saturated fat. (In fact, eating too much saturated fat is one way to sabotage your weight-loss goals.) But if you follow the portion-size guidelines I gave you, your diet will be perfectly healthy.

COCONUT 101: A QUICK PRIMER

I'm sure you're noticing that lots of recipes in this book use forms of coconut—especially coconut milk. That's because coconut is packed with nutrition, and it makes an excellent replacement for dairy milk or cream.

But I know that when it comes to coconut products, things can get confusing. What's the difference between canned and refrigerated coconut milk? Between coconut milk and coconut cream? Between coconut cream and coconut oil?

If all this has you baffled, I understand—and I'm here to help. Here's a quick look at the different forms of coconut you'll come across at the grocery story or health food store, and how to count the fat content in each.

Coconut milk in a can—count ⅓ cup as a fat serving

This form of coconut milk has much the same consistency as cow's milk. Whether a recipe calls for full-fat or low-fat coconut milk, always reach for full-fat; it tastes better, and it's better for you.

Canned coconut milk typically separates in the can, creating a thick layout of cream on top and a thinner layer of milk on the bottom. That's why it's a good idea to shake the can vigorously before opening it.

Refrigerated coconut milk—doesn't count as a fat serving

This is a thin liquid that contains very little fat and makes a great base for smoothies. If you buy refrigerated coconut milk, make sure it's free of added sugars and carrageenan, an additive that's highly inflammatory. You don't need to count refrigerated coconut milk as a fat on your diet.

Coconut cream in a can—count ¼ cup as a fat serving

Coconut cream is much like canned coconut milk. However, it's thicker and contains less water, so it's a great swap for dairy cream.

If you're shopping for coconut cream, be sure you don't buy cream of coconut instead. This is coconut cream mixed with lots of sugar—the coconut version of condensed milk.

Coconut oil—count 1 tablespoon as a fat serving

This is oil pressed from the coconut. It's great for cooking and baking, and it's rich in medium chain triglycerides (MCTs), which stimulate your metabolism so you burn fat faster.

You can buy virgin or refined coconut oil. The virgin type has more nutrients, while the refined version has no coconut taste or aroma.

LUNCH OR DINNER ENTRÉES: Chicken and Turkey

Some of these are stand-alone recipes, while others go well with the vegetable sides and condiments in Chapter 8 or with a big tossed salad.

CREAMY CHICKEN CURRY

PREP TIME: 20 MINUTES • COOK TIME: 4–6 HOURS

Yield: Makes 4 servings • *Portions: 1 protein, negligible fat*

2 sweet potatoes or yams, peeled and cut into 2" cubes

1 pound boneless, skinless chicken breasts

1 can (14.5 ounces) diced tomatoes

¼ cup tomato paste

½ cup Chicken Bone Broth (page 98)

1 sweet onion, finely chopped

2 red or yellow bell peppers, finely chopped

2 cloves garlic, minced

2 teaspoons chili powder

2 teaspoons ground cumin

1 teaspoon curry powder

¾ teaspoon Celtic or pink Himalayan salt

⅛ teaspoon ground black pepper

⅔ cup full-fat canned coconut milk

In a slow cooker, combine the sweet potatoes or yams, chicken, tomatoes, tomato paste, broth, onion, bell peppers, garlic, chili powder, cumin, curry powder, salt, and black pepper. Cook on low for 6 hours or on high for 4 hours. Before serving, shred the chicken with a fork, stir in the coconut milk, and warm through.

> **NOTE:**
>
> *This is excellent as leftovers, and you can easily double the recipe. If you do double it, don't double the herbs and spices; instead, use 1½ times the amount for each of the herbs, spices, salt, and black pepper. You can double all other ingredients.*

VARIATIONS:

Use a combination of white and dark meat for a heartier dish.

Add 1 to 2 cups cauliflower or broccoli florets 30 minutes before the curry is ready if you're cooking on high or 45 minutes before the curry is ready if you're cooking on low.

Spoon the curry over Cauliflower Rice (page 222) and sprinkle with coarsely chopped cilantro.

CHICKEN CUTLETS WITH FRENCH HERBS AND CREAMY ROASTED RED PEPPER SAUCE

PREP TIME: 20 MINUTES • COOK TIME: VARIES WITH METHOD

Yield: 4 servings • Portions: 1 protein

CHICKEN

- 4 boneless, skinless chicken breasts, 4–6 ounces each (see *Notes* for slicing technique)
- 2 tablespoons melted ghee or avocado oil
- 2 tablespoon fresh tarragon leaves, chopped or 1 tablespoon dried
- 2 teaspoons fresh thyme leaves or 1 teaspoon dried
- ½ teaspoon paprika
- ¼ teaspoon garlic powder
- 1 teaspoon Celtic or pink Himalayan salt
- ½ teaspoon ground black pepper

RED PEPPER SAUCE

- 1 (12-ounce) jar roasted red peppers, drained
- 1 small garlic clove
- 2 teaspoons lemon juice, freshly squeezed
- ¼ teaspoon Hungarian paprika
- ½ teaspoon Celtic or pink Himalayan salt
- ⅛ teaspoon ground black pepper
- ⅛ teaspoon ground nutmeg (optional)
- ¾ cup full-fat coconut milk

Rinse chicken in cold water and pat dry with paper towels.

OVEN METHOD:

Preheat oven to 450°F. Place the chicken on a baking sheet and brush both sides with melted ghee. In a small bowl, combine the tarragon, thyme, paprika, garlic powder, salt, and pepper. Sprinkle the herb mixture evenly over the chicken. Place pan in middle rack of oven and roast the chicken for 8 to 12 minutes, depending on thickness. Test for doneness with an instant-read thermometer. Internal temperature should be 165°F. Remove the chicken from the oven, tent with foil, and let rest for at least 5 minutes.

STOVETOP METHOD:

Heat ghee in a large skillet over medium heat. In a small bowl, combine the tarragon, thyme, paprika, garlic powder, salt, and pepper. Sprinkle the herb mixture evenly over the chicken and place it in the pan with the ghee. Cook for 3 to 4 minutes on each side until the chicken is golden and the internal temperature reaches 165°F. Remove the skillet from the heat, tent the chicken with foil, and let rest for 5 or more minutes. It's very easy to overcook chicken using the stovetop method, so stay close to the stove while it cooks.

FOR THE RED PEPPER SAUCE:

Put all of the ingredients in a food processor or blender and process until smooth, stopping a few times to scrape down the sides. Pour the sauce over the roasted chicken or serve on the side. Optionally garnish with fresh herbs.

NOTES:

Slicing technique for large chicken breasts: When chicken breasts are large, 8 to 10 ounces each, the best way to cook them to an internal temperature of 165°F without overcooking is by slicing them horizontally into cutlets so you have two thinner breast fillets. To do so, be sure the chicken is very cold or just thawed. Place the breasts in a single layer on a plate and freeze for 10 to 20 minutes if they aren't cold enough. Place a cold chicken breast on a cutting board with the smooth side up. Hold it in place with the palm of your hand. Starting at the thickest end, slice the breast in half horizontally, cutting toward the thinner end. You will end up with two fairly even chicken breast cutlets that will be 4 to 5 ounces each.

You don't need to slice smaller (4- to 5-ounce) chicken breasts.

You will likely have extra red pepper sauce. If you are serving the chicken with cauliflower or cauliflower rice, the sauce is fabulous on it also. Store any leftover sauce in a sealed container in the refrigerator for up to 7 days.

CHICKEN SHAWARMA

PREP TIME: 20 MINUTES • COOK TIME: 20 MINUTES

Yield: 4 servings • Portions: 1 protein, 1 fat

- 1 tablespoon ground cumin
- 2 teaspoons turmeric
- 1 tablespoon ground coriander
- 2 garlic cloves, minced
- 2 teaspoons paprika
- ¼–½ teaspoon cayenne (optional, depending on how much heat you want)
- 2 teaspoons Celtic or pink Himalayan salt
- 2 pounds boneless, skinless chicken thighs (about 8 depending on size)
- 1 large onion, sliced
- Juice of 1 lemon, about 2 tablespoons
- ¼ cup extra-virgin olive oil
- Avocado, coconut, or olive oil pan spray

Put the cumin, turmeric, coriander, garlic, paprika, cayenne, salt, onion, lemon juice, and olive oil in a large non-aluminum bowl or in a 1-gallon zip-top plastic bag. Pat the chicken dry and slice across the grain into ½" strips. Add to the spice mixture and coat the chicken. Cover and let marinate in the refrigerator for at least 4 hours, ideally overnight.

Preheat the oven to 425°F and spray a sheet pan with pan spray. When ready to bake, take the chicken out of the refrigerator and let come to room temperature, 15 to 20 minutes. Spread the marinated chicken and onion on the prepared sheet pan and roast for about 18 to 20 minutes. If you want crispier chicken, put it under the broiler for a few minutes and watch carefully so it doesn't burn. The chicken is done when the internal temperature reaches 165°F.

NOTES:

Chicken shawarma is delicious grilled. If you are grilling the chicken for a salad, do not slice until after it is grilled. If you are making shawarma kabobs, cut the meat into 1" chunks that will easily skewer. Skewer the meat, adding vegetables like sliced bell peppers, mushrooms, onion wedges, cherry tomatoes, and so on, if desired. Heat a grill to medium-high. Cook for 4 to 5 minutes on one side, turn, and grill on the second side for 3 to 4 minutes.

If you don't have time to marinate for at least 4 hours, the recipe is still very good, but the flavors are heightened after marinating for a longer time.

The chicken can easily be reheated if you have leftovers or if you want to do batch cooking for the week. Reheat chicken in a sauté pan with 1 or 2 tablespoons of water or chicken bone broth and cook over medium heat to warm through.

EASY ROAST CHICKEN BREASTS

PREP TIME: 5 MINUTES • COOK TIME: 40 MINUTES

Yield: Makes 4 servings • *Portions: 1 protein, negligible fat*

4 teaspoons ghee or coconut oil, divided

4 palm-size boneless, skinless chicken breasts (about 1 pound total)

Celtic or pink Himalayan salt

Ground black pepper

⅛–¼ teaspoon garlic powder (optional)

Any herbs or spices you like (optional)

Move an oven rack to the center of the oven. Preheat the oven to 400°F. Cut a piece of parchment to lie flat inside an ovenproof baking dish, making sure the parchment reaches edge to edge.

Rub the bottom of the baking dish with about 2 teaspoons of the ghee or oil. Rub 1 side of the parchment with about 1 teaspoon of ghee.

Pat the chicken dry with a paper towel and rub the remaining ghee on the top of the chicken. Season with salt, pepper, garlic powder (if using), and any other herbs, as desired. Transfer the chicken to the prepared baking dish, leaving room between the pieces.

Place the parchment, buttered side down, on top of the chicken and press down. The parchment should completely cover the chicken and reach to the inside edges of the pan.

Bake for 30 to 40 minutes, or until an instant-read thermometer inserted in the thickest portion registers 165°F and the juices run clear.

NOTES:

This technique is called dry poaching because it doesn't use additional liquid to cook the chicken. Dry poaching is an excellent way to cook lean meats because they remain moist and juicy. Follow the directions exactly to get the best results. Don't use foil; only use parchment.

In addition to your favorite herbs and spices, you can add lemon slices to flavor the chicken.

This recipe is adaptable to any number of chicken breasts. Calculate 1 teaspoon of fat per piece of chicken, and don't crowd the chicken in the baking dish.

EASY ROAST CHICKEN

PREP TIME: 10 MINUTES • COOK TIME: VARIES WITH WEIGHT

Yield: Varies by the weight of the chicken • Portions: 1 protein for a palm-size portion without skin or bones

- 1 tablespoon fresh lemon peel
- 1 tablespoon fresh rosemary leaves + 2 or 3 sprigs for the cavity (optional)
- 1 teaspoon fresh thyme (optional)
- 1 clove garlic, minced
- ½ teaspoon Celtic or pink Himalayan salt
- ¼ teaspoon ground black pepper
- 1 whole chicken
- 1 lemon, sliced into rounds

Move an oven rack to the center of the oven. Preheat the oven to 450°F.

In a small bowl, mix the lemon peel, 1 tablespoon rosemary leaves, thyme (if using), garlic, salt, and pepper. Gently loosen the skin around the breast, legs, and thighs and rub the herb mixture under the skin. Place the rosemary sprigs (if using) and lemon slices in the cavity. Lightly rub or spray ghee or coconut oil over the chicken.

Roast for 10 to 15 minutes at 450°F. Reduce the heat to 350°F and continue roasting for approximately 20 minutes per pound, or until an instant-read thermometer inserted in a breast registers 180°F and the juices run clear.

Remove from the oven, tent with foil, and let stand for 10 to 15 minutes before carving.

IN-A-HURRY NO-PREP STIR-FRY

PREP TIME: 20 MINUTES • COOK TIME: 15–20 MINUTES

Yield: 4 servings • *Portions: 1 protein, 1 fat*

SAUCE

2 tablespoons toasted sesame oil

3 tablespoons coconut aminos

1–2 tablespoons coconut or apple cider vinegar

2 teaspoons fish sauce (optional)

2 or 3 garlic cloves, minced

2" knob of ginger, peeled and grated on a Microplane

Small bunch of cilantro leaves, loosely packed (about ½ cup), coarsely chopped

1–2 teaspoons toasted sesame seeds (optional)

STIR-FRY

2 tablespoons avocado, coconut, or olive oil

1 pound fresh or frozen cauliflower rice or 1 medium head of cauliflower, finely chopped

1 pound or more frozen or precut stir-fry vegetables

3 green onions, white and green parts, sliced into ¼" pieces

12–16 ounces cooked chicken (from a rotisserie chicken) or 8 eggs

Avocado, coconut, or olive oil pan spray, if you are serving with eggs

Sriracha (optional), for serving

FOR THE SAUCE

In a small bowl or a jar with tight-fitting lid, combine the oil, aminos, vinegar, fish sauce (if using), garlic, ginger, cilantro, and sesame seeds (if using) in a small bowl or lidded jar and set aside.

FOR THE STIR-FRY

Heat the oil in a large skillet or wok over high heat. When the oil shimmers, add the cauliflower rice and cook for about 3 minutes so some of the water evaporates. Reduce the heat to medium-high and sauté for 5 to 6 minutes, stirring occasionally, until the cauliflower begins to brown. Add the stir-fry vegetables and sauté for another 3 to 4 minutes or 7 to 8 minutes if the vegetables are still frozen. Add the green onions and toss to combine.

If you are serving with chicken, cut or shred the chicken and add the chicken and sauce to the vegetable mixture and warm through for 1 to 2 minutes. Serve with Sriracha.

If you are serving topped with sunny-side up eggs, in a separate skillet generously spray the pan with pan spray. Cook the eggs to desired doneness. While the eggs are cooking, pour the sauce over the vegetable mixture and warm through for 1 to 2 minutes. Serve the eggs over the vegetable stir-fry. Serve with Sriracha.

NOTES:

If you don't purchase the cauliflower rice premade, it's simple to make using a food processor. Cut the cauliflower, including the core, into chunks, then put a third to a half of the chunks into the bowl of a food processor and pulse until it is the size of rice. Transfer the cauliflower rice to a bowl and repeat with the remaining chunks.

You can make this stir-fry without chicken or eggs and enjoy as a vegetable dish.

If you like your stir-fry sauce with a bit of sweetness, add stevia or monk fruit sweetener to equal 2 teaspoons sugar to the sauce.

This dish makes a great leftover. The next day, enjoy it for lunch by reheating it in the microwave.

LOUISIANA CREOLE JAMBALAYA

PREP TIME: 30 MINUTES • COOK TIME: 55 MINUTES

Yield: 8 to 10 servings • *Portions:* 1 protein, negligible fat

- 2 tablespoons avocado or olive oil
- 12 ounces sugar- and nitrate-free andouille sausage or kielbasa, cut into ¼"-thick rounds
- 3 boneless, skinless chicken thighs, cut into 1" pieces
- 1 medium yellow onion, chopped
- 3 celery stalks, chopped
- 1 green bell pepper, chopped
- 2 garlic cloves, minced
- 1 teaspoon dried thyme or 1 tablespoon fresh thyme leaves
- 1 teaspoon oregano or 1 tablespoon fresh oregano leaves
- 2 teaspoons smoked paprika
- ¼–½ teaspoon cayenne or chile flakes
- 1 teaspoon coarsely ground black pepper
- 1 (28-ounce) can diced or crushed tomatoes, preferably fire-roasted
- 2 cups Chicken Bone Broth (page 98)
- 18 large shrimp, peeled and deveined
- 8 cups raw cauliflower rice, about 1 large head cut into rice-size pieces
- 1 teaspoon Celtic or pink Himalayan salt
- Parsley, chopped, for garnish (optional)

In a Dutch oven, heat the oil over medium heat. When the oil shimmers, add the sausage and sauté for about 5 minutes, until it starts to brown. Transfer the sausage to paper towels to drain. Set aside. Add the chicken to the same Dutch oven and cook for 3 to 4 minutes, or until the chicken easily releases on its own. Flip and cook for another 3 to 5 minutes, depending on the thickness of the chicken thighs. Transfer the chicken to the paper towels with the sausage.

Add the onion, celery, bell pepper, and garlic to the Dutch oven and sauté 2 to 3 minutes, until aromatic. Stir in the thyme, oregano, paprika, cayenne, and black pepper. Stir in the tomatoes and chicken broth. Return the sausage and chicken to the Dutch oven, reduce the heat to low, cover, and simmer, stirring occasionally, for 30 minutes.

Add the shrimp, cauliflower rice, and salt to the Dutch oven and simmer for 10 to 15 minutes, or until the cauliflower is soft. Garnish with parsley, if desired.

NOTES:

If you prefer not to use shrimp, add additional chicken thighs and/or sausage.

SPICY CHICKEN DRUMSTICKS OR THIGHS

PREP TIME: 10 MINUTES • COOK TIME: 30–40 MINUTES

Yield: 4 servings • *Portions: 1 protein, ½ fat*

- 8–10   chicken drumsticks or 4 or 5 thighs or some combination of the two (about 2½ pounds total)
- 2–3   tablespoons avocado, coconut, olive oil, or melted ghee
- 1   teaspoon cumin
- 1   teaspoon coriander
- 1   teaspoon sweet or smoked paprika
- ⅛–¼   teaspoon cayenne
- ½   teaspoon garlic powder
- ½   teaspoon Celtic or pink Himalayan salt
- ½   teaspoon white pepper
- Juice of half a lemon
- 3–4   tablespoons fresh parsley or cilantro, coarsely chopped

Preheat the oven to 400° F, and line a sheet pan with aluminum foil or parchment paper (see Notes). Rinse the chicken with cold water, dry with paper towels, and set aside. In a bowl large enough to hold all the chicken, make a spice rub by combining the oil, cumin, coriander, paprika, cayenne, garlic powder, salt, and white pepper. Add the chicken and toss to coat evenly. Place the chicken in one layer on the prepared sheet pan and bake for 25 to 35 minutes, depending on the size of the pieces. Test for doneness with an instant-read thermometer. The internal temperature should reach 165°F. If they are not done, return to the oven and test for doneness every 3 to 5 minutes. If the chicken gets too brown, cover lightly with aluminum foil. For a crispier finish, place the pan on the lower rack of a preheated broiler for 2 to 3 minutes. Sprinkle with the lemon juice and parsley before serving.

> **NOTES:**
>
> *Don't use parchment to line the pan if you are finishing the chicken in the broiler to crisp it; the parchment will catch on fire.*
>
> *This dish is great served with a cooling side dish such as coleslaw or a salad with ranch dressing.*
>
> *Thighs may take a little longer to cook than drumsticks.*

CHICKEN WITH ORANGE-ROSEMARY SAUCE

PREP TIME: 10 MINUTES • COOK TIME: 15 MINUTES

Yield: Makes 8 servings • **Portions:** *1 protein, negligible fat, 1 fruit*

- 2¼ pounds boneless, skinless chicken breast halves (about 4 large halves or 6 medium halves), pounded to about ½" thickness and cut into 4" pieces or sliced into cutlets
- 1–1½ teaspoons Celtic or pink Himalayan salt
- ¼ teaspoon ground black pepper
- 1 teaspoon coconut oil or ghee
- 1 cup fresh orange juice (about 2 large oranges)
- 1 teaspoon fresh rosemary or ½ teaspoon dried, very finely chopped
- 1 teaspoon Dijon mustard
- 1 tablespoon ghee

Pat the chicken dry with paper towels and sprinkle lightly on both sides with the salt and pepper. Generously brush or spray a large nonstick skillet with the oil or ghee.

Heat the skillet over medium-high heat. When hot, arrange the chicken pieces in the skillet without crowding. You may need to cook in 2 batches.

Cook for about 3 minutes on each side, turning only once, or until the chicken pieces are a rich golden brown and the juices run clear. Remove from the skillet and set aside.

In a small bowl, combine the orange juice with the rosemary and mustard. Pour into the hot skillet and reduce to ½ cup. Tilt the skillet and whisk in the ghee until melted.

Spoon the pan sauce over the chicken pieces and serve.

NOTE:

This recipe can be made ahead and refrigerated.

CHOPPED BALSAMIC CHICKEN SALAD

PREP TIME: 10 MINUTES

Yield: Makes 4 servings • Portions: 1 protein, 1 fat

- **4 cooked boneless, skinless chicken breast halves (3–4 ounces each), cut into cubes (use leftover chicken or turkey)**
- **½ cup shredded carrots (about 2 medium)**
- **⅓ cup shredded beet (about 1 medium)**
- **4 cups finely shredded purple or green cabbage (¼ large–½ small cabbage or 1½–2 bags prepared shredded cabbage)**
- **¼ cup Balsamic Vinaigrette (page 252)**

In a large bowl, toss together the chicken, carrots, beets, cabbage, and dressing. (Alternatively, put the cut chicken into the dressing and let it marinate for at least 15 minutes before tossing with the vegetables.) Season to taste with salt and pepper. Serve chilled.

NOTE:

A chopped Granny Smith apple would add a nice tartness to the salad, but remember to calculate the fruit into your day.

CHICKEN STIR-FRY

PREP TIME: 20 MINUTES • COOK TIME: 15 MINUTES

Yield: Makes 4 servings • *Portions:* 1 protein, ½ fat

MARINADE

- 1 tablespoon coconut oil, melted
- 3 tablespoons fresh lime juice
- ¼ cup + 2 tablespoons coconut aminos, divided
- 2 tablespoons finely chopped fresh ginger
- 2–3 cloves garlic, minced
- 1 teaspoon ground cumin
- ½ jalapeño, seeded and finely chopped (wear plastic gloves when handling)
- ¼ cup cilantro, finely chopped
- ¼ teaspoon paprika
- ¼ teaspoon ground white pepper

STIR-FRY

- 1 tablespoon coconut oil, melted, or coconut oil spray
- 4 boneless, skinless chicken breast halves (about 4–5 ounces each), cut into ½" strips
- 1 head broccoli, broken or cut into florets (don't use the stems unless you peel them)
- 1 small head bok choy or 3–4 baby bok choy
- 1 red bell pepper, cut into strips
- ½ pound snow peas (about 2 cups)
- 6 scallions, white and green parts, cut into ½" pieces
- 1 package (8–10 ounces) mushrooms (1½–2 cups)
- 1 can (8 ounces) water chestnuts, drained
- ½ cup fresh basil
- ½ cup fresh cilantro

To make the marinade: In a medium bowl, mix together the oil, lime juice, ¼ cup of the coconut aminos, the ginger, garlic, cumin, jalapeño, cilantro, paprika, and white pepper. Divide this marinade in half; there should be about ¼ cup in each half. Set aside half for the chicken.

Add the remaining 2 tablespoons coconut aminos to the other half of the marinade and refrigerate. (You will use this portion just before serving.)

Place the chicken in a nonmetallic bowl or in a large resealable plastic bag. Pour in the reserved marinade. Mix well, cover the bowl or seal the bag, and marinate in the refrigerator for 1 to 2 hours.

To make the stir-fry: Heat a large skillet or a wok over high heat. Brush or spray with the oil. Repeat brushing or spraying with oil before cooking each batch of chicken or vegetables.

To test if the skillet or wok is hot enough, put in a strip of chicken. It should sizzle immediately. If it doesn't, wait to begin cooking. When the pan is hot, place half the chicken in the pan and cook, moving the meat around with tongs or a wooden spoon, for 3 to 4 minutes, or until the chicken is lightly browned and no longer pink inside. Remove from the pan and set aside. Repeat with the remaining chicken strips. Discard the chicken marinade.

To the hot skillet or wok, add the broccoli and cook for 2 to 3 minutes, or until tender but still crisp, and remove from the pan. Repeat with the bok choy and bell pepper, cooking for 1 to 2 minutes, or until tender but still crisp. Follow the same procedure for the snow peas and scallions, then for the mushrooms. Add the water chestnuts and cook for about 1 minute to heat through. Combine the chicken and vegetables and toss in the reserved coconut aminos marinade. Garnish with basil and cilantro.

NOTES:

You can use whatever combination of vegetables you like. Select vegetables that will keep their crunch.

If you're making this for 1 or 2 people, with a large enough skillet or wok, you can prepare the stir-fry by cooking the meat in one batch and then the vegetables in the second batch.

The secret to making a good stir-fry is to cook at a very high heat and never crowd the skillet or wok. Don't be intimidated by the instructions. They may sound difficult, but actually, all you're doing is cooking in small batches in a very hot pan so the meat and vegetables can sauté (not steam) and remain crunchy.

It's worth doubling the recipe for leftovers; the vegetables won't stay quite as crisp as when they're freshly prepared, but they're still yummy.

Serve with Cauliflower Rice (page 222).

This can be prepared ahead and refrigerated.

VARIATION:

Make this recipe with 1 pound of lean beef or 48 to 52 medium to large shrimp, peeled and deveined. Beef cooking time should be about the same as chicken. Shrimp will cook in about 2 minutes; cook only until they turn opaque. You can marinate beef as long as overnight. Chicken and shrimp absorb the marinade in 1 to 2 hours.

BRAISED CHICKEN WITH LEEKS AND MUSHROOMS

PREP TIME: 15 MINUTES • COOK TIME: 25 MINUTES

Yield: Makes 4 servings • Portions: 1 protein, ½ fat

   2 tablespoons ghee

   4 boneless, skinless chicken thighs, trimmed of fat

   1 teaspoon Celtic or pink Himalayan salt, divided

⅛–¼ teaspoon ground black pepper

   4 leeks, white part only, cut into rounds

   1 package (8–10 ounces) mushrooms, sliced (1½–2 cups)

1–2 cloves garlic, minced

   ½ cup Chicken Bone Broth (page 98), more as needed

Spray or brush a large skillet with 1 tablespoon of the ghee. Sprinkle the chicken with ½ teaspoon of the salt and the pepper and cook over medium-high heat for 3 to 4 minutes per side, or until browned. Remove from the pan and set aside.

To the hot skillet add the leeks, mushrooms, and the remaining 1 tablespoon ghee and cook for about 5 minutes, or until the vegetables are lightly browned. Season with the remaining ½ teaspoon salt.

Stir in the garlic and place the chicken on top of the vegetables. Add the broth, cover, and reduce the heat to medium or medium-low. Simmer for about 25 minutes, or until an instant-read thermometer inserted in the thickest portion of a thigh registers 165°F.

   NOTES:

   This is an easy and luscious recipe you'd be proud to serve company. You might want to double the recipe to have leftovers.

   It's great served with Garlic Mashed Cauliflower "Potatoes" (page 223) or Cauliflower Rice (page 222).

   This recipe can be made ahead and refrigerated.

CHICKEN SALAD WITH CRUNCH

PREP TIME: 10 MINUTES

Yield: Makes 4 servings • Portions: 1 protein, 1 fat

4   cooked boneless, skinless chicken breast halves (3–4 ounces each), cut
     into cubes (use leftover chicken or turkey breast)

4   ribs celery, finely chopped

1   red or yellow bell pepper, finely chopped

1   carrot, cut into ⅛" pieces or shredded

1   small red onion, finely chopped (optional)

1   small jicama, peeled and finely chopped (optional)

¼   cup Balsamic Vinaigrette (page 252)

     Celtic or pink Himalayan salt

     Ground black pepper

1   large or 2 small heads romaine lettuce, chopped (about 8 cups)

In a large bowl, combine the chicken, celery, bell pepper, carrot, onion (if using),
and jicama (if using). Toss with the dressing and season to taste with salt and
black pepper. Serve on top of the lettuce.

NOTES:

*Jicama adds a great crunch to the salad. If you haven't tried this juicy root, I think
you'll like it. It's also known as Mexican yam or Mexican turnip, although it
tastes like neither a yam nor a turnip.*

This recipe can be made ahead and refrigerated.

VARIATION:

I love tarragon in this salad along with French Vinaigrette (page 255).

ORANGE-ROSEMARY CHICKEN SALAD

PREP TIME: 10 MINUTES

Yield: Makes 4 servings • Portions: 1 protein, 1 fat

4   cooked boneless, skinless chicken breast halves (about 3–4 ounces each), sliced into ½" strips (you can use leftover Chicken with Orange-Rosemary Sauce, page 155; see Note)

1   cup snap peas

½   English cucumber, sliced

½   small red onion, sliced

¼   cup Orange Vinaigrette (page 257)

About 8 cups lettuce, your choice

In a medium bowl, toss the chicken, peas, cucumber, and onion with the dressing. Serve on a bed of the lettuce.

VARIATION:

Add a handful of fresh blueberries for a fruitier salad or a handful of radishes for more crunch.

ONE-SKILLET ZUCCHINI PASTA WITH SAUSAGE

PREP TIME: 15 MINUTES • COOK TIME: 15 MINUTES

Yield: Makes 4 servings • **Portions:** *1 protein, ½ fat*

2 tablespoons coconut oil or ghee

½ onion, finely chopped

6–8 Roma tomatoes, seeded and finely chopped

2 cloves garlic, minced

1 pound ground turkey or chicken

2 teaspoons dried Italian seasoning

1 teaspoon Celtic or pink Himalayan salt

¼ teaspoon ground black pepper

⅛ teaspoon red-pepper flakes (optional)

Zucchini Wide-Cut Pasta (page 231)

4–6 leaves fresh basil, cut into chiffonade ribbons (see Notes) or coarsely chopped

Melt the oil or ghee in a large skillet over medium-high heat. Cook the onion and tomatoes for about 8 minutes, or until softened. Add the garlic, turkey, Italian seasoning, salt, black pepper, and red-pepper flakes (if using) and cook for about 10 minutes, or until the meat is no longer pink. Serve over the prepared pasta and top with the basil.

NOTES:

Chiffonade simply means "cut into very thin ribbons." To do this, pile basil leaves on top of one another. Roll them together the long way and slice through the roll at a perpendicular angle to create very fine strips.

Serve with additional red-pepper flakes, if desired.

TURKEY OR CHICKEN SAVORY SAUSAGE

PREP TIME: 5 MINUTES • COOK TIME: 10 MINUTES

Yield: Makes 4 servings • *Portions: 1 protein*

- 1¼ pounds ground turkey or chicken
- 1½ teaspoons Bell's Seasoning or a combination of your favorite herbs
- Pinch of garlic powder or 1 clove garlic, minced
- 1 teaspoon Celtic or pink Himalayan salt
- ⅛–¼ teaspoon ground black pepper

Brush or spray a skillet with coconut oil. Add the turkey or chicken, herb seasoning, garlic, salt, and pepper and cook over medium-high heat for about 10 minutes, or until the meat is no longer pink. Alternatively, mix the ingredients in a bowl and form into 4 patties and sauté or grill for about 5 minutes on each side, or until an instant-read thermometer inserted in the center registers 165°F and the meat is no longer pink.

> **NOTE:**
>
> *Turkey or chicken sausage is great on its own; you'll also find it in a number of recipes in this chapter.*

TURKEY OR CHICKEN ITALIAN SAUSAGE

PREP TIME: 5 MINUTES • COOK TIME: 10 MINUTES

Yield: Makes 4 servings • *Portions: 1 protein*

- 1¼ pounds ground turkey or chicken
- 1½ teaspoons dried Italian seasoning (salt-, sugar-, dextrose-, and gluten-free)
- Pinch of garlic powder or 1 clove garlic, minced
- Pinch of fennel seed (optional)
- ⅛ teaspoon crushed red-pepper flakes (optional)
- 1 teaspoon Celtic or pink Himalayan salt
- ⅛–¼ teaspoon ground black pepper

Brush or spray a skillet with coconut oil. Add the turkey or chicken, Italian seasoning, garlic powder, fennel seed, red-pepper flakes (if using), salt, and black pepper and cook over medium-high heat for about 10 minutes, or until the meat is no longer pink. Alternatively, you can mix the ingredients in a bowl and form into 4 patties and sauté or grill for about 5 minutes on each side, or until an instant-read thermometer inserted in the center registers 165°F and the meat is no longer pink.

TURKEY OR CHICKEN CHORIZO

PREP TIME: 5 MINUTES • COOK TIME: 10 MINUTES

Yield: Makes 4 servings • Portions: 1 protein

- 1¼ pounds ground turkey or chicken
- 2 tablespoons apple cider vinegar
- 1–2 tablespoons ground dried chiles (ancho, California, or New Mexico; not chili powder)
- ½ tablespoon Celtic or pink Himalayan salt
- 1 teaspoon garlic powder
- 1 teaspoon onion powder
- ½ teaspoon ground cumin
- ½ teaspoon dried oregano
- ¼ teaspoon ground cinnamon
- ⅛–¼ teaspoon ground black pepper

Brush or spray a skillet with coconut oil. Add the turkey or chicken, vinegar, ground chiles, salt, garlic powder, onion powder, cumin, oregano, cinnamon, and pepper and cook over medium-high heat for about 10 minutes, or until the meat is no longer pink. Alternatively, mix the ingredients in a bowl and form into 4 patties and sauté or grill for about 5 minutes on each side, or until an instant-read thermometer inserted in the center registers 165°F and the meat is no longer pink.

EASY ROAST TURKEY BREAST

PREP TIME: 10 MINUTES • COOK TIME: VARIES WITH WEIGHT

Yield: *Varies with the weight of the turkey* • **Portions**: *1 protein (for palm-size portion without skin or bones), ½ fat*

3½–4 pounds turkey breast, bone in and skin on

  2 tablespoons ghee, softened

  2 teaspoons fresh thyme leaves or 1 teaspoon dried

  1 clove garlic, minced

  ½ teaspoon Celtic or pink Himalayan salt

  ¼ teaspoon ground black pepper

Move an oven rack to the lower third of the oven. Preheat the oven to 450°F.

Rinse the turkey under cold water. Blot dry with paper towels. In a small bowl, mix the ghee, thyme, garlic, salt, and pepper. Gently loosen the skin around the breast and rub about three-quarters of the ghee mixture under the skin. Pull the skin tightly to cover as much of the breast as possible. Rub the remaining ghee mixture on the skin.

Place the turkey on a rack in a shallow roasting pan and reduce the heat to 350°F. Roast for 1½ to 2 hours for a 3½- to 4-pound breast. Check at 1 hour to see if the skin is getting too dark; if so, tent with foil. At 1½ hours, begin testing for doneness. The turkey is done when an instant-read thermometer inserted in the thickest portion registers 170°F and the juices run clear.

Remove the turkey from the oven and let it stand on the rack in the pan, covered with foil, for at least 20 minutes before carving. This gives the juices time to redistribute and the turkey time to firm up.

NOTE:

Turkey breasts vary in size, but your portion size should be a palm-size piece of boneless turkey, which is approximately 3 to 4 ounces for a woman and 4 to 5 ounces for a man.

EASY TURKEY BURGERS

PREP TIME: 10 MINUTES • COOK TIME: 15 MINUTES

Yield: Makes 4 servings • Portions: 1 protein

1–1¼ pounds lean ground turkey

¼ cup onion, finely chopped

½ teaspoon garlic powder

1 teaspoon Dijon mustard

2–3 tablespoons coarsely chopped flat-leaf parsley or cilantro (optional)

½ teaspoon Celtic or pink Himalayan salt

⅛–¼ teaspoon ground black pepper

Spray or brush a skillet or grill pan with coconut oil.

In a medium bowl, mix together the turkey, onion, garlic powder, mustard, parsley or cilantro, salt, and pepper. Form into 4 patties. Heat the skillet or grill pan over medium-high heat. Cook or grill the burgers for 5 to 6 minutes per side (depending on their thickness), or until an instant-read thermometer inserted in the center registers 165°F and the meat is no longer pink.

NOTES:

Burgers will be soft until fully cooked, so turn only once and do so carefully. These are also great prepared on an outdoor grill. Clean the grill and brush the burgers with coconut oil before grilling.

Try topping your burgers with Creamy Avocado Sauce (page 253), Ketchup (page 262), Homemade Mayonnaise (page 260), or Roasted Sweet Onions (page 229), or serve them on Roasted Portobello Burger "Buns" (page 229).

These can be made ahead and refrigerated.

MIDDLE EASTERN MEATBALLS

PREP TIME: 25 MINUTES • COOK TIME: 40 MINUTES

Yield: Makes 4 servings • Portions: 1 protein

1¼ pounds ground turkey

1 egg

½ onion, finely chopped

¼ cup chopped fresh cilantro

1 clove garlic, minced

1 teaspoon ground cumin

1 teaspoon paprika

¼ teaspoon ground cinnamon

½ teaspoon ground coriander (optional)

½ teaspoon Celtic or pink Himalayan salt

¼ teaspoon ground black pepper

Preheat the oven to 425°F. Line a baking sheet with parchment.

In a large bowl, mix the turkey, egg, onion, cilantro, garlic, cumin, paprika, cinnamon, coriander (if using), salt, and pepper. Form into golf-ball-size meatballs; you should end up with 16 meatballs. Place on the prepared baking sheet.

Bake at 425°F for 10 minutes. Reduce the heat to 350°F and bake for 15 to 20 minutes, or until an instant-read thermometer inserted in the center registers 165°F and the meat is no longer pink.

NOTES:

This can be prepared ahead and refrigerated.

Serve with roasted vegetables (see pages 224–225), Lemon-Roasted Asparagus (page 226), or a large garden salad with one of the Bone Broth Diet dressings (see Chapter 8).

VARIATION:

You can also make this dish with lamb.

RICH AND HEARTY TURKEY CHILI

PREP TIME: 15 MINUTES • COOK TIME: 60 MINUTES

Yield: Makes about eight 1½-cup servings (about 10 cups) • **Portions:** *1 protein, negligible fat*

2 tablespoons coconut oil

1 red bell pepper, finely chopped

1 green bell pepper, finely chopped

1 small jalapeño, seeded and finely chopped (optional; wear plastic gloves when handling)

3 cloves garlic, minced, or ½ teaspoon garlic powder

1 large sweet onion, finely chopped

2¼ pounds coarsely ground turkey

2–3 tablespoons chili powder

1 tablespoon smoked paprika

2 teaspoons ground cumin

1 can (28 ounces) diced tomatoes, drained

1 can (6 ounces) tomato paste

1 cup Chicken Bone Broth (page 98) or Beef Bone Broth (page 100)

1½ teaspoons Celtic or pink Himalayan salt

¼ teaspoon ground black pepper

Warm the oil in a large pot over medium-high heat. Add the bell peppers, jalapeño (if using), garlic, and onion. Reduce the heat to medium-low and cook for about 10 minutes, or until tender. Add the turkey, chili powder, paprika, and cumin and gently stir, trying not to break up the meat. Cover and cook for about 10 minutes, or until the meat is no longer pink. Add the tomatoes, tomato paste, broth, salt, and pepper. Stir to combine. Cover and bring to a simmer. Reduce the heat to low and simmer, partially covered, for at least 1 hour, stirring occasionally.

NOTES:

This can be prepared ahead and refrigerated or frozen; the recipe is doubled to save cooking time.

You can also make this in a slow cooker. Put everything together and cook for about 4 hours on high or 6 hours on low.

Serve with sliced limes, chopped onions, coarsely chopped cilantro, and hot sauce, if desired.

TURKEY MEATLOAF LOADED WITH VEGETABLES

PREP TIME: 10 MINUTES • COOK TIME: 50–55 MINUTES

Yield: *Makes 4 servings* • **Portions:** *1 protein*

1 sweet onion, cut into large chunks

2 ribs celery, cut into large chunks

2 carrots, cut into large chunks

1 small green bell pepper, seeded and cut into chunks

8 ounces mushrooms

Handful of fresh parsley (about ⅓ cup)

1¼ pounds ground turkey

1 egg

1 teaspoon ground sage

½ teaspoon ground thyme

½ teaspoon garlic powder

1½ teaspoons Celtic and pink Himalayan salt

½ teaspoon ground black pepper

Preheat the oven to 350°F.

In a food processor, pulse the onion, celery, and carrots for 1-second intervals until the vegetables are finely chopped. Transfer to a large bowl. Add the bell pepper, mushrooms, and parsley to the food processor and pulse in 1-second intervals until they reach a small dice. Transfer to the vegetable bowl.

Add the turkey, egg, sage, thyme, garlic powder, salt, and pepper to the bowl and mix together. Form into a loaf and place on a baking sheet. Brush or spray with coconut oil. Bake for 50 to 55 minutes, or until an instant-read thermometer inserted in the center registers 165°F and the meat is no longer pink. Let stand for 10 minutes before slicing.

NOTES:

You can hand-cut all the vegetables if you choose, but the food processor makes the process much faster.

Serve with Roasted Red Pepper Sauce (page 268).

This recipe easily doubles for fabulous leftovers. It can be prepared ahead and refrigerated.

VARIATIONS:

Dress up cold meatloaf with Ketchup (page 262) or make into a lettuce-wrap turkey meatloaf sandwich.

KALE SALAD WITH TURKEY

PREP TIME: 10 MINUTES

Yield: Makes 4 servings • **Portions:** 1 protein, 1 fat

8 cups fresh baby kale or kale mix or 1½ packages (5 ounces each) triple-washed baby kale

½ English cucumber, sliced

1 pound snap peas (about 2 cups)

4 scallions, white and green parts, sliced

1 can (8 ounces) water chestnuts, drained

¼ cup Orange Vinaigrette (page 257)

1 pound turkey breast (sugar-, dextrose-, nitrite-, and gluten-free), sliced (use roasted turkey leftovers or deli turkey)

In a large bowl, toss the kale, cucumber, peas, scallions, and water chestnuts with the dressing. Plate the salad and top with the turkey.

NOTE:

For salads, I prefer baby kale because it's more tender than regular kale. If you do use regular kale, slice it in very fine ribbons, place it in a large bowl, and knead it with your hands for about 2 minutes to break down some of the fibers.

TURKEY TACO SALAD

PREP TIME: 5 MINUTES

Yield: Makes 4 servings • *Portions: 1 protein, ½ fat*

6 cups Rich and Hearty Turkey Chili (page 168) (1½ cups per person)

1 large or 2 small heads romaine lettuce, torn or cut into bite-size pieces (about 8 cups)

1 small bell pepper, cut into thin strips

1 small jicama, peeled and cut into strips (optional)

1 small red onion, thinly sliced

2 tablespoons fresh lime juice

1 avocado, pitted and quartered

Celtic or pink Himalayan salt

Ground black pepper

Lime wedges (optional)

In a small saucepan, heat the chili. In a bowl, toss the lettuce, bell pepper, jicama (if using), and onion with the lime juice. Top each salad serving with 1½ cups chili and 1 avocado quarter. Season with salt and black pepper. Garnish with the lime wedges (if using).

NOTE:

Serve with hot sauce or any of the salsas (pages 267, 269, and 272).

ASIAN TURKEY BURGERS

PREP TIME: 10 MINUTES • COOK TIME: 12 MINUTES

*Yield: Makes 8 servings • **Portions:** 1 protein*

2 pounds lean ground turkey

4 scallions, white and green parts, thinly sliced

2 teaspoons fresh ginger, grated

1 small jalapeño, seeded and finely chopped (wear plastic gloves when handling)

1½ teaspoons Celtic or pink Himalayan salt

⅛–¼ teaspoon ground black pepper

Pinch of cayenne

Toasted sesame oil (optional but tasty)

Spray or brush a skillet with coconut oil.

In a large bowl, mix together the turkey, scallions, ginger, jalapeño, salt, black pepper, and cayenne. Heat the skillet over medium-high heat. Cook the burgers for 5 to 6 minutes per side (depending on how thick you make them), or until an instant-read thermometer inserted in the center registers 165°F and the meat is no longer pink. Brush the burgers with a few drops of toasted sesame oil (if using).

NOTES:

Burgers will be soft until fully cooked, so turn only once and do so carefully.

These are also great grilled. Clean the grill and brush the burgers with coconut oil before grilling.

Serve with Lemony Cucumber Salad (page 226) or Napa Slaw with Creamy Ginger Dressing (page 227).

These can be made ahead and refrigerated.

LUNCH OR DINNER ENTRÉES: Beef, Bison, and Pork

EASY BEEF OR BISON BURGERS

PREP TIME: 5 MINUTES · COOK TIME: 10 MINUTES

Yield: Makes 4 servings • *Portions: 1 protein*

1 **pound lean ground beef, sirloin, or bison**

¼ **cup finely chopped onion (optional)**

½ **teaspoon garlic powder**

½ **teaspoon Celtic or pink Himalayan salt**

⅛–¼ **teaspoon ground black pepper**

Spray or brush a skillet or grill pan with coconut oil.

In a bowl, mix the beef, onion (if using), garlic powder, salt, and pepper. Form into 4 patties. Heat the skillet or grill pan over medium-high heat. Cook the burgers for about 4 minutes per side (depending on how thick you make them), or until an instant-read thermometer inserted in the center registers 160°F and the meat is no longer pink.

NOTES:

These are also great grilled. Clean the grill and brush the burgers with coconut oil before grilling.

Try topping your burgers with Creamy Avocado Sauce (page 253), Ketchup (page 262), Homemade Mayonnaise (page 260), or Roasted Sweet Onions (page 229), or serve them on Roasted Portobello Burger "Buns" (page 229).

These can be made ahead and refrigerated.

BOLOGNESE

PREP TIME: 30 MINUTES • COOK TIME: 6 HOURS ON LOW IN SLOW COOKER OR
4 HOURS ON STOVETOP

Yield: 8 to 9 servings • *Portions:* 1 protein, negligible fat

- 2 tablespoons olive oil
- 1 tablespoon ghee
- 1 medium onion, finely chopped
- 2 carrots, finely chopped
- 2 celery stalks, finely chopped
- 2 garlic cloves, minced
- 1 pound ground beef
- 1 pound ground pork
- 4 ounces bacon or pancetta, nitrate- and sugar-free, diced and cooked
- 1 (24-ounce) jar store-bought sugar-free tomato sauce
- ¼ teaspoon nutmeg
- ⅓–½ cup full-fat canned coconut milk
- ½ teaspoon Celtic or pink Himalayan salt
- 1 teaspoon ground black pepper
- Wide-cut zoodles, for serving (see Note)

Hear 2 tablespoons oil and 1 tablespoon ghee in a large pot over medium heat. Add the onion, carrots, and celery to the pot and cook for 7 to 8 minutes, stirring frequently. Add the garlic and cook for 2 more minutes. Transfer the vegetables to a slow cooker or set them aside on a plate if you are using the stovetop method. (If you are using the slow cooker mode on an Instant Pot, you can use the sauté function to sauté the vegetables. When done, remove them from the Instant Pot before browning the meat.)

In the same large pot or using the sauté function on an Instant Pot, increase the heat to medium-high and add the beef, pork, and bacon or pancetta, cooking for 5 to 8 minutes, until browned. In a slow cooker, Instant Pot, or large pot, combine the sautéed vegetables, browned meat, tomato sauce, and nutmeg and cook on low for about 6 hours in the Instant Pot or slow cooker or 4 hours on low heat on the stovetop. Just before serving, add ⅓ cup coconut milk, salt, and pepper and stir to combine. Taste and add the remaining coconut milk if desired. (You don't want to add any coconut flavor to the Bolognese; you just want to add a bit of creaminess.) Serve over wide-cut zoodles.

NOTES:

The key to good Bolognese is low and slow. Let it simmer at a very low tempera-ture for a long time for the richest flavor.

Since Bolognese is traditionally served with wide, flat pasta, use a vegetable peeler and slice the zucchini vertically to create wide zoodles. You will need one small to medium zucchini per person. Heat in a microwave for about 30 seconds, or in a skillet for 1 to 2 minutes per zucchini to warm. The sauce is also good on cauli-flower rice.

20 Cooking Shortcuts

Leanne Ely, nutritionist and bestselling author of _Part-Time Paleo_
SavingDinner.com

When it comes to putting healthy meals on the table in a hurry, no one's more of an expert than Leanne. Here are some of her best tricks for getting you out of the kitchen fast.

1. Make your own mixes.

Instead of measuring out spices at meal prep time, make your own mixes ahead of time, and just measure out one serving at a time. An example would be our Italian Seasoning.

ITALIAN SEASONING
(Makes 1 cup)

½ cup + 2 tablespoons dried oregano

¼ cup dried basil

1 tablespoon dried marjoram

1 tablespoon garlic powder

In a small bowl, combine the oregano, basil, marjoram, and garlic powder. Transfer to a sandwich-size resealable plastic bag. Seal the bag and mark "Italian Seasoning" and the date prepared on the bag. Use 1 tablespoon for every 2 cups of sauce.

Other spice blends you could mix ahead of time include Tex-Mex, Indian, and Chicken Soup. By taking a few minutes in 1 day to mix up these spice blends, you'll save all kinds of time when it comes to dinnertime.

2. Use your egg slicer.

Use a simple egg slicer to slice mushrooms, strawberries, and any other soft foods you can chop in there!

3. Make stock cubes.

A muffin pan is perfect for freezing leftover broth portions. These frozen servings of stock can be tossed into resealable plastic freezer bags and thawed for later use.

4. Funnel it.

If you need to funnel dry ingredients, rather than fussing with packaging and looking for a plastic funnel, simply snip the end off of a coffee filter.

5. Use rotisserie chicken.

If you watch the prices on your grocery store's rotisserie chickens, you can get them at quite a bargain. I generally buy two at a time if the price is right. You can use the meat for dinner and freeze the leftovers in 2-cup portions. Great to haul out for a quick meal.

6. Grate and juice lemons.

If you have some time on your hands, grate the peel of a few lemons at once, and freeze the grated peel for future use. Same with the juice. If you're going to use it up within a couple of days, leave it in the fridge. If it will be around longer, you probably should freeze it.

7. Prep herb olive oil.

Freeze fresh herbs and olive oil or melted clarified butter in ice cube trays. Then when you need to sauté something with herbs and oil, simply pop one out and you're good to go.

8. Process ginger.

Grating fresh ginger can be a pain, so I like to peel a couple of ginger roots at once and pop them in the food processor. Generally, recipes call for 1-tablespoon measures, so freeze several portions on waxed paper or in ice cube trays. Then put those portions in freezer bags.

9. Make smoothie packs.

If you have a standard smoothie that you love and enjoy every day, why not do a whole week's worth of prep at once? All you need is seven freezer bags and a week's worth of ingredients. Put your berries, greens, protein powder, etc., in the bag and refrigerate or freeze. When it's time to blend it up, simply toss the smoothie pack in the blender with your liquid and off you go!

10. Use kitchen shears.

It's so much quicker to snip herbs with shears than cut them with a knife. You can use shears for all kinds of things, but try to use a separate set of shears for meats and another set for other purposes.

11. Quickly warm eggs.

If you need to bring eggs to room temperature in a hurry, simply place them in a bowl of warm water.

12. Measure oil first.

If you're making a recipe that calls for oil and sticky ingredients, measure the oil first so the remaining ingredients slide out of the measuring cup.

13. Freeze tomato paste.

Most recipes requiring tomato paste will call for only 1 tablespoon. Rather than wasting the rest of the can, freeze in 1-tablespoon amounts on a sheet of waxed paper or in ice cube trays. Once frozen, toss the paste clumps in a freezer bag and take out when needed.

14. Bake bacon.

Nothing is quite as delicious as baked bacon! Simply place on a parchment-lined baking sheet, sprinkle with black pepper, and bake at 350°F until cooked. It should take 10 to 15 minutes, which gives you plenty of time to do other things (instead of standing and watching the skillet).

15. Think outside the waffle iron.

If you own a waffle iron, you can prepare omelets in there!

16. Separate eggs carefully.

If you're separating a bunch of eggs, all you need is one drop of yolk in your whites to ruin your plans. I separate my

(continued)

20 Cooking Shortcuts—*cont.*

eggs one at a time into a small ramekin before adding to the larger bowl. This way, if I get a speck of yolk, I don't have to dump the whole lot. And if you're not a great egg separator using the shell method, just use your fingers! The white slides through your fingers while the yolk sits on your palm.

17. Slice peppers easily.

When slicing a bell pepper, make things easy on yourself. Slice the top off the pepper first and pull out the core and seeds. Then slice the pepper from the inside (because the outside is slippery).

18. Mix in a jar.

Use mason jars for dressings and other types of sauces and marinades. Simply measure, shake, and pour! Saves you from having to whisk.

19. Skim the fat.

When you have to skim the fat off of a soup or stock, rather than chasing the fat globules around with a spoon, put a couple of ice cubes in the pot. This will help solidify the fat for easy removal.

20. Freeze before slicing.

When cutting chicken breasts or steak into thin slices, the job will be easier if the meat is partially frozen first.

EASY POT ROAST

PREP TIME: 15 MINUTES • COOK TIME: 3–8 HOURS
(DEPENDING ON METHOD OF COOKING)

Yield: Makes 6 or more servings • Portions: 1 protein (for a palm-size portion)

2½–3 pound beef roast (see Note)

1 teaspoon Celtic or pink Himalayan salt

½ teaspoon ground black pepper

2 cloves garlic, smashed

1 bay leaf

2–3 sprigs fresh thyme or ¼ teaspoon dried

1 sprig fresh rosemary or ¼ teaspoon dried (optional)

1 onion, cut into wedges

2 carrots, cut into 2" slices

2 ribs celery, cut into 2" slices

1 cup Beef Bone Broth (page 100)

Spray or brush a large skillet with coconut oil and heat over medium-high heat. When the pan is hot, sear the meat for 4 to 7 minutes, or until browned on all sides.

To use a slow cooker: Put all the ingredients in the cooker, cover, and cook on low for 6 to 8 hours.

To use the oven: Preheat the oven to 300°F. Put all the ingredients in an ovenproof Dutch oven or roasting pan, cover, and bake for 3 or more hours for a 3-pound roast or 4 or more hours for a 4- to 5-pound roast, or until fork-tender.

Reduce the heat to 200°F. Remove the meat from the pan, pull it apart with a fork, and return it to the pan immersed in juices. Return the pan to the oven for about 20 minutes. Remove and discard the bay leaf before serving.

NOTE:

The leanest cut is a rump roast; other cuts include chuck roast, bottom round, and brisket. Because the cuts used for pot roast tend to be tougher than other cuts, they should be cooked on low heat so the fibers get broken down, which softens the meat.

SLOW COOKER SOUTHWEST PULLED PORK

PREP TIME: 25 MINUTES • COOK TIME: 6–8 HOURS

Yield: 5 to 7 servings • *Portions:* 1 protein, negligible fat

3–4 pounds boneless pork shoulder or butt

¾ teaspoon salt

½ teaspoon pepper

1–2 tablespoons avocado oil

4 garlic cloves, minced

1½ teaspoons cumin

1½ teaspoons oregano

1½ teaspoons chili powder

1 cup salsa, sugar- and dextrose-free

⅓ cup Chicken Bone Broth (page 98) or water

7-ounce can mild green chilies, drained and diced

Juice of 1 lime

½ cup green onions, thinly sliced

1 jalapeño, seeded and minced (wear plastic gloves when handling)

½–¾ cup cilantro, chopped

Cauliflower rice or lettuce leaves, for serving

Cut the pork into 4 to 6 pieces and sprinkle with the salt and the pepper. In a Dutch oven, heat the oil on medium-high, until shimmering. Add the pork and cook, 5 to 7 minutes, until browned on all sides. Transfer the pork to a slow cooker. Add the garlic, cumin, oregano, chili powder, salsa, broth, green chilies, lime juice, green onions, jalapeño, and cilantro. Cook on low for 6 to 8 hours. Using 2 forks, shred the pork directly in the cooker, discarding any pieces of fat. Serve on cauliflower rice or on a bed of lettuce.

NOTES:

There are a number of optional toppings you can add: chopped tomatoes, shredded lettuce, chopped avocado or guacamole, green or red onions, cilantro, or sliced black olives.

Pork shoulder and pork butt, or Boston butt, both come from the shoulder of the pig. The butt is higher on the front leg.

With so many kinds of salsas on the market, you could vary the recipe to your liking. For example, salsa verde (green salsa made with tomatillos) will flavor the pork differently than a fire-roasted-tomato salsa. Don't be shy about trying salsa verde if you've never had green salsa. It sings in this recipe!

FIESTA BEEF FAJITAS

PREP TIME: 15 MINUTES • COOK TIME: 15 MINUTES

*Yield: Makes 8 servings • **Portions:** 1 protein, ¼ fat*

⅔–1 cup fresh orange juice

⅓ cup apple cider vinegar

2 cloves garlic, minced, or 1½ teaspoons garlic powder

1½–2 teaspoons dried oregano

1 teaspoon Celtic or pink Himalayan salt

¾ teaspoon ground cumin

½ teaspoon ground black pepper

2 pounds lean beef, cut into ½" strips (skirt, flank, top round, or sirloin works well; see Notes)

2 tablespoons coconut oil

4 red bell peppers, cut into strips

4 yellow or orange bell peppers, cut into strips

2 onions, sliced

In a medium bowl or resealable plastic bag, combine the orange juice, vinegar, garlic, oregano, salt, cumin, and black pepper. Add the beef and marinate for at least 2 hours in the refrigerator. (For more flavor, marinate the beef overnight.)

Spray or brush a nonstick skillet with some of the oil and heat over medium-high heat. Cook the bell peppers and onions until tender but still crisp. Remove from the pan and set aside. You may need to do this in 2 batches, depending on the size of your skillet. (Spray or brush the skillet with oil between each batch of vegetables or meat.)

Drain the beef. Discard the marinade. In the same skillet, cook the beef for 4 to 6 minutes, or until it reaches the desired doneness. You may need to do this in 2 batches; it's best not to crowd the meat, so it will cook quickly and evenly. Return the vegetables to the skillet to heat through.

> **NOTES:**
>
> *If you use top round, it's best to marinate it overnight to tenderize the meat.*
>
> *This fajita recipe is another favorite—it's doubled so you can have it for lunch the next day.*
>
> *Serve with Garlic Mashed Cauliflower "Potatoes" (page 223) or Cauliflower Rice (page 222).*
>
> *This recipe can be prepared ahead and refrigerated.*

VARIATIONS:

Serve the beef at room temperature piled into lettuce cups. Bibb lettuce or romaine works very well.

Use chicken and make chicken fajitas. Marinate the chicken for 1 to 2 hours.

GREEK-STYLE BEEF OR BISON BURGERS

PREP TIME: 15 MINUTES • COOK TIME: 10 MINUTES

Yield: Makes 8 servings • *Portions: 1 protein, ½ fat*

- 2 pounds ground sirloin, lean ground beef, or ground bison, pasture-raised/grass-fed if possible
- 2–3 cloves garlic, minced
- ½ onion, finely chopped
- 1 teaspoon dried marjoram
- 1 teaspoon dried oregano
- ¼ cup chopped fresh flat-leaf parsley
- ½ cup kalamata olives, pitted and chopped
- 1 jar (10 ounces) roasted red peppers, drained well, blotted with paper towels, and chopped
- 1 egg
- 1 teaspoon Celtic or pink Himalayan salt
- ½ teaspoon ground black pepper

In a large mixing bowl, combine the meat, garlic, onion, marjoram, oregano, parsley, olives, red peppers, egg, salt, and black pepper. Form into 8 patties, making them thicker around the outside edge. (Burgers puff up in the center when cooked; forming them with a thinner center makes them cook evenly.)

Spray or brush a grill pan or grill rack with coconut oil and heat to high. When the pan or rack is hot, add the burgers. Turn the burgers once to cook on both sides, grilling 4 to 5 minutes per side, or until an instant-read thermometer inserted in the center registers 160°F and the meat is no longer pink.

NOTE:

It's not necessary to cook these in a grill pan or on the grill. You can cook them in a skillet or broil them in the oven. The timing should be about the same.

VARIATION:

To offer a burger as a "sandwich," serve in a Roasted Portobello Burger "Bun" (page 229) or wrapped in lettuce.

PORK TENDERLOIN WITH APPLES AND ONIONS

PREP TIME: 15 MINUTES • COOK TIME: 20 MINUTES

Yield: *Makes 4 servings* • **Portions**: *1 protein, 1 fruit*

1 teaspoon garlic powder

1 teaspoon dried marjoram

1 teaspoon ground cumin

1 teaspoon ground coriander

1 teaspoon dried thyme

½ teaspoon Celtic or pink Himalayan salt

¼ teaspoon ground black pepper

1 large pork tenderloin (about 1 pound)

1 large sweet onion, sliced

2 Granny Smith apples, peeled, cored, and sliced

Pinch of ground cinnamon

Preheat the oven to 425°F.

In a small bowl, mix the garlic powder, marjoram, cumin, coriander, thyme, salt, and pepper. Blend well to create a dry rub. Sprinkle the rub evenly over the tenderloin and pat it into the meat so the tenderloin is entirely covered.

Spray or brush a large nonstick skillet with coconut oil and place over medium-high heat. When the pan is hot, add the pork and sear for 5 to 8 minutes, or until all sides are brown. Transfer the pork to a roasting pan and roast for 15 to 20 minutes, or until an instant-read thermometer inserted in the center reaches 145°F and the juices run clear.

Meanwhile, in the hot skillet used for the pork, cook the onion and apples over medium heat for about 5 minutes, or until golden. Remove from the heat and season with salt, pepper, and cinnamon.

When the pork is done, transfer to a platter and tent with foil. Let stand for 5 minutes before carving. Cut the pork into ½" slices. Serve with the apples and onion.

BALSAMIC ROAST PORK LOIN

PREP TIME: 10 MINUTES • COOK TIME: 45–60 MINUTES

*Yield: Varies with the size of the roast • **Portions:** 1 protein (for a palm-size portion; 3–4 ounces cooked)*

2½–3 pound pork loin

4–6 cloves garlic, minced

¼ cup balsamic vinegar

1 tablespoon Dijon mustard

½ teaspoon Celtic or pink Himalayan salt

½ teaspoon ground black pepper

2 tablespoons fresh rosemary, thyme, or tarragon (remove leaves from stem and finely chop) or 2 teaspoons dried

Pat the pork dry with paper towels. In a small bowl or a food processor, mix or pulse the garlic, vinegar, mustard, salt, pepper, and herbs. Rub all over the loin. Or place the loin and garlic mixture in a resealable plastic bag and shake to thoroughly coat. Let the coated pork sit at room temperature for 15 to 20 minutes, or cover and refrigerate for several hours or overnight.

Preheat the oven to 350°F.

Generously spray or brush a large skillet with coconut oil and heat on medium-high heat. When the pan is hot, sear the pork for 3 to 4 minutes per side on all sides, or until browned. Place in a roasting pan and roast for 45 to 60 minutes, or until an instant-read thermometer inserted in the center reaches 145°F and the juices run clear. Let stand for 5 minutes before slicing.

NOTES:

Pork loin is very easy to prepare and makes great leftovers. Pork and Eggs (page 133) uses leftovers.

Since you'll have the oven on, it's a great time to make roasted vegetables, too. See "Roasting and Sautéing Vegetables" (pages 224–225).

ROASTED SALMON GREMOLATA

PREP TIME: 5 MINUTES • COOK TIME: 20 MINUTES

Yield: *Makes 4 servings* • **Portions**: *1 protein, ½ fat*

1 pound salmon fillet

2 tablespoons coconut oil or ghee, melted

Celtic or Pink Himalayan salt

Ground black pepper

⅓–½ cup fresh lemon juice

½ cup chopped flat-leaf parsley

Preheat the oven to 425°F. Line a baking sheet with parchment.

Rub both sides of the salmon with the oil or ghee and place on the prepared baking sheet. (If the salmon has skin, place it skin side down.)

Lightly salt and pepper the fillet, drizzle with the lemon juice, and sprinkle with the parsley. Bake for 20 to 25 minutes, or until the fish is opaque.

NOTES:

Perfectly done fish flakes easily, and the cooked inner flesh is opaque. Under-cooked fish resists flaking, and the inside is translucent.

To test fish for doneness, poke the tines of a fork into the thickest portion of the fish at a 45-degree angle. Then gently pull up some of the fish. If it easily flakes and the inside is opaque, it is done. If it does not flake when you insert the fork and/or the inside flesh is still translucent, it is not done. If your fish is underdone, just continue cooking it until it is done. Keep in mind that fish cooks fast, so 1 to 3 minutes can make a big difference.

AIR FRYER FISH AND ZUCCHINI "FRIES" (WITH OVEN COOKING INSTRUCTIONS INCLUDED)

PREP TIME: 30 MINUTES • COOK TIME: VARIES WITH METHOD

Yield: 4 *servings* • *Portions:* 1 *protein, negligible fat*

2 small to medium zucchini

1 or 2 eggs

½ cup almond flour

¼ cup coconut flour

1 tablespoon arrowroot

¼ teaspoon onion powder

¼ teaspoon garlic powder

¼ teaspoon dried parsley

¼ teaspoon paprika

⅛ teaspoon cayenne

1 teaspoon Celtic or pink Himalayan salt

¼–½ teaspoon ground black pepper

1–1½ pounds cod of uniform thickness, if possible

Avocado, coconut, or olive oil pan spray

PREPARATION FOR ZUCCHINI FRIES:

In a shallow bowl or a pie plate, beat the eggs until frothy. In a second shallow bowl or pie plate, mix the almond flour, coconut flour, arrowroot, onion powder, garlic powder, dried parsley, paprika, cayenne, salt, and pepper.

Slice off both ends of the zucchini and cut into steak-fry-size spears. Dip each spear into the egg mixture, letting excess drip off, and lightly sprinkle with the flour mixture. The zucchini should not be heavily coated with the flour mixture.

If using the air fryer method for cooking, place the coated fries on a plate and skip to *Air fryer method for fries.* You can begin cooking them while preparing the fish.

If you are using the *Oven method for fish and fries,* lay the spears evenly on a sheet pan, lightly spray with pan spray, and set aside until the fish is prepped.

AIR FRYER METHOD FOR FRIES:

Preheat the oven to 200°F and an air fryer to 400°F. Place the zucchini fries into the air fryer basket without overlapping any pieces, spray with pan spray, cook for 5 to 7 minutes until lightly browned, and flip to cook second side. Cook for an additional 5 to 7 minutes. Depending on your air fryer, you may have to cook in 2 batches. Transfer the fries to the oven while cooking the remaining fries and fish.

PREPARATION FOR FISH:

If the cod is a whole fillet or loin, cut into 4 individual pieces. Fish will cook more evenly if all pieces are approximately the same thickness. Rinse the fish in cold water and pat dry with a paper towel. One piece at a time, dip the fish into the beaten eggs so both sides are covered, letting the excess drip off. Gently place the fish in the flour mixture and flip to cover both sides. The fish will not be heavily coated with the flour mixture. Transfer to a plate and repeat with remaining fish.

AIR FRYER METHOD FOR FISH:

Preheat the oven to 200°F and an air fryer to 400°F. Line the air fryer basket with parchment. Lightly spray both sides of each piece of fish with pan spray and place into the air fryer's basket. Do not crowd the fish; you may have to cook in 2 batches based on the size of your air fryer. Cook for 7 minutes, flip, and cook the second side for 3 to 4 minutes. You may need to vary the time a bit based on the thickness of the fish. Place the fish on the same sheet pan where you are holding the fries and return to the oven until you have completed cooking. Do not cover the zucchini or fish; it will make the coating soggy.

OVEN METHOD FOR FISH AND FRIES:

Fish and fries can cook at the same time in the oven and will be done approximately at the same time. Preheat the oven to 425°F. Place zucchini fries on the bottom rack and bake for about 8 to 10 minutes. Meanwhile, line a baking sheet with parchment and spray the parchment with pan spray. Preheat the pan for 5 to 7 minutes on the top oven rack.

Carefully flip the zucchini and bake for about 8 to 10 minutes more.

Add the fish to the preheated pan, spray the top of the fish with pan spray and bake for 5 to 7 minutes, depending on thickness. Gently flip and bake for 3 to 5 minutes more. Do not cover the zucchini or fish; it will make the coating soggy.

NOTES:

Timing is important when putting a meal together, especially when using an air fryer. Because of its limited capacity, you often need to cook in small batches. Cook the fries first because they take longer than the fish. If using the oven method, they will be done at approximately the same time.

Fish should be cooked to an internal temperature of 145°F. Test with an instant-read thermometer. You can also test fish for doneness with a fork. Insert the fork into the thickest part of the fish and gently twist the fork so you can see the internal flesh. The fish will flake easily when it's done, and the flesh will lose its translucence, or raw appearance, and appear opaque.

Read the label before you buy coconut flour and select one that has less than 9 grams of carbohydrates per a 2 tablespoon serving, for example, Bob's Red Mill.

BUTTERY SALMON AND ASPARAGUS

PREP TIME: 15 MINUTES • COOK TIME: 15–20 MINUTES

Yield: 2 servings • *Portions:* 1 protein, 1 fat

¼ pound or more fresh asparagus, tough ends removed

2 (4–6 ounce) salmon fillets

2 tablespoons or more fresh dill

1 tablespoon capers, rinsed

2 tablespoons ghee or grass fed butter

1 lemon + zest from ½ lemon

¼ teaspoon Celtic or pink Himalayan salt

⅛ teaspoon ground black pepper

Preheat the oven to 325°F. Cut two 8- to 9-inch squares of parchment and cut two pieces of foil a little larger. Place foil on sheet pan. Top each piece of foil with parchment, asparagus, salmon, dill, capers, and ghee. Squeeze the juice of half of the lemon over each and sprinkle with lemon zest. Season with salt and pepper. Tightly wrap the parchment and foil over the salmon to create a sealed packet and set them on a rimmed baking sheet. Bake for 15 to 20 minutes, depending on the thickness of the salmon. Remove from the oven and let the parcels steam for 2 minutes before serving.

NOTES:

This is delicious served with cauliflower rice. It will soak up all the buttery juices.

You can also make this dish with any fish, but you'll have to adjust the cooking time. You might want to omit or reduce the capers if you are using a more delicate white fish such as cod or halibut.

Fish should be cooked to an internal temperature of 145°F. Test with an instant-read thermometer. You can also test fish for doneness with a fork. Insert the fork into the thickest part of the fish and gently twist the fork so you can see the internal flesh. The fish will flake easily when it's done. The flesh will lose its translucence, or raw appearance, and appear opaque.

To make a delicious Dijonnaise sauce, combine 2 tablespoons avocado mayonnaise, 1 teaspoon Dijon mustard, and ½ to 1 teaspoon fresh dill. Using 1 tablespoon Dijonnaise per serving will add 1 serving of fat to the meal. This Dijonnaise is also a great spread for lettuce roll ups.

SHRIMP CEVICHE

PREP TIME: 30 MINUTES • CURE TIME: 30 MINUTES (IF USING RAW SEAFOOD)

Yield: 4 servings • *Portions:* 1 protein, ½ fat

- 1 pound shrimp, peeled and deveined
- ⅔ cup freshly squeezed lime juice (5–6 limes)
- 2 plum tomatoes, seeded and diced into ½" cubes (about 1 cup)
- 1 small red onion, minced (about ½ cup)
- 1 small to medium cucumber, peeled, seeded, and diced into ½" cubes (about 1 cup)
- ½ bunch cilantro leaves, coarsely chopped (about ¼ cup)
- 1 medium jalapeño, seeded if you want less heat, minced (wear plastic gloves when handling)
- ½ teaspoon Celtic or pink Himalayan salt
- ⅛ teaspoon ground black pepper
- 1 avocado, pitted, peeled, and cut into ½" cubes (about ½ cup)
- Bibb lettuce leaves, for serving (optional)

Prepare an ice water bath. To steam the shrimp, fill a large pot with enough water to come just below the bottom of a steamer basket. The water should not touch the bottom of the basket. Bring the water to a boil, add the shrimp, turn the heat to medium high, cover, and steam for about 2 minutes, depending on the size of the shrimp. Remove one shrimp and cut in half to test for doneness. The shrimp should be totally opaque in the center. If not fully cooked, steam for another minute or two. Immediately remove shrimp and put into the ice bath to stop the cooking. Blot dry with paper towels and cut into ½" pieces. You can also boil the shrimp if you don't have a steamer basket. Timing will be about the same.

Place shrimp pieces in a nonreactive bowl and add the lime juice. Add the tomatoes, onion, cucumber, cilantro, jalapeño, salt, and pepper and gently toss together. Cover and chill in the refrigerator and for 30 to 60 minutes, stirring halfway through. Just before serving, gently stir in the avocado. Serve chilled, in Bibb lettuce cups, if desired, on the day it was prepared.

NOTES:

Only use fresh lime juice. Bottled juice is bitter and contains preservatives.

Aluminum, copper, iron, and steel (not "stainless" steel) are all reactive to acidic or alkaline foods. Glass, stainless, and ceramic are nonreactive.

Ceviche should be eaten the same day it is prepared.

You can also use firm, non-fatty white saltwater fish, scallops, or lobster. Examples of firm and semi-firm fish include mahi-mahi, cod, halibut, sea bass, and snapper.

For guidelines on sustainability, check out Seafood Watch, published by the Monterey Bay Aquarium, at www.seafoodwatch.org.

Using raw seafood:

Ceviche is traditionally made with raw seafood. Should you decide to prepare it without cooking, remember to use only wild-caught saltwater seafood. Never use fish from a freshwater source. When selecting the seafood, talk with the vendor and inquire what is the freshest.

To prepare, use peeled and deveined shrimp and cut them into ½" pieces. Use 1 full cup of lime juice (8–9 limes). Pour the lime juice into a nonreactive bowl and add the shrimp. Cover and refrigerate for at least 30 minutes. Be sure to cure the seafood in the lime juice until it has become completely opaque. To test, remove one piece of shrimp and cut it in half to test for doneness. The shrimp should be totally opaque in the center. If not fully cured, return to the lime juice and refrigerate for 10 more minutes more before retesting.

When the shrimp is fully cured, add the remaining ingredients and gently toss together. Refrigerate if not serving immediately. Serve on the day it is prepared.

POKE BOWL

PREP TIME: 15 MINUTES

Yield: 4 to 6 servings • *Portions:* 1 protein, negligible fat

POKE MARINADE

- ¼ cup coconut aminos + more for serving
- 1 tablespoon toasted sesame oil
- 2 tablespoons freshly squeezed lime juice
- 1 tablespoon freshly squeezed orange juice
- 1 teaspoon or more Sriracha or ½ teaspoon or more crushed red-pepper flakes
- 1 tablespoon toasted sesame seeds
- 1 green onion, white and green parts, very thinly sliced
- 1 pound fresh ahi tuna, preferably sushi grade, cut into ¼ to ½" chunks

ACCOMPANIMENTS (SELECT AS MANY OF THESE INGREDIENTS AS YOU LIKE):

Cauliflower rice

Cucumber, diced

Jalapeño, sliced into rounds or minced (wear plastic gloves when handling)

Radishes, sliced into rounds

Avocado, diced

Red or green onions, thinly sliced

Tomatoes, diced

Cabbage, shredded

Broccoli florets, blanched and chilled

Coconut aminos

Whisk together the aminos, oil, lime juice, orange juice, Sriracha, sesame seeds, and green onions in a nonreactive bowl (see Notes). Add the tuna and mix together so all the tuna is coated with the sauce. You can serve immediately or marinate in the refrigerator for up to 2 hours.

Build a poke bowl by starting with ½ cup or more cold or room temperature cauliflower rice. Sprinkle with coconut aminos, if desired. Top with poke and serve as is or add any combination of sliced or diced vegetable accompaniments. Enjoy the poke on the day that it is made.

NOTES:

Aluminum, copper, iron, and steel (not "stainless" steel) are all reactive to acidic or alkaline foods. Glass, stainless, and ceramic are nonreactive.

Buy your tuna fresh from a reputable market. If possible, purchase sushi grade ahi. Tell the vendor you will be serving the fish raw. Don't be shy about asking questions so you get the freshest fish possible. Almost all fish is frozen on the fishing boat as soon as it is caught, so it's best not to refreeze it after purchasing.

Poke is sometimes accompanied by a spicy mayonnaise. To make this sauce, combine ½ cup avocado mayonnaise and 1½ tablespoons Sriracha. Add 1 teaspoon coconut aminos for more umami flavor, if desired.

Raw fish should be eaten on the day it was prepared.

SEARED SCALLOPS

PREP TIME: 15 MINUTES • COOK TIME: 15 MINUTES

Yield: Makes 4 servings • *Portions:* 1 protein, ½ fat

1 **pound sea scallops**

2 **tablespoons ghee or coconut oil (see Note)**

  Celtic or Pink Himalayan salt

  Ground black pepper

1 **very small clove garlic, minced (about ¼ teaspoon)**

  Chopped fresh parsley, as garnish (optional)

  Lemon wedges, as garnish (optional)

Rinse the scallops well. Blot on paper towels to thoroughly dry. Blot a second time. You want the scallops as dry as possible so they sear, not steam.

Heat a large nonstick skillet over medium-high heat for 1 to 2 minutes. Add the ghee or oil and heat until very hot. Put the scallops in the pan in a single, uncrowded layer. (If you are cooking for 4, cook the scallops in 2 batches; overcrowding the pan will prevent a good sear.) Season with salt and pepper and let sear undisturbed for 2 to 4 minutes, or until one side is browned and crisp. Don't move the scallops in the pan; barely lift the edge of a scallop to check the color. Using tongs, turn the scallops and sear for 2 to 4 minutes, or until the second side is well browned and the scallops are almost firm to the touch. Their centers should be slightly translucent because the scallops will continue to cook when you remove them from the heat. Using tongs, transfer the scallops to dinner plates, leaving the ghee or oil in the skillet.

Add the garlic to the hot skillet, reduce the heat to medium-low, and cook for 1 to 2 minutes, or until the garlic softens. Pour the garlic mixture over the plated scallops. Top with parsley and serve with lemon wedges (if using).

NOTE:

To get the richest flavor, use ghee. Because there are no milk solids in ghee, it works well at a very high heat.

ZESTY SALMON PATTIES

PREP TIME: 15 MINUTES · COOK TIME: 10 MINUTES

Yield: Makes 4 servings • *Portions: 1 protein, negligible fat*

1 can (14.75 ounces) red salmon or just under 1 pound cooked salmon, flaked into small pieces

¼ cup finely chopped red onion

¼ cup finely chopped celery

¼ cup coarsely chopped parsley

2 teaspoons coconut oil, melted

1 egg + 1 egg yolk, slightly beaten

1 teaspoon paprika

½ teaspoon mustard powder

¼ teaspoon ground black pepper

⅛ teaspoon cayenne

1 lemon, cut into wedges

Spray or brush a large nonstick skillet with coconut oil. In a medium bowl, thoroughly combine the salmon, onion, celery, parsley, oil, egg and egg yolk, paprika, mustard, black pepper, and cayenne. Mix thoroughly. Form into 4 patties. Heat the skillet over medium-high heat and cook the patties for 4 to 5 minutes on each side, or until they are lightly browned. Serve with the lemon wedges.

NOTES:

Serve with Napa Slaw with Creamy Ginger Dressing (page 227).
These can be prepared ahead and refrigerated.

TUNA-STUFFED TOMATOES

PREP TIME: 10 MINUTES

Yield: Makes 4 servings • *Portions: 1 protein, ½ fat*

4 cans (4–5 ounces each) water-packed chunk white or albacore tuna, drained well

⅓ cup chopped celery

¼ cup chopped red onion

⅓ cup Creamy Avocado Sauce or Salad Dressing (page 253)

4 large tomatoes

4–8 cups lettuce of your choice

Celtic or pink Himalayan salt

Ground black pepper

In a medium bowl, break apart the tuna with a fork and add the celery, onion, and dressing. Mix well. Cut each tomato into 8 wedges, but do not cut all the way through. Place each tomato on a plate of greens and gently spread the wedges open. Fill each tomato with the tuna mixture. Season with salt and pepper.

VARIATION:

Add ¾ cup finely chopped roasted red peppers.

GRAB-AND-GO MEALS

In a big hurry? Here are superquick meals you can toss together in minutes. Most of them use leftovers from the entrée recipes.

Grab-and-Go Turkey Meatloaf (1 protein, 1 fat): Place leftover Turkey Meatloaf Loaded with Vegetables (page 169) in 1 or 2 lettuce leaves and top with Ketchup (page 262).

Grab-and-Go Zesty Salmon Patty (1 protein, 1 fat): Place a leftover Zesty Salmon Patty (page 195) on 2 or more large lettuce leaves. Top with ½ avocado, 1 serving of any Bone Broth Diet dressing (see Chapter 8), Creamy Avocado Sauce or Salad Dressing (page 253), Napa Slaw with Creamy Ginger Dressing (page 227), or Lemony Cucumber Salad (page 226). Add lemon wedges for the salmon and 1 or 2 handfuls of crispy vegetables as a side.

Grab-and-Go Avocado Egg Salad (1 protein, 1 fat, 1 fruit): Cut 2 or 3 hard-cooked eggs in half. Scoop out the yolks into a small bowl, mix with Creamy Avocado Sauce or Salad Dressing (page 253) or avocado, and refill the eggs. Sprinkle with a little paprika, salt, and pepper, if desired. Add a handful of berries on the side.

Grab-and-Go Eggs and Salmon (1 protein, 1 fat, 1 fruit): Scramble 1 or 2 eggs. When they're almost done, toss them with a palm-size portion of smoked salmon (sugar-, nitrite-, and dextrose-free); add a handful of berries on the side.

Grab-and-Go Chicken à la Carte (1 protein, 1 fat): Start with 1 serving of leftover chicken. Add your choice of ½ avocado, ⅓ cup Creamy Avocado Sauce or Salad Dressing (page 253), 1 tablespoon Homemade Mayonnaise (page 260), ¼ cup Roasted Red Pepper Sauce (page 268), or ¼ cup Pesto (page 267). Add 2 handfuls of fresh, crunchy vegetables to enjoy as a crudité.

Grab-and-Go Quick Egg Drop Soup (1 protein, 1 fat, if you add the avocado): Heat 3 cups Chicken Bone Broth (page 98) to a simmer. In a bowl, whisk together 2 or 3 eggs and ½ teaspoon Celtic or pink Himalayan salt. Pour the eggs into the broth in a slow, steady stream, whisking constantly. Toss in fresh baby spinach and (optionally) a few drops of chili oil. Finely chop ½ avocado to use as a garnish.

Grab-and-Go Rich and Hearty Turkey Chili (1 protein, 1 fat): Top 2 or 3 handfuls of prepared lettuce or cabbage with 1½ cups Rich and Hearty Turkey Chili (page 168). Optional: Dress the lettuce or cabbage with a little lime juice just before topping with the chili.

Grab-and-Go Instant Salad (1 protein, 1 fat): Combine 2 to 3 handfuls of triple-washed greens of your choice with a handful of cherry tomatoes and a protein—for instance:

1 chicken breast

1 turkey burger or beef burger

4 ounces sliced roast turkey (sugar-, nitrite-, dextrose-, and gluten-free)

5–6-ounce can water-packed tuna or salmon

4 ounces smoked salmon (sugar-, nitrite-, and dextrose-free)

2–3 hard-cooked eggs

Toss with 1 serving of any Bone Broth Diet salad dressings (see Chapter 8) or 1 tablespoon olive oil and (optional) vinegar or lemon juice.

Alternative: Place 1 serving of protein on a lettuce leaf and top with avocado, any Bone Broth Diet salad dressings, or 1 tablespoon olive oil and (optional) vinegar or lemon juice. Roll or fold the lettuce to make a wrap.

You can also add any of the vegetables on the Bone Broth Diet vegetables list (Chapter 4) to your salad or wrap.

Grab-and-Go Quick Bone Broth Soup (1 protein, 1 fat): Bring 3 cups bone broth to a simmer and add 1 portion of leftover meat, 2 or 3 handfuls of fresh spinach or other leftover vegetables, and 1 tablespoon ghee. (*Note:* You can make this ahead of time. It's great with leftover roasted vegetables.)

Grab-and-Go Roast Turkey Breast (1 protein, 1 fat): Toss 1 portion of sliced Easy Roast Turkey Breast (page 165) with 2 or 3 handfuls of prepared lettuce or cabbage slaw and a handful of cherry or grape tomatoes (or a large slicing tomato) *or* 2 handfuls of fresh, crunchy raw vegetables to enjoy as a crudité. Top with your favorite Bone Broth Diet salad dressing or sauce (see Chapter 8) or ½ avocado. (*Note:* The Creamy Ginger Dressing on page 254 is excellent with the cabbage slaw.)

Grab-and-Go Tuna or Salmon (1 protein, 1 fat): Mix a 5- to 6-ounce can of water-packed tuna or salmon with 2 or 3 handfuls of prepared lettuce or cabbage and a handful of cherry or grape tomatoes (or a large slicing tomato) *or* 2 handfuls of fresh, crunchy vegetables to enjoy as a crudité. Top with your favorite Bone Broth Diet salad dressing or sauce (see Chapter 8) *or* ½ avocado *or* 1 tablespoon Homemade Mayonnaise (page 260).

Grab-and-Go Burger (1 protein, 1 fat): Place a leftover burger on 2 or more large lettuce leaves. Top with a slice of a large sweet onion, Ketchup (page 262) and/ or Dijon mustard, and ½ avocado. Sprinkle with your favorite Bone Broth Diet salad dressing or sauce, or use the dressing as a dip for 2 handfuls of fresh, crunchy vegetables. (*Note:* Beef burgers are also excellent with the Creamy Chimichurri on page 266. A ½ fat serving is ¼ cup chimichurri.)

Grab-and-Go Fiesta Beef Fajita Lettuce Wraps (1 protein, 1 fat): Place half of the Fiesta Beef Fajitas recipe (page 181), left over from a previous meal, on 8 to 12 large lettuce leaves such as green leaf, red leaf, or Bibb lettuce. Top with ¼ avocado, sliced. Roll up like a burrito. (*Note:* This is good with any of the salsa recipes in Chapter 8. You can warm up the leftover fajitas before assembling the wraps, if desired.)

Other great grab-and-go leftovers:

Sausage and Apple Frittata (page 136)

Baked Egg Cups with Spinach (page 125)

Breakfast Egg Muffins with Italian Sausage (page 128)

Tips to make grab-and-go meals as simple as possible:

Don't run out of food. Keep lean meats and lots of fresh vegetables in the refrigerator.

Buy prewashed and precut vegetables or prep them ahead of time and store in containers or plastic bags in the refrigerator ready to grab and go.

Keep canned tuna, salmon, and smoked salmon on hand.

Make your favorite salad dressings using the recipes in this book and store them in the refrigerator in small jars with tight-fitting lids.

Keep berries in the freezer and apples on hand.

Keep avocados on hand.

COOKING METHODS: A QUICK PRIMER

Not used to cooking? If you're a newbie in the kitchen, here are quick tips that will turn you into a pro.

Cooking methods fall into two basic categories: dry heat or moist heat.

Dry-heat methods include baking, roasting, grilling, and sautéing. (And deep-frying—but not on this diet!) Sautéing falls into the "dry" category because you use fat instead of a liquid.

In dry-heat cooking, heat—for instance, the hot air in your oven or the heat from a pan on the stove—gets transferred directly to your food. Since vegetables contain little to no fat, you'll typically add a bit of fat when you cook them with dry heat.

Here are three ways to cook with dry heat.

■ *On the stovetop*: To sauté, add some fat to your pan, heat it to a fairly high temperature (usually medium-high), and add your meat or vegetables. Because of the high heat, vegetables cook quickly. This is a simple and quick method of cooking.

■ *In the oven*: Roasting is a common way to cook meat. The fat in the meat usually doesn't need to be supplemented with another fat. You can toss veggies with a little fat and roast them at a high temperature with no added liquid. Make sure they're not crowded or piled on the pan, or they'll steam as they release moisture and get soggy. Keep your vegetables in one layer, and roast them at

Store leftovers in individual servings in plastic containers ready to grab and go.

Keep natural sliced deli turkey that is sugar-, dextrose-, nitrite, and gluten-free (such as Applegate brand).

Keep hard-cooked eggs in the refrigerator.

Whenever you cook, make extra to freeze or refrigerate, especially if it's burgers, meatloaf, individual pieces of chicken, or chili. Pack in individual serving-size containers.

Roast a whole chicken or turkey breast and/or bake, broil, or grill 6 or more boneless, skinless chicken breasts at least once a week.

Keep fresh eggs on hand.

Keep 1 or 2 yams or sweet potatoes in the pantry.

Keep ghee or grass-fed butter, coconut oil, and olive oil on hand.

Use your bone broth to make a big pot of soup with meat, poultry, or seafood and lots of vegetables.

a high temperature: between 400° and 450°F.

■ *On the grill:* Grilling is a fabulous method for cooking meat. If you like to grill, go for it! You can put veggies directly on the grill if the pieces are large enough that they won't fall through the grates. Skewer them if they're smaller. You can also use a grill basket. Again, a bit of fat is helpful.

Moist-heat cooking involves a liquid, whether it's water, broth, or wine. Moist heat uses a lower temperature than dry heat because water can't get hotter than 212°F, its boiling point.

Moist-heat methods include steaming—I'll tell you two ways to do that later—as well as boiling, poaching, and braising.

Braising is when you briefly sauté the food on the stovetop and then add a liquid, cover the pan, and let the food steam or simmer.

Braising is a great choice when you're cooking tougher cuts of meat, such as pot roasts. It breaks the connective tissue down into gelatin, which tenderizes the meat and thickens the cooking liquid. It's also a good way to cook fibrous veggies like kale and collard greens.

Slow cookers use moist heat at a very low temperature. Usually you'll sear meat on the stovetop before you pop it into the slow cooker, where you'll cook it very gradually in water or broth. The process of searing the meat first and then finishing it in a slow cooker mimics braising.

ENTRÉE SOUPS

COCONUT CURRIED CHICKEN SOUP

PREP TIME: 15 MINUTES • COOK TIME: 30 MINUTES

Yield: *Makes eight 1–1½ cup servings** • **Portions:** *½ protein, negligible starchy vegetable,*
½ fat

8-10 cups Chicken Bone Broth (page 98), divided

1 onion, chopped

1½ tablespoons finely chopped fresh ginger

2 cloves garlic, minced

1 pound cooked chicken, finely chopped

1½ cups seeded and chopped butternut squash

½ cup finely chopped fresh cilantro

1⅓ cups coconut milk

3 tablespoons tomato paste

1½ teaspoons curry powder

½ teaspoon ground coriander

¼ teaspoon cayenne

¼ teaspoon ground nutmeg

Pinch of fenugreek (optional)

Celtic or pink Himalayan salt

Ground black pepper

Heat ½ cup of the broth in a large pot over medium heat. Add the onion, ginger, and garlic, cooking until the onion is softened. Stir in the chicken, squash, and cilantro. Add 4 cups of the broth, the coconut milk, tomato paste, curry powder, coriander, cayenne, nutmeg, and fenugreek (if using). Bring to a boil and immediately reduce the heat to low. Simmer for 20 to 30 minutes, or until the squash is tender.

Remove from the heat. Puree with a handheld immersion blender or in batches in a food processor or blender until very smooth. Return to the pot. Add as much of the remaining 3½–5½ cups broth as desired to achieve the consistency you like, and simmer for 5 to 10 minutes. Season with salt and pepper.

Serving size will vary slightly depending on how much broth you use.

CREAM OF WILD MUSHROOM SOUP

PREP TIME: 10 MINUTES • COOK TIME: 45 MINUTES

Yield: Makes eight 1-cup servings • Portions: negligible fat

- 2 teaspoons ghee
- 1 cup finely chopped yellow onion
- ½ cup chopped celery
- ¼ teaspoon cayenne
- 1 large clove garlic
- 6 ounces shiitake mushrooms, wiped clean (about 2 cups)
- 9 ounces cremini mushrooms, wiped clean (about 3 cups), divided
- 6 ounces white mushrooms, wiped clean (about 2 cups)
- 2 teaspoons fresh thyme or 1 teaspoon dried
- 1 teaspoon Celtic or pink Himalayan salt
- ½ teaspoon ground black pepper
- 6 cups Chicken Bone Broth (page 98) or Beef Bone Broth (page 100)
- ⅔ cup coconut milk

Melt the ghee in a large pot over medium-high heat. Add the onion, celery, and cayenne and cook, stirring frequently, for about 4 minutes, or until the vegetables are soft. Add the garlic and cook for 30 seconds. Add the shiitakes, 6 ounces (about 2 cups) of the cremini, the white mushrooms, thyme, salt, and black pepper. Continue to cook, stirring, for 7 to 10 minutes, or until the mushrooms give off their liquid and start to brown.

Add the broth and bring to a boil. Immediately reduce the heat to medium-low and simmer uncovered, stirring occasionally, for about 15 minutes, or until the mushrooms are soft.

Remove from the heat. Add the coconut milk and the remaining 3 ounces cremini. Puree with a handheld immersion blender or in batches in a food processor or blender. Return to the pot and simmer for 10 minutes. Adjust the seasoning to taste and serve.

NOTE:

Substitute additional cremini if shiitakes are not available.

GREEK-STYLE LEMONY CHICKEN SOUP

PREP TIME: 15 MINUTES • COOK TIME: 30 MINUTES

Yield: Makes eight 1½-cup servings • Portions: 1 protein

- 3 cloves garlic, minced
- 1 large onion, chopped
- 2 carrots, chopped
- 2 leeks, white part only, chopped
- 1 tablespoon chopped fresh parsley
- 1 teaspoon fresh thyme or ½ teaspoon dried
- 1 teaspoon lemon peel
- 1 bay leaf
- 9 cups Chicken Bone Broth (page 98)
- 1 pound cooked chicken, chopped
- 4 eggs
- ½ cup fresh lemon juice
- 1 teaspoon Celtic or pink Himalayan salt
- ¼ teaspoon ground black pepper

Brush or spray a large, heavy pot with coconut oil. Add the garlic, onion, carrots, and leeks and cook over medium-high heat until the vegetables are softened and starting to brown. Add the parsley, thyme, lemon peel, and bay leaf and cook for a minute or two. Add the broth and bring to a boil. Immediately reduce the heat to medium-low and simmer for 20 to 25 minutes. Add the chicken. Reduce the heat to the lowest possible setting and cook for about 5 minutes more. Remove and discard the bay leaf.

In a small bowl, beat the eggs with a whisk until they are starting to get frothy, then whisk in the lemon juice. Remove 1 cup of hot broth from the soup, let the broth cool slightly, and whisk in ½ cup broth and then another ½ cup into the egg mixture, beating well between each addition.

Whisk this mixture into the soup (be sure the temperature is very low) and let the soup heat gently. *Do not boil* after the egg mixture has been added. This soup cannot be frozen and must be reheated carefully or the eggs will curdle the broth. It will keep in the fridge for a few days, but it is best freshly made.

HEARTY BEEF AND VEGETABLE SOUP

PREP TIME: 20 MINUTES • COOK TIME: 30 MINUTES

*Yield: Makes eight 1½-cup servings • **Portions:** 1 protein*

- 2 pounds lean beef (stew meat, top round, flank steak, or sirloin), cut into small cubes
- 1 large onion, finely chopped
- ½ cup finely chopped celery
- 5 cups Beef Bone Broth (page 100)
- 1 can (28 ounces) diced tomatoes
- 1 cup peeled and finely chopped carrots
- 1 cup green beans, trimmed and cut into thirds
- ½ cup peeled and finely chopped parsnips
- ½ cup chopped fresh parsley
- 2 bay leaves
- 1 teaspoon fresh thyme or ½ teaspoon dried
- 1 teaspoon Celtic or pink Himalayan salt
- ½ teaspoon ground black pepper

Brush or spray a large pot with coconut oil. Place over medium-high heat and add the beef. Stir occasionally until well browned.

Add the onion and celery and cook until softened.

Add the broth, tomatoes, carrots, green beans, and parsnips and bring to a boil. Immediately reduce the heat to medium-low and add the parsley, bay leaves, thyme, salt, and pepper.

Simmer for 30 minutes. Remove and discard the bay leaves before serving.

HERB-INFUSED CHICKEN SOUP

PREP TIME: 20 MINUTES · COOK TIME: 45 MINUTES

Yield: Makes eight 1½-cup servings • **Portions**: 1 protein

1 pound boneless, skinless chicken breast or thighs, cut into ½" pieces

1 pound Turkey or Chicken Italian Sausage (page 163)

1 yellow onion, chopped

1 red bell pepper, chopped

1 rib celery, chopped

3 cloves garlic, minced

12 cups Chicken Bone Broth (page 98)

2 tablespoons tomato paste

1 teaspoon finely chopped fresh oregano or ½ teaspoon dried

½ teaspoon finely chopped fresh rosemary or ¼ teaspoon dried, crushed

½ teaspoon finely chopped fresh thyme or ¼ teaspoon dried

1 teaspoon Celtic or pink Himalayan salt

¼ teaspoon ground black pepper

3 cups fresh baby spinach

Place a large pot over medium-high heat. Lightly brush or spray with coconut oil and brown the chicken and sausage for 8 to 10 minutes.

Add the onion, bell pepper, celery, and garlic and cook until the vegetables have softened.

Add the broth, tomato paste, oregano, rosemary, thyme, salt, and black pepper and bring to a boil. Immediately reduce the heat, cover, and simmer on medium-low heat for 30 minutes.

Add the spinach and simmer for 5 or 10 minutes, or until the spinach softens.

ITALIAN WEDDING SOUP

PREP TIME: 20 MINUTES · COOK TIME: 40 MINUTES

Yield: Makes eight 1½-cup servings · *Portions: 1 protein*

MEATBALLS

2 pounds ground turkey

¼ cup finely chopped onion

¼ cup finely chopped parsley

¼ cup finely chopped red bell pepper

1 tablespoon dried Italian seasoning or a combination of your favorite herbs

1 teaspoon Celtic or pink Himalayan salt

½ teaspoon garlic powder or 2 cloves garlic, minced

¼ teaspoon ground black pepper

Pinch–⅛ teaspoon ground fennel seeds (optional)

Pinch–⅛ teaspoon crushed red-pepper flakes (optional)

SOUP

12 cups (1½ quarts) Chicken Bone Broth (page 98)

1 pound curly endive, coarsely chopped (escarole may be substituted)

1 teaspoon Celtic or pink Himalayan salt

¼ teaspoon ground black pepper

2 eggs

Preheat the oven to 350°F. Line a baking sheet with parchment.

To make the meatballs: Combine the turkey, onion, parsley, bell pepper, Italian seasoning or herbs, salt, garlic, and black pepper. Add the fennel seeds and red-pepper flakes (if using). Mix well. Form into tiny meatballs about the size of a large marble. Arrange in a single layer on the prepared baking sheet and bake for 15 to 20 minutes, or until no longer pink. Set aside.

To make the soup: In a large pot over medium-high heat, bring the broth to a boil. Immediately reduce the heat to medium and add the meatballs. Add the endive, salt, and pepper and simmer for 5 to 8 minutes, or until the greens are tender.

In a medium bowl, whisk the eggs. Stir the soup in a circular motion and gradually drizzle the eggs into the moving broth, stirring gently with a fork to form thin strands of egg, about 1 minute.

PORTUGUESE KALE AND SWEET POTATO SOUP

PREP TIME: 25 MINUTES · COOK TIME: 35 MINUTES

Yield: *Makes eight 1½-cup servings* • **Portions**: *½ protein, ½ starchy vegetable, negligible fat*

- 2 tablespoons coconut oil
- 1 pound Turkey or Chicken Chorizo (page 164)
- 1 onion, finely chopped
- 2 cloves garlic, minced
- 12 cups Chicken Bone Broth (page 98)
- 1 bunch fresh kale, washed, stems removed, and cut into ½"-thick chiffonade (see Notes, page 162) ribbons (about 2 cups)
- 1 teaspoon Celtic or pink Himalayan salt
- ¼ teaspoon ground black pepper
- 2 sweet potatoes, cut into ½" cubes (about 1 pound or less)

Place a large pot over medium-high heat. Add the oil, chorizo, onion, and garlic. Cook for 8 to 10 minutes, crumbling the chorizo as it cooks.

Add the broth, kale, salt, and pepper. Cover and cook for about 5 minutes, or until the kale begins to soften.

Add the sweet potatoes. Simmer, covered, for 20 to 30 minutes, or until the sweet potatoes are soft.

NOTE:

Both the kale and the sweet potatoes will absorb a great deal of broth as they cook, so you may want to add more broth.

BONE BROTH EGG DROP SOUP

PREP TIME: 15 MINUTES • COOK TIME: 15 MINUTES

Yield: Makes 4 servings • *Portions:* 1 protein, negligible fat

12 cups Chicken Bone Broth (page 98)

6 or more cups fresh baby spinach

8 eggs

1 teaspoon Celtic or pink Himalayan salt

⅛ teaspoon ground white pepper

2–3 scallions, white and green parts, minced

1 tablespoon ghee

4–6 drops chili oil (optional; see Notes)

In a large pot, bring the broth to a simmer over medium-high heat. Reduce the heat to medium, add the spinach, and cook for 1 to 2 minutes.

In a medium bowl, whisk the eggs, salt, and pepper. Pour the eggs into the broth in a very slow, steady stream, whisking constantly.

Remove the pan from the heat and toss in the scallions, ghee, and chili oil (if using).

Cover the pan and wait for 1 to 2 minutes, or until the eggs have set.

NOTES:

If you use chili oil, be sure the only ingredients are olive oil, chile peppers, and seasonings.

You can add a few drops of coconut aminos if you like the flavor of soy sauce.

This can be made ahead and refrigerated.

SPICY CHICKEN SOUP

PREP TIME: 15 MINUTES • COOK TIME: 60 MINUTES

*Yield: Makes eight 1½-cup servings • **Portions:** 1 protein, negligible fat*

- 2 tablespoons coconut oil
- 2 pounds boneless, skinless chicken breasts, chopped
- 1½ cups peeled and sliced carrots
- 1½ cups finely chopped celery
- 1½ cups finely chopped onion
- 1 jalapeño, seeded and finely chopped (wear plastic gloves when handling)
- 4 cloves garlic, minced
- 1 teaspoon chili powder
- 1 teaspoon ground cumin
- 1 teaspoon Celtic or pink Himalayan salt
- 1 teaspoon ground black pepper
- ¼ teaspoon cayenne
- ¼ teaspoon dried oregano
- 8 cups (2 quarts) Chicken Bone Broth (page 98)
- 1 can (14.5 ounces) diced tomatoes

Heat the oil in a large pot over medium-high heat. When the oil is hot, add the chicken and cook for about 8 minutes, or until no longer pink and the juices run clear.

Add the carrots, celery, onion, jalapeño, and garlic. Simmer for about 5 minutes and add the chili powder, cumin, salt, black pepper, cayenne, and oregano, stirring well to blend the seasonings.

Add the broth and tomatoes and bring to a boil. Immediately reduce the heat to low and simmer for about 1 hour.

NOTE:

Serve with 1 avocado, chopped, and ⅓ cup chopped cilantro as a garnish.

TOMATO, BASIL, AND ITALIAN SAUSAGE SOUP

PREP TIME: 30 MINUTES • COOK TIME: 30 MINUTES

Yield: Makes eight 1½-cup servings • *Portions: 1 protein, negligible fat*

2 pounds Turkey or Chicken Italian Sausage (page 163)

5 carrots, peeled and finely chopped

1 large onion, finely chopped

2 cans (28 ounces each) tomatoes in puree
   (San Marzano type is best—see Note)

4 cups Chicken Bone Broth (page 98)

½ cup roughly chopped fresh basil

1 cup coconut milk

1 teaspoon Celtic or pink Himalayan salt

½ teaspoon ground black pepper

¼ cup fresh basil, cut into fine chiffonade (see Notes, page 162) ribbons

Preheat the oven to 350°F. Line a baking sheet with parchment.

Prepare the sausage according to the directions on page 163, increasing the Italian seasoning quantity to 1 tablespoon. Form into small meatballs about the size of a large marble and place in a single layer on the prepared baking sheet. Bake for 20 to 25 minutes, or until tender and the meat is no longer pink.

While the meatballs are baking, lightly spray or brush a large saucepan with coconut oil. Cook the carrots and onion over medium heat for about 10 minutes, or until softened. Add the tomatoes with puree, broth, and chopped basil. Bring to a boil. Immediately reduce the heat to medium-low and simmer, uncovered, for 20 minutes.

Remove from the heat. Puree with a handheld immersion blender or in batches in a blender or food processor. Return the soup to the pan. Add the coconut milk and meatballs and place over medium heat. Warm until heated through and season with the salt and pepper. Serve warm, garnished with the basil ribbons.

NOTE:

San Marzano tomatoes are thinner than Romas and have thicker flesh and fewer seeds. Their flavor is stronger, sweeter, and less acidic than Romas. Canned San Marzano tomatoes are available in most grocery stores.

TUSCAN SEAFOOD SOUP

PREP TIME: 20 MINUTES · COOK TIME: 60 MINUTES

Yield: Makes eight 1¾–2-cup servings of broth + seafood divided among servings
• Portions: 1 protein, negligible fat

2 tablespoons ghee

1 small onion, finely chopped

1 large leek, white part only, thinly sliced (about ½ cup)

1 small green bell pepper, finely chopped

2 carrots, finely chopped

3 cloves garlic, minced

8 cups (2 quarts) Fish Bone Broth (page 103)

1 can (28 ounces) diced tomatoes

2 teaspoons fresh oregano or 1 teaspoon dried

2 teaspoons fresh basil or 1 teaspoon dried

1 teaspoon fresh thyme or ½ teaspoon dried

1 bay leaf

Pinch of cayenne (optional)

1½ pounds littleneck clams or green mussels (8 clams or mussels yield about 4 ounces meat)

1 pound firm whitefish (halibut, cod, red snapper), cut into 1" cubes

½ pound large shrimp, peeled and deveined (6–8 shrimp)

¼ pound sea scallops (6–8 scallops)

¼ pound lobster or crabmeat (6-ounce lobster tail yields 4 ounces meat)

3 tablespoons finely chopped fresh parsley

1 teaspoon Celtic or pink Himalayan salt

½ teaspoon ground black pepper

In a large pot, heat the ghee over medium heat. Add the onion, leek, and bell pepper and cook for about 5 minutes, or until softened. Add the carrots and garlic and cook for 3 minutes.

Stir in the broth, tomatoes, oregano, basil, thyme, bay leaf, and cayenne (if using) and bring to a boil. Immediately reduce the heat to medium-low and simmer, covered, for 30 to 40 minutes.

Add the clams to the pot, cover, and simmer about 10 minutes, or until the clams begin to open. Gently add the fish, shrimp, scallops, lobster, and parsley. (You can put an entire lobster tail into the soup, and when it's done, remove the meat from the shell and cut into 1" pieces, or you can remove the meat from the shell and cut into pieces before cooking.)

Cover and simmer for 5 to 10 minutes, or until the fish flakes with a fork and the shrimp turn opaque. Remove and discard the bay leaf and serve.

NOTE:

This is a suggested combination of seafood, but you can modify it to suit your tastes. Plan for about 5 ounces of seafood (excluding the shells) per person.

Bone Broth Bonus: It's Easy on the Budget!

Diane Sanfilippo, certified nutrition consultant, owner and founder of Balanced Bites, and *New York Times* **bestselling author of** *Practical Paleo* **and** *The 21-Day Sugar Detox*

balancedbites.com

My friend Diane Sanfilippo points out yet another big plus of adding bone broth to your diet: At a time when grocery costs keep soaring, it's inexpensive (and it can even be free).

"While there are many amazing health benefits to drinking bone broth, what's often overlooked are the remarkable cost-saving benefits to making it at home. In fact, bone broth can be made from what we might otherwise consider waste: bones from which we've already eaten the meat. Of course, you can make broth from meaty bones that are roasted and then cooked in water to create a rich-tasting soup or stew base, but bones that have already been a part of a meal are perfect as well.

"The best ways to make broth from ingredients you might otherwise throw away: Save your bones (and even vegetable scraps, like carrot ends, celery leaves, and onion pieces) in the freezer. You can freeze bones in a resealable plastic bag or other container until you fill up a gallon-size portion, then simply place the bones into water and allow it all to simmer to create your broth. You can easily follow specific recipes like the ones in this book, or use what you have on hand. Your family's chicken wings remains, or a carcass left from roasting a whole chicken, make perfect bases for future broths."

CALL-TO-ACTION SOUPS

You're already burning fat and erasing wrinkles like crazy. But if you want to take your results to a higher level, check out these power-packed soups! I've designed them to address specific health and fitness issues. The soups with meat make great entrées, while the meatless soups are excellent side dishes.

MARY'S HOT-AND-SOUR SOUP
For Fighting Cellulite

PREP TIME: 30 MINUTES • COOK TIME: 15 MINUTES

Yield: Makes eight 2-cup servings with 1 cup vegetables and 1 cup broth • *Portions: 1 protein*

1 large carrot, peeled and grated

1 can (8 ounces) bamboo shoots, drained

1 cup snow peas, cut into matchsticks

1 small or ½ large red bell pepper, cut into matchsticks

2 heads baby bok choy, chopped or shredded into fine ⅛" ribbons

8 cups (2 quarts) Chicken Bone Broth (page 98)

6 or more slices fresh ginger

6 cloves garlic, chopped

1–2 jalapeños, seeded and chopped (wear plastic gloves when handling)

2 pounds cooked chicken, chopped

10 ounces cremini mushrooms, cut into thirds

¼ cup coconut vinegar or white wine vinegar

¼ cup coconut aminos

½ teaspoon salt

¼ teaspoon ground white pepper

8 scallions, white and green parts, thinly sliced

1 cup chopped cilantro

Toasted sesame oil (optional)

Hot chili oil (optional)

In a large bowl, combine the carrot, bamboo shoots, snow peas, bell pepper, and bok choy. Set aside.

Place the broth in a large pot over high heat. Add the ginger, garlic, and jalapeño and bring to a boil. Immediately reduce the heat and simmer for 10 minutes.

Add the chicken, mushrooms, vinegar, and coconut aminos and simmer for 5 minutes.

Place a serving of vegetables in each individual soup bowl and ladle the broth over the vegetables so they stay nice and crunchy.

Garnish each bowl with scallions, cilantro, and 1 or 2 drops each of sesame oil and hot chili oil (if using).

SHIITAKE MUSHROOM SOUP
For Healing

PREP TIME: 15 MINUTES • COOK TIME: 30 MINUTES

Yield: Makes eight 1-cup servings • *Portions: No protein or fat*

1 ounce dried shiitake mushrooms

¼ cup wakame seaweed

3 cups very warm brewed green tea

1 white onion, quartered and thinly sliced

3 cloves garlic, chopped

2 tablespoons chopped fresh ginger

1 teaspoon finely chopped fresh turmeric or ½ teaspoon ground

4 cups (1 quart) Chicken Bone Broth (page 98)

1 tablespoon dulse seaweed flakes

1 tablespoon coconut aminos

½ tablespoon coconut vinegar or white wine vinegar

2 cups thinly sliced napa cabbage

¼ cup scallions, white and green parts, sliced

Rinse the mushrooms and wakame seaweed and, in a small bowl, soak in the tea for 15 to 20 minutes, or until soft.

Meanwhile, heat 2 tablespoons of the soaking liquid in a large pot. Add the onion, garlic, ginger, and turmeric and cook until soft.

Add the broth and dulse seaweed.

Cut off and discard the mushroom stems. Slice the mushroom caps into thin strips. Add the mushrooms, wakame seaweed, and soaking liquid to the pot and bring to a boil over high heat.

Immediately reduce the heat to medium. Add the coconut aminos, vinegar, and cabbage and simmer for about 10 minutes.

Serve with a sprinkling of scallions.

NOTE:

This soup has a deep, woodsy aroma and flavor from the shiitakes. The seaweed is delicious in the soup, but wakame has a slippery texture that you may not be used to. You can omit it and just use the dulse.

RED BELL PEPPER SOUP
For Healthy Hormones

PREP TIME: 25 MINUTES • COOK TIME: 30 MINUTES

Yield: Makes ten 1-cup servings • *Portions: negligible fat*

- 2 tablespoons ghee
- 6 red bell peppers, seeded and chopped
- 2 carrots, peeled and chopped
- 1 large onion, chopped
- 2 ribs celery, chopped
- 4 cloves garlic, minced
- 6 cups (1½ quarts) Chicken Bone Broth (page 98)
- 2 tablespoons fresh thyme, chopped, or 1 tablespoon dried
- 1 teaspoon chopped fresh turmeric or ½ teaspoon ground

  Pinch of cayenne

  Pinch of red-pepper flakes
- 1 teaspoon Celtic or pink Himalayan salt
- ½ teaspoon ground black pepper
- 2½ medium avocados, pitted, peeled, and chopped

Heat the ghee in a large pot over medium-high heat. Stir in the bell peppers, carrots, onion, celery, and garlic and cook for about 10 minutes, stirring occasionally.

Stir in the broth, thyme, turmeric, cayenne, red-pepper flakes, salt, and black pepper and bring to a boil. Immediately reduce the heat, cover, and simmer for about 15 minutes, or until the vegetables are very tender.

Remove from the heat and cool for 30 minutes.

Add the avocados to the mixture. Puree with a handheld immersion blender or in batches in a food processor or blender until very smooth.

Return to the pot and simmer for 5 to 10 minutes before serving.

COOL AND CREAMY AVOCADO-PUMPKIN SOUP
For Healthy Skin

PREP TIME: 15 MINUTES

Yield: Makes ten 1-cup servings • Portions: ½ starchy vegetable, 1 fat

8 cups (2 quarts) Chicken Bone Broth (page 98), divided

1 cup brewed green tea

4–5 firm, ripe avocados (6–7 ounces each), pitted, peeled, and chopped (about 3 cups)

1 can (15 ounces) pumpkin puree

½ cup coconut milk

¼ cup fresh lime juice (about 3 limes)

1 small jalapeño, seeded and chopped (wear plastic gloves when handling)

4 scallions, white and green parts, chopped

¼ cup chopped cilantro

1 clove garlic, chopped

½–1 teaspoon ground dried chiles (ancho, New Mexico, or California; not chili powder)

½–1 teaspoon ground cumin

1 teaspoon Celtic or pink Himalayan salt

¼ teaspoon ground black pepper

1 red bell pepper, finely chopped

Combine 4 cups of the broth and the tea with the avocados, pumpkin, coconut milk, lime juice, jalapeño, scallions, cilantro, garlic, chiles, cumin, salt, and black pepper in a food processor or blender and process until smooth and creamy. Transfer to a large bowl.

Gradually whisk in the remaining 4 cups broth until fully combined. Taste and adjust seasoning.

Cover and place in the refrigerator to allow the flavors to meld. When ready to serve, whisk again.

You may add more broth, a small amount at time, until the desired consistency is reached.

Serve in bowls and garnish with a sprinkling of the bell pepper.

NOTE:

This is a chilled soup. No cooking!

WATERCRESS SOUP
For Weight Loss

PREP TIME: 5 MINUTES · COOK TIME: 5–10 MINUTES

Yield: Makes eight 1-cup servings • *Portions: No protein or fat*

8 cups (2 quarts) Chicken or Turkey Bone Broth (page 98 or 99)

1" piece fresh ginger, peeled and finely chopped

2 cloves garlic, chopped

1 teaspoon chopped fresh turmeric or ½ teaspoon ground

Pinch of cardamom

Pinch of cayenne

Pinch of ground cumin

Celtic or pink Himalayan salt

2 cups fresh baby spinach

2 cups fresh watercress, chopped

½ cup fresh parsley, chopped

2–3 scallions, white and green parts, minced (optional)

1–2 drops chile oil (see Notes) or toasted sesame oil (optional)

In a large pot over medium-high heat, combine the broth, ginger, garlic, turmeric, cardamom, cayenne, cumin, and salt and bring to a boil.

Immediately reduce the heat to medium-low and simmer for 10 to 20 minutes.

Add the spinach, watercress, parsley, and scallions.

Remove from the heat and serve with the chile oil (if using).

NOTES:

If you use chile oil, be sure its only ingredients are olive oil, chile peppers, and seasonings.

You can also add a few drops of coconut aminos if you like the flavor of soy sauce.

VARIATIONS:

Add 1 cup cooked, chopped chicken meat; this will yield ¼ portion of protein per serving.

Add 6 eggs. Whisk the eggs in a medium bowl. After adding the spinach, watercress, and scallions to the soup, pour in the eggs in a very slow, steady stream, whisking constantly. Remove the pot from the heat and toss in the scallions and chile oil. Cover the pot and wait for 1 to 2 minutes, or until the eggs have set; this will yield a little less than ½ portion of protein per serving.

YOUR SKIN ON BONE BROTH

My absolute favorite "plus one" about bone broth is its ability to give you dewy, healthy, supple skin. If you ever meet me or one of the thousands of patients I've worked with, you'll see that we're all living proof.

It's amazing what drinking bones can do to de-age your skin. It simply erases the years and lets you step into sexier.

Did you ever notice that as you "mature" (or as I like to say, "evolve"), your skin gets thinner and less elastic? The protein, healthy fat, minerals, and collagen components in bone broth make your skin smooth and give it a beautiful fullness, much in the same way that fillers do.

In short, fillers and Botox are not your only way to tackle physical imperfections. The nutrients in bone broth can replenish your body's own collagen.

Here's what Botox doesn't treat: the wrinkles caused by loss of collagen in your skin over time. Botox focuses on freezing the muscles of problem areas, but it does nothing to replenish the collagen that makes your skin look so smooth and young and bouncy.

Bottom line: Whether you make the choice to shoot stuff in your face or not, the only permanent way to plump your skin and make it firmer is to replenish your body's own collagen. And the best "medicine" for that is bone broth.

Five Fabulous Foods for Your Skin

Dr. Trevor Cates, naturopathic physician

drtrevorcates.com

Dr. Trevor Cates was the first woman licensed as a naturopathic doctor in the state of California and was appointed by former governor Arnold Schwarzenegger to California's Bureau of Naturopathic Medicine Advisory Council. Also known as the Spa Dr., Dr. Cates sees patients at world-renowned spas and in her Park City, Utah, private practice, where she focuses on anti-aging, hormonal balance, and glowing skin. She's the host of the *The Spa Dr. Secrets to Smart, Sexy, and Strong* podcast and the online Glowing Skin Summit and the author of the ebook *Glowing Skin from Within*. Here's her take on superfoods for your skin.

"If your skin is dry, discolored, or lacking in tone—or worse, you develop acne, eczema, rosacea, or premature wrinkles—it's a sign that something is off balance within your body. Often, this imbalance stems from a poor diet.

"An increasing amount of research is debunking the claim that what we eat doesn't affect our skin quality. For example, we know that eating high glycemic index foods (like pastas and breads) causes glucose and insulin levels to increase. And research shows that high insulin stimulates sebum production and androgen activity, which play a role in the development of acne. Conversely, there are many nutrients and foods that nourish skin from the inside out.

"Here are five of my favorite foods for glowing skin."

1. Avocado

Avocados contain monounsaturated

fats and antioxidants. Because antioxidants help fight oxidative damage that speeds the aging of our skin, and good fats help nourish our cells, both are essential for optimal skin health.

2. Wild salmon

Wild salmon is rich in omega-3 fatty acids, which are anti-inflammatory. These fats are crucial to the health of your skin, because many skin problems stem from inflammation. Salmon's pink color means it has astaxanthin, which helps protect your skin from sun damage.

3. Coconut

Coconut contains lauric acid, which has powerful immune-enhancing and antimicrobial properties, so it's great for skin health. The coconut's water, milk, meat, and oil are all good for you!

And coconut isn't only ideal as a food; you can use it to moisturize and soothe your skin.

4. Kale

Kale is part of the brassica and cruciferous veggie family, known for their liver detox—enhancing properties (diindolylmethane and indole-3-carbinole). These veggies have a higher anticancer phytochemical content than any other vegetable family.

5. Bone broth

Bone broth is filled with the building blocks of collagen, which is essential for healthy skin and avoiding premature skin aging. Be sure to follow a good recipe and use bones of organic animals if possible.

SALMON AND LEEK CHOWDER
For a Healthy Brain

PREP TIME: 20 MINUTES • COOK TIME: 20 MINUTES

Yield: Makes eight 1-½ cup servings (12 cups) • *Portions: 1 fat*

½ yellow onion, finely chopped

1 carrot, peeled and finely chopped

1 rib celery, finely chopped

½ green bell pepper, finely chopped

2 leeks, white part only, thinly sliced

2 cloves garlic, minced

6 cups (1½ quarts) Fish Bone Broth (page 103) or Chicken Bone Broth (page 98)

2 tablespoons tomato paste

¼ teaspoon cayenne

1 teaspoon Celtic or pink Himalayan salt

¼ teaspoon ground black pepper

1–2 teaspoons adobo sauce from canned chipotle chile peppers in adobo sauce

2 pounds fresh salmon, cut into ½" cubes

1 bag (5 ounces) fresh baby spinach (about 4 cups loosely packed), cut into ½" chiffonade (see Notes, page 162) ribbons

2⅔ cups coconut milk

¼ cup fresh dill, finely chopped (optional)

1 lemon, cut into wedges (optional)

Spray or brush a large pot with coconut oil and heat over medium-high heat.

Cook the onion, carrot, celery, bell pepper, leeks, and garlic until softened.

Add the broth, tomato paste, cayenne, salt, and black pepper.

Add the adobo sauce ½ teaspoon at a time, tasting the broth after each addition until the desired flavor is achieved. Bring to a boil.

Immediately reduce the heat and add the salmon. Stir gently and simmer for 5 minutes.

Gently stir in the spinach and coconut milk and simmer for 5 to 10 minutes.

Serve with a sprinkling of dill and a lemon wedge (if using).

CHAPTER 8

Luscious Sides, Condiments, and "Extras" for Your Nonfasting Days

NOW THAT I'VE GIVEN you dozens of entrée and soup recipes, it's time to introduce you to the supporting cast! In this chapter, I'll serve up mouthwatering recipes for vegetable side dishes, condiments, salad dressings, shakes, and desserts—along with "mocktails" for a diet-friendly happy hour.

As you're planning which sides and extras to complement your meals, here's one reminder: Really load up on the low-carb veggies. They're filling, they're packed with inflammation-fighting nutrients, and they help heal your gut. (And they're delicious, too.) Aim to fill the edges of your plate with them at every meal.

And here's one more tip: If the Sugar Demon tries to derail you, check out the shakes and fruit desserts toward the end of this chapter. They'll satisfy your sweet tooth in a sin-free way.

And now, on to the recipes. It's time to check out everything from show-stealing Cauliflower Rice to my amazing Creamy Avocado Salad Dressing to Sweet Black Cherry Gummies. (Gummies on a real-food diet? You bet.) Enjoy!

REMINDER
Each recipe includes portion sizes so you can easily calculate a serving size.

LOW-CARB VEGGIES

CAULIFLOWER RICE

PREP TIME: 10 MINUTES • COOK TIME: 10 MINUTES

Yield: Makes 4 servings • *Portions: No protein or fat*

1 large head cauliflower

½ onion, finely chopped

1 clove garlic, minced

Celtic or pink Himalayan salt

Ground black pepper

Break the cauliflower into florets, removing the stems. Place the florets in a food processor or blender and pulse or blend for ten to fifteen 1-second intervals, or until the cauliflower looks like rice. You may need to do this step in 2 or more batches, depending on the size of the cauliflower.

Spray a nonstick skillet with coconut oil and place over medium heat. When the pan is hot, add the onion and garlic and cook for about 7 minutes, or until the onion is translucent.

Add the cauliflower to the pan and cook for 5 to 7 minutes, or until tender. Season with salt and pepper.

NOTE:

This can be made ahead and refrigerated.

GARLIC MASHED CAULIFLOWER "POTATOES"

PREP TIME: 15 MINUTES • COOK TIME: 12 MINUTES

Yield: Makes 4 servings • **Portions**: No protein or fat

1 large head cauliflower, broken or cut into florets

2 cloves roasted garlic

¼ cup almond milk or coconut milk (not canned), sugar-free (see Notes)

¼ teaspoon Celtic or pink Himalayan salt

⅛ teaspoon ground black pepper

¼ cup chopped fresh parsley (optional)

Steam the cauliflower in a saucepan for 10 to 12 minutes, or until soft. Drain well.

Return it to the pan and add the garlic, almond or coconut milk, salt, and pepper.

Mash with a potato masher or transfer to a food processor and puree. Garnish with the parsley (if using).

NOTES:

If you use coconut milk, select the milk in a carton—not the coconut milk in a can. This can be prepared ahead and refrigerated.

ROASTING AND SAUTÉING VEGETABLES: A DRY-HEAT COOKING METHOD

Roasted and sautéed vegetables stand on their own as a flavorful side dish, and they're also great with eggs for breakfast or added to a salad. You can roast or sauté any of your favorite vegetables on the Bone Broth Diet vegetables list.

Keep in mind that softer vegetables, such as mushrooms, roast or sauté faster than very dense vegetables, such as broccoli. When you're roasting a variety of vegetables at one time, you can toss in the softer vegetables after the first 10 minutes of baking. Similarly, if you're sautéing, you can cook vegetables of the same density together and add the softer vegetables after the first few minutes. You can also sauté them separately, but it's really not necessary.

Make a big batch of roasted or sautéed vegetables on your batch-cooking day and you'll have veggies for several days. They're a great grab-and-go option with any meat, seafood, or poultry.

To roast or sauté vegetables, start with these ingredients.

- Any vegetables on the Bone Broth Diet vegetables list
- 1–2 tablespoons approached oil or liquid fat
- Celtic or pink Himalayan salt and ground black pepper to taste
- Your choice of dried or fresh herbs (optional)

Here's an example.

- 1–2 tablespoons oil or fat
- 1 large sweet onion, cut into rounds or wedges
- 1 bell pepper, any color, cut into strips or wedges
- 1 bunch asparagus, cut into 2" pieces
- 1 zucchini, cut into rounds
- 1 teaspoon garlic powder
- ½ teaspoon Celtic or pink Himalayan salt

- ¼ teaspoon ground black pepper
- 2 or more teaspoons dried or fresh herbs of your choice (optional)

Directions for Roasting

Preheat the oven to 425°F. Line 1 or more sheet pans with parchment, depending on how many vegetables you're roasting. You can also spray your pans lightly with coconut oil.

Mix all of your vegetables and seasonings in a large bowl. Add 1 to 2 tablespoons oil or fat and toss well. Spread the vegetables evenly in 1 layer and bake for 10 to 15 minutes. Don't crowd the vegetables or they'll steam instead of roast.

Remove the vegetables from the oven and toss them with tongs or a spatula. Return them to the oven to bake for 10 to 20 minutes, or until they're done to your liking.

Directions for Sautéing

Preheat a skillet over medium-high heat. Add oil or fat to the pan and wait a minute until the oil is hot. Toss in your vegetables, being careful not to overcrowd the pan (which will cause the vegetables to steam because of their high moisture content).

When you're sautéing, it's a good idea to remain at the stove because vegetables cook quickly. Using tongs, flip the vegetables so they cook evenly. Remove them from the pan when they're done to your liking.

A Note about Portions

It's easy to calculate portions for your sautéed or roasted vegetables. One handful of nonstarchy vegetables, or about a softball-size portion, is 1 serving. One tablespoon of oil or fat is equal to 1 serving of fat.

If you're roasting vegetables for 4 people and you use approximately 8 handfuls of vegetables and 2 tablespoons oil or fat, you'll have 2 servings of vegetables per person and ½ serving of fat per person. Simple.

LEMON-ROASTED ASPARAGUS

PREP TIME: 5 MINUTES • COOK TIME: 20 MINUTES

Yield: Makes 4 servings • *Portions:* Negligible fat

- 1 or more pounds asparagus, tough ends trimmed
- 1 clove garlic, minced
- 2–3 teaspoons lemon peel
- 2 teaspoons coconut oil, melted
- Celtic or pink Himalayan salt
- Ground black pepper
- 1 cup lemon juice (optional)

Preheat the oven to 425°F. Line a baking sheet with parchment.

Place the asparagus in a single layer on the prepared baking sheet. Sprinkle with the garlic and lemon peel, then drizzle with the oil and season with salt and pepper. Bake for 15 to 20 minutes.

When you remove the asparagus from the oven, top it with the lemon juice (if using).

NOTE:

This is a great recipe to double. It's quick and easy, and the leftovers are terrific with eggs or tossed into a salad.

LEMONY CUCUMBER SALAD

PREP TIME: 5 MINUTES

Yield: Makes 4 servings • *Portions:* ½ fat

- 2 cups thinly sliced cucumber (about 1 large English cucumber or 2 traditional cucumbers)
- ½ red onion, thinly sliced
- 2 tablespoons coarsely chopped fresh mint leaves or cilantro
- ⅛ teaspoon Celtic or pink Himalayan salt
- 4 tablespoons Lemon Vinaigrette or Creamy Lemon Dressing (page 254)

In a large bowl, toss together the cucumbers, onion, mint or cilantro, salt, and dressing.

NAPA SLAW WITH CREAMY GINGER DRESSING

PREP TIME: 10 MINUTES

Yield: Makes four 1¼–1½ cup servings • **Portions:** *½ fat*

5 cups shredded napa cabbage (about 1 head)

Large handful of snow peas, strings removed and thinly sliced on the diagonal (about 1 cup)

4 scallions, green and white parts, sliced

½ cup thinly sliced radishes

¼–½ cup coarsely chopped cilantro (optional)

⅓ cup + 2 tablespoons Creamy Ginger Dressing (page 254)

Celtic or pink Himalayan salt

Ground black pepper

In a large bowl, toss together the cabbage, peas, scallions, radishes, cilantro (if using), and dressing. Season with salt and pepper. Refrigerate until serving.

NOTE:

This is especially good after the flavors have had time to meld. As the slaw sits in the refrigerator, it will decrease in bulk because the cabbage absorbs the liquids.

ROASTED CURRY CAULIFLOWER

PREP TIME: 10 MINUTES • COOK TIME: 35 MINUTES

Yield: Makes 8 servings • *Portions: Negligible fat*

- 2 tablespoons coconut oil, melted
- ¼ cup fresh orange juice
- 1 teaspoon orange peel
- ½ teaspoon ground coriander
- ½ teaspoon ground cumin
- 2 teaspoons curry powder
- 1 tablespoon Hungarian paprika
- 1 teaspoon Celtic or pink Himalayan salt
- ¼ teaspoon ground black pepper
- 8 cups cauliflower florets (from about 2½ pounds cauliflower)
- 1 large onion, sliced
- Cilantro for garnish (optional)

Preheat the oven to 450°F. Line 2 sheet pans with parchment.

In a large bowl or a resealable plastic bag, mix together the oil, orange juice, orange peel, coriander, cumin, curry powder, paprika, salt, and pepper. Add the cauliflower and onion to the bowl and toss to coat; alternatively, put the cauliflower and onion in the plastic bag with the marinade and shake well to distribute seasonings.

Spread the vegetables in a single layer on the prepared sheet pans. Roast for about 35 minutes, stirring occasionally, until tender, or longer if you like your cauliflower softer.

Garnish with cilantro (if using). Serve warm or at room temperature.

NOTE:

To make the spices more flavorful, place them in a small ungreased skillet and toast for 3 to 5 minutes over low heat, or until they become aromatic and you see a light puff of smoke rise from the pan. Then add them to the recipe.

ROASTED SWEET ONIONS

PREP TIME: 10 MINUTES · COOK TIME: 45–60 MINUTES

Yield: Makes 4 servings • *Portions: Negligible fat*

3–4 large sweet onions, very thinly sliced into rounds

Celtic or pink Himalayan salt

Ground black pepper

2 teaspoons coconut oil or ghee, melted

Preheat the oven to 350°F. Line 2 sheet pans with parchment.

Spread the onion rounds evenly on the prepared sheet pans; don't crowd the onions. You want them to roast and caramelize, not steam. Sprinkle with salt and pepper. Brush or spray with the oil or ghee.

Bake for 20 to 25 minutes. About halfway through the cooking time, flip the onions when the tops are golden brown.

NOTE:

It's easy to pop these in the oven when you're roasting meat. If Vidalia onions are in season, be sure to roast some. They are unbelievably delicious!

ROASTED PORTOBELLO BURGER "BUNS"

PREP TIME: 5 MINUTES · COOK TIME: 10 MINUTES

Yield: Makes 4 servings • *Portions: No protein or fat*

4 portobello mushrooms

Preheat the oven to 350°F. Line a sheet pan with parchment.

Gently wipe the mushroom caps to clean. Break off the stems and reserve for another use. Using a spoon, carefully scoop out all the gills on the underside of the mushroom caps. Place the caps on the prepared pan. Bake for 5 to 7 minutes on each side, or until the caps soften.

NOTE:

Alternatively, you can grill the mushroom caps. Spray them with coconut oil before grilling.

RATATOUILLE

PREP TIME: 15 MINUTES • COOK TIME: 45 MINUTES

Yield: Makes 8 or more 1-cup servings • *Portions: Negligible fat*

- 2 teaspoons coconut oil
- ½ large yellow onion, finely chopped
- 1 can (28 ounces) petite dice tomatoes
- 1 can (6 ounces) tomato paste
- 1 eggplant, finely chopped
- 2 zucchini, finely chopped
- 1 package (8 ounces) mushrooms, cut into thirds (2 or more cups)
- 2–3 cloves garlic, minced
- 1 tablespoon balsamic vinegar
- 1 teaspoon fresh thyme or ½ teaspoon dried
- 1 teaspoon Celtic or pink Himalayan salt
- ¼ teaspoon ground black pepper
- 1 cup fresh basil, cut into chiffonade (see Notes, page 162) ribbons
- ¼ cup chopped fresh parsley

Heat the oil in a large skillet or pot over medium-high heat.

Cook the onion until soft. Add the tomatoes, tomato paste, eggplant, zucchini, mushrooms, garlic, vinegar, thyme, salt, and pepper.

Reduce the heat and simmer for about 45 minutes. Remove from the heat, stir in the basil and parsley, and adjust the salt and pepper to taste.

NOTES:

The vegetables should be cut into about ¾" pieces.

As the flavors meld overnight, the ratatouille gets even better. Serve hot, at room temperature, or cold.

ZUCCHINI WIDE-CUT PASTA

PREP TIME: 5 MINUTES • COOK TIME: 5 MINUTES

Yield: Makes four 1-cup servings • *Portions:* No protein or fat

4–6 zucchini

Coconut oil spray or a smidge of coconut oil

Celtic or pink Himalayan salt

Ground black pepper

Using a vegetable peeler, peel long, wide, thin ribbons of zucchini (see Note). Heat a nonstick skillet over medium-high heat, then spray or brush with oil.

When the pan is hot, add the zucchini and toss for 2 to 3 minutes, or until warmed through and just tender. Depending on the size of your skillet, this could take a minute or two longer, but it's best not to crowd the zucchini. You want the zucchini to cook very quickly so it doesn't get soggy.

Use tongs to remove the zucchini from the skillet so you don't pick up any liquid from the bottom of the skillet. Sprinkle with salt and pepper. Serve immediately, topped with your favorite sauce or ghee.

> **NOTE:**
>
> *You are not cutting the zucchini into spaghetti strands. You are using a vegetable peeler to cut long, wide ribbons. To do this, cut off the top stem and the very bottom, and slice vertically, from top to bottom. You want thin zucchini "noodles," so don't press hard on the slicer. Use just as much pressure as you would to peel a carrot.*

VARIATIONS:

This recipe was prepared with virtually no fat. You can also cook the zucchini with coconut oil or ghee and, optionally, 1 to 2 cloves minced garlic and your favorite herbs. Remember to count the fat.

MEDITERRANEAN PEASANT SALAD

PREP TIME: 10 MINUTES

Yield: Makes 4 servings • *Portions:* ½ fat

- 2 cups multicolored cherry or grape tomatoes, cut in half, or 2 heirloom tomatoes, sliced into wedges
- 1 cucumber, peeled, seeded, and finely chopped
- ½ onion, finely chopped
- 2–3 tablespoons chopped fresh basil leaves
- ½ teaspoon Celtic or pink Himalayan salt
- ⅛ teaspoon ground black pepper
- 1 tablespoon + 1 teaspoon olive oil
- 2 teaspoons red wine vinegar

In a large bowl, combine the tomatoes, cucumber, onion, and basil. Season with the salt and pepper. Drizzle with the oil and vinegar and toss gently.

> **NOTE:**
>
> *This salad gets even better as it marinates, so if you can make it a few hours ahead of time, all the better. It's also terrific the next day, and it's a great base for a luncheon salad. Finely chop 1 palm-size piece of roasted chicken breast per person and add to the salad.*

MAC AND CHEESE (OR JUST MAKE THE CHEESE SAUCE TO USE AS A DIP OR SAUCE)

PREP TIME: 20 MINUTES • COOK TIME: 15 MINUTES

Yield: 4 *servings* • *Portions:* Negligible fat

PASTA:
  2 (14-ounce) cans or 2 (9-ounce) packages hearts of palm pasta

CHEESE SAUCE:
  1 cup unsweetened almond milk
  ⅓ cup nutritional yeast
  ½ teaspoon dried mustard or Dijon mustard
  ¼ teaspoon Celtic or pink Himalayan salt
  ⅛ teaspoon paprika
  2 tablespoons arrowroot
    Pinch or more cayenne (optional)
  2 tablespoons pasture-raised butter or ghee

FOR THE PASTA:

In a large pot, bring about 2 quarts of water to a boil. Rinse and drain the pasta.

Add the pasta to the boiling water and cook for about 10 minutes to tenderize. Drain when the cheese sauce is done.

FOR THE CHEESE SAUCE:

In a blender, combine the almond milk, nutritional yeast, mustard, salt, paprika, arrowroot, and cayenne (if using) and blend until smooth and creamy. Pour into a saucepan over medium-low heat and add the butter. Stir with a wooden spoon or whisk until it begins to thicken, 2 to 3 minutes. Test with a spoon. When sauce clings to the back of the spoon, it's ready.

Pour the sauce over the pasta and stir to combine. Serve immediately.

  NOTES:

  If you've never had hearts of palm pasta, this is an easy recipe to give it a try. Keep in mind the pasta will be al dente. It's loaded with fiber and very low in carbohydrates. Hearts of palm pasta comes in cans or in sealed plastic pouches.

  This cheese sauce also stands on its own. Although it's great in mac and cheese, it's also fabulous as a dip or drizzled over steamed or roasted vegetables! Think broccoli and cauliflower with cheese sauce.

  Store cooled leftover sauce in a sealed container in the refrigerator for 3 to 4 days. Reheat the sauce on the stovetop, not in the microwave. The consistency of the reheated sauce will likely be thinner, and you may need to add a bit more arrowroot to thicken it.

ASIAN SESAME NOODLE SALAD

PREP TIME: 35 MINUTES • COOK TIME: 3 MINUTES

Yield: 4 entrée servings or 6 to 8 side servings • *Portions*: Negligible fat

SALAD:

- 2 (7-ounce) packages angel hair shirataki noodles (also called "miracle noodles")
- 6 cups julienned vegetables, such as carrots; red, yellow, and/or orange bell peppers; zucchini; cucumbers; radishes; snow peas
- ½ cup or more cilantro leaves, lightly packed
- 3 scallions, thinly sliced

DRESSING:

- 2 tablespoons tahini
- 2 tablespoons coconut aminos
- 1 tablespoon coconut or white vinegar
- 2 teaspoons toasted sesame oil
- 2 teaspoons freshly squeezed lime juice, about ½ lime
- 2" piece ginger, peeled and shredded on a Microplane, about 1 tablespoon
- 1 teaspoon or more chile-garlic sauce or Sriracha, to taste
- ¼–½ teaspoon Celtic or pink Himalayan salt
- Stevia or monk fruit sweetener equal to 1 to 2 teaspoons sugar
- 3 tablespoons sesame seeds, toasted (optional)

Correct preparation of the shirataki is very important. On high heat set a pot of water large enough for both packages of shirataki noodles. Drain the noodles in a colander or large sieve and rinse in cool water for 15 seconds. (Konjac has a unique smell, but it will go away as the noodles are dried.) Boil the noodles for 2 minutes, drain well, and place them in a non-oiled skillet over medium heat until they are dry. In a large bowl, combine the noodles and the julienned vegetables.

In a medium bowl, whisk all of the dressing ingredients together. Taste and adjust the seasoning, if necessary. Pour the dressing over the noodles and vegetables, add the sesame seeds (if using), and toss. Serve chilled or at room temperature.

NOTES:

To make this a complete meal, add 4 to 6 ounces of cooked shrimp, scallops, or chicken to add protein.

This salad is best eaten within 2 days of preparation.

BALSAMIC ROASTED BRUSSELS SPROUTS

PREP TIME: 10 MINUTES • COOK TIME: 20 MINUTES

Yield: 4 servings • Portions: ½ fat

1 pound Brussels sprouts

2 tablespoons olive or avocado oil

⅛ teaspoon ground black pepper

2 ounces pancetta or bacon, nitrate- and sugar-free, diced

2–3 tablespoons balsamic vinegar

To prepare the Brussels sprouts, wash, remove any tough or discolored outer leaves, trim the bottoms, and slice in half vertically. Preheat the oven to 425°F and put a rack in the middle of the oven. Toss the Brussels sprouts in oil and pepper and place them on a sheet pan. Add the pancetta or bacon to the pan and roast, stirring once after 10 minutes. Cook until the Brussels sprouts are tender and golden brown, about 20 minutes. When done, drizzle with the balsamic vinegar and toss to coat.

NOTES:

If the Brussels sprouts are large, cut into quarters.

Since the pancetta or bacon is already quite salty there is no additional salt in this recipe. If desired, you can salt after tasting.

BROCCOLI SALAD WITH CREAMY POPPYSEED DRESSING

PREP TIME: 15 MINUTES

Yield: 4 *servings* • *Portions:* 1 *fat,* ½ *fruit*

SALAD:

- 1 pound fresh broccoli, cut into small florets (see Notes)
- 1 cup fresh blueberries
- ⅛ cup red onion, thinly sliced
- ¼ cup hulled sunflower or pumpkin seeds, toasted

DRESSING:

- ¼ cup avocado mayonnaise
- Stevia or monk fruit sweetener equal to 1 tablespoon sugar
- 1 tablespoon apple cider or red wine vinegar
- 1 teaspoon poppy seeds
- ¼ teaspoon Celtic or pink Himalayan salt
- ⅛ teaspoon ground black pepper

If blanching the broccoli, do that first. Toss all the salad ingredients together in a bowl.

Combine all the dressing ingredients in a small bowl or a jar with a tight-fitting lid and whisk or shake well to blend. Pour over the salad and toss.

NOTES:

After trimming the broccoli you'll end up with 10 to 12 ounces of florets. If you're enjoying this for breakfast you can add another cup of blueberries to the recipe to get your full serving of fruit.

I've never been a fan of raw broccoli. I prefer to blanch it to heighten the color and tenderize it. To blanch the broccoli set a pot of water to boil. Immerse the broccoli florets in the water for 1 to 2 minutes, or until the color heightens to a bright green. Immediately drain and put into an ice bath to stop the cooking process.

To toast the sunflower or pumpkin seeds, heat a skillet on medium-low heat. Do not add any oil. Add the seeds, stirring or shaking the pan frequently until the seeds become fragrant and lightly browned. Sunflower seeds will brown in about 3 minutes. Pumpkin seeds will take a bit longer, 5 to 7 minutes. Watch carefully because seeds, like nuts, can burn easily.

BRUSSELS SPROUTS SALAD WITH A SWEET AND TANGY VINAIGRETTE

PREP TIME: 20 MINUTES • COOK TIME: 12–17 MINUTES (FOR BACON)

Yield: 4 to 6 servings • Portions: ½ protein, 1 fat, ¼ fruit

SALAD:

- 1 pound Brussels sprouts, shaved or thinly sliced
- 1 tart apple, julienned
- ¼ cup red onion, very thinly sliced
- ¼ cup pecans or walnuts, toasted and coarsely chopped
- 4 strips bacon, well done so they are crispy, diced

VINAIGRETTE:

- ¼ cup extra-virgin olive oil
- 1–2 tablespoons apple cider or red wine vinegar
- ½ teaspoon dry ground mustard or Dijon mustard
- Stevia or monk fruit sweetener to equal 1 teaspoon sugar
- ¼ teaspoon Celtic or pink Himalayan salt
- ⅛ teaspoon ground black pepper

Toss all the salad ingredients together in a large bowl. Put all the vinaigrette ingredients in a bowl or glass jar with a tight-fitting lid and whisk or shake to fully blend. Pour the vinaigrette over the salad and toss.

> **NOTES:**
>
> *To prepare the Brussels sprouts, wash, remove any tough or discolored outer leaves, trim the bottoms, and slice in half vertically. Lay each half cut side down and thinly slice to create shreds. You can use a mandolin to shred the Brussels sprouts, but you will need a protective no-cut glove. A food processor fitted with the shredding disk will also work, but it will produce a finer shred that is not advisable for this recipe. Often you can find shredded Brussels sprouts in bags in the supermarket.*
>
> *Here's a great tip for cutting the pungency from uncooked red onion: soak in ice water for about 10 minutes, drain, and pat dry with paper towels.*

BUFFALO CAULIFLOWER (WITH AIR FRYER AND OVEN COOKING METHODS)

PREP TIME: 10 MINUTES • COOK TIME: 15–20 MINUTES, VARIES WITH METHOD

Yield: 5 servings • *Portions*: *negligible fat*

1 tablespoon pasture-raised butter, melted

⅓–½ cup Frank's RedHot sauce

½ teaspoons garlic powder

½ teaspoon salt

1 head cauliflower, cut into florets (4 to 5 cups)

⅓ cup finely ground almond flour

Avocado, coconut, or olive oil pan spray

Ranch Dressing for dipping, optional (page 239)

Combine the melted butter, hot sauce, garlic powder, and salt in a bowl. Add the cauliflower and toss to coat.

Place the almond flour in another bowl. Using a slotted spoon or tongs transfer the florets into the almond flour mixture and toss to coat. Don't pour the almond flour mixture over the cauliflower because there will be excess hot sauce in the bottom of the cauliflower bowl that will absorb part of the almond flour.

AIR FRYER METHOD:

Preheat the air fryer to 350°F. Line the basket with parchment and spray with pan spray. Place half the florets on one tray and the other half on the other tray. Spray the florets with pan spray. Cook for about 15 minutes, checking for doneness twice during the cooking process, once after 6 minutes and again after another 6 minutes. The florets are done when they are a bit browned and can be pierced easily with a skewer or fork. The florets should not be mushy. Remove the florets from the fryer and repeat with the second batch.

OVEN METHOD:

Preheat the oven to 400°F, place a rack in the middle of the oven, and line a baking sheet with parchment. Spray the parchment with pan spray. Add the florets to the pan, leaving space between them, and spray with pan spray. Bake for 10 minutes. Turn the florets and bake for 10 more minutes. The florets are done when they are a bit browned and can be pierced easily with a skewer or fork. The florets should not be mushy.

NOTE:

Do not preheat the air fryer with the parchment paper in the basket or tray. Most manufacturers note that the paper could ignite.

These should be eaten right when they come out of the air fryer or oven. They will get soggy if refrigerated.

DAIRY-FREE CREAMY RANCH DRESSING

PREP TIME: 10 MINUTES

Yield: *About 1 cup* • *Portions*: *1 tablespoon = 1 fat*

½ cup avocado oil mayonnaise

1 teaspoon fresh thyme leaves or ⅓ teaspoon dried

1–2 garlic cloves, smashed

¼ cup chives, coarsely chopped or 1 tablespoon + 1 teaspoon dried

1 tablespoon dill, coarsely chopped or 1 teaspoon dried

2 tablespoons fresh Italian parsley or 2 teaspoons dried

½ cup full-fat coconut milk

1 tablespoon white wine or champagne vinegar

½ teaspoon dried mustard

¼ teaspoon Celtic or pink Himalayan salt

Freshly ground black pepper

In a food processor, combine the mayonnaise, thyme, garlic, chives, dill, and parsley. If using fresh herbs, process until the herbs are finely chopped. If using dried herbs, pulse a few times to thoroughly mix the ingredients.

With the motor running, slowly pour in the coconut milk, and then add the vinegar, mustard, salt, and pepper. Taste and adjust seasonings. Transfer to a jar or airtight container and refrigerate up to 1 week.

ROASTED KOHLRABI

PREP TIME: 15 MINUTES • COOK TIME: 30 MINUTES

Yield: 4 servings • *Portions:* No protein or fat

4 to 6	small kohlrabi (1–1½ pounds)
	Avocado, coconut, or olive oil pan spray
¼–½	teaspoon Celtic or pink Himalayan salt
	Sprinkling of ground black pepper
2	teaspoons chopped parsley, as garnish (optional)

Preheat the oven to 450°F and place the rack in the middle of the oven. Peel the kohlrabi with a paring knife or vegetable peeler. Cut into small wedges. Place on a parchment lined baking sheet, spray with pan spray, and season with salt and pepper. Roast for about 30 minutes, flipping half way through roasting. To serve, sprinkle with chopped parsley (if using).

NOTES:

When peeling kohlrabi, cut off the bottom woody part and peel until you get to the lighter flesh. The outside is tough and will not soften when cooked.

When buying fresh kohlrabi, choose small, firm bulbs about the size of a tennis ball. If the leaves are still attached, they should be fresh and not wilted.

There is so much you can do with kohlrabi. It is great sliced and served with a dip. Try it with the Roasted Cauliflower Hummus on page 248 or the Roasted Red Pepper Hummus on page 249. You can also slice it paper thin on a mandolin or cut it into matchsticks and add it to your salad. Cut into small wedges, it's a wonderful addition to soups and stews. Use it as a substitute for potatoes.

Shred it and add it to slaws or use it to enhance a creamy soup.

You can experiment with other seasonings, such as paprika or garlic powder.

ZUCCHINI FRITTERS (AIR FRYER AND STOVETOP METHODS)

PREP TIME: 20 MINUTES • COOK TIME: 14–20 MINUTES,
VARIES BY COOKING METHOD

Yield: 4 servings • *Portions: Negligible fat in air fryer, ½ fat on stovetop*

- 4 cups zucchini (2 to 3 medium), shredded
- ½ teaspoon salt
- 1 egg, beaten
- 2 tablespoons arrowroot
- 2 tablespoons almond flour
- 1 teaspoon baking powder
- 1 teaspoon dried dill or chives
- ¼ teaspoon ground black pepper
- Pinch cayenne (optional)
- Avocado, olive, or coconut pan spray, if you are using an air fryer
- 2 tablespoons coconut oil, avocado oil, or ghee, if you are cooking on the stovetop

Shred the zucchini on a box grater using the large holes or in a food processor using the shredding disk. Put the zucchini in a large fine-mesh sieve placed over a bowl. Salt the zucchini, toss to disperse, and let sit in the sieve for 15 to 20 minutes to remove some of the water. Using your hand or a rubber spatula, press the zucchini against the sieve to remove some of the water. Then place the zucchini in a clean dish towel or several layers of paper towels and very thoroughly wring out any remaining water. Repeat with a clean towel or paper towels. The key to good fritters is getting the zucchini as dry as possible so they crisp.

In a large bowl combine the zucchini, egg, arrowroot, almond flour, baking powder, dill or chives, pepper, and cayenne.

If you are cooking in an air fryer, set it to 400°F and lightly spray the air fryer basket with pan spray. Pack ¼-cup measuring cup with the mixture, flip the measuring cup of fritter batter into the basket, and gently flatten the batter with a spatula or the back of a measuring cup so the fritter is about ½" thick. Lightly spray the top. Cook in batches so you don't overcrowd the basket. Cook for about 6 to 7 minutes, flip, lightly spray the top with pan spray, and cook another 6 to 7 minutes. Serve warm.

If you are cooking on the stovetop, use a heavy skillet on medium heat. Add 2 teaspoons oil or ghee to the pan and heat until a tiny bit of batter sizzles when you put it in the pan. Pack ¼-cup measuring cup with the mixture, flip the measuring cup of fritter batter into the pan, and gently flatten the fritter with a spatula or the back of a measuring cup so it is about ½" thick. Sauté for 3 to 4 minutes, or until the edges start to crisp. Very carefully flip the fritter and cook the second side for 3 to 4 minutes. Remove the fritter from the pan and place it on a paper towel–lined plate. Add 2 more teaspoons oil or ghee to the pan and repeat. Serve warm.

NOTES:

I can't emphasize enough how important it is to dry the zucchini as much as you possibly can. Zucchini contain a lot of water, and too much water will create a soggy fritter.

Cook in batches and don't crowd the air fryer or pan, so you will get crispy fritters.

If you have leftovers, refrigerate in a sealed container layering with paper towels to absorb any excess moisture.

For the stovetop method do not use butter; it will burn. Ghee is fine because the milk solids have been removed from the butter.

STARCHY VEGETABLES

REMINDER

Eat these vegetables sparingly—only after a workout, or if you're feeling weak and tired and you know it's not due to the carb flu (see "Troubleshooting Tips" in Chapter 4).

BAKED OR MASHED SWEET POTATOES

PREP TIME: 3 MINUTES • COOK TIME: 45 MINUTES

Yield: Makes 4 servings • *Portions:* 1 starchy vegetable, ½ fat

4 sweet potatoes

Celtic or pink Himalayan salt

Ground black pepper

2 tablespoons ghee (optional)

Ground cinnamon and/or nutmeg (optional)

Preheat the oven to 400°F. Line a baking sheet with parchment.

Pierce each sweet potato several times with the tines of a fork. Place on the prepared baking sheet. Bake for about 45 minutes, or until very tender. Remove from the oven, slit the top of each potato, and top with butter and spices (if using).

You can also scrape all the flesh from the inside of the potatoes and serve as mashed sweet potatoes. If the potatoes are baked until the inside is soft and creamy, you can mash them with a fork; otherwise, use a potato masher.

NOTES:

It's easy to pop these in the oven when you're roasting meat.

Although the oven method is better, you can also use the microwave method if you're in a hurry. Pierce each sweet potato several times with the tines of a fork. Place the sweet potatoes on a microwaveable plate. Use the "potato" button on your microwave oven or cook for 5 to 10 minutes. Because each oven heats food differently, check at 5 minutes and continue for a minute at a time.

VARIATION:

For a Mexican sweet potato, top with Pico de Gallo (page 267).

OVEN-STEAMED WINTER SQUASH

PREP TIME: 3 MINUTES • COOK TIME: 1 HOUR

Yield: Makes 4 or more 1-cup servings • *Portions:* 1 starchy vegetable, ½ fat

1 butternut or acorn squash

Celtic or pink Himalayan salt

Ground black pepper

2 tablespoons ghee (optional)

Cinnamon and/or nutmeg (optional)

Preheat the oven to 350°F.

Carefully cut the squash in half. Remove and discard the seeds. Place the squash cut side down in a shallow baking dish. Add ½" to ¾" water or bone broth and cover very tightly with foil.

Bake for about 1 hour. The flesh should be very tender. Scrape all the flesh from the inside of the squash and serve. The consistency will be like very moist mashed potatoes. Season with salt and pepper. Top with the ghee and spices (if using)

NOTE:

It's easy to pop these in the oven when you're roasting meat.

ROASTED WINTER SQUASH

PREP TIME: 10 MINUTES • COOK TIME: 35 MINUTES

Yield: Makes 4 or more 1-cup servings • *Portions:* 1 starchy vegetable, ½ fat

1 butternut or acorn squash

2 tablespoons coconut oil, melted, or coconut oil spray

Celtic or pink Himalayan salt

Ground black pepper

Cinnamon and/or nutmeg (optional)

Preheat the oven to 425°F. Line a baking sheet with parchment.

Carefully cut the squash in half. Remove and discard the seeds. Use a vegetable peeler to remove the skin. Lay the squash cut side down on a cutting board and cut into 1" cubes. In a large bowl or a resealable plastic bag, toss or shake the squash with the oil. Season with salt and pepper. Sprinkle with cinnamon or nutmeg (if using).

Place the squash on the prepared baking sheet in 1 layer and roast for 15 to 20 minutes. Flip the pieces with a spatula or tongs and bake for 15 minutes, or until the flesh is very tender.

TWO TECHNIQUES FOR STEAMING VEGETABLES

Steamed vegetables are quick and easy to make, and you don't need a fancy electric steamer to get the job done. Here are two speedy ways to steam your veggies.

Steaming on the stove: Prepare the vegetables for cooking. Place a steamer or metal colander inside a pot with a cover. Add ½" to 1" water. Be sure the steamer or colander is above the water level and covers the pan. When the water boils, add the vegetables to the steamer basket or colander, cover the pot, and reduce the heat.

Steaming always takes less time than you think, so keep your eyes on the pot. You want your veggies to have some crunch and not to turn to mush! When they're done, remove the pot from the stove and place the vegetables on a tray or sheet pan in a single layer to cool. They'll continue to cook for a few minutes. If you want the vegetables to remain very crispy and bright green, plunge them into an ice water bath to stop the cooking process immediately. Salt to taste.

Steaming in the oven: Preheat the oven to 350°F and put the vegetables in a roasting pan or ovenproof Dutch oven with about ½" bone broth (preferred) or water. Cover tightly with foil or the pan lid. Check the progress after about 5 minutes and continue to check every few minutes. (If you're cooking in broth, it will be full of vitamins and minerals from the vegetables, so be sure to save it and drink it.) If you are not serving the veggies immediately, place them on a tray or sheet pan in a single layer to cool. They will continue to cook for a few minutes after you take them from the oven. Salt to taste.

Tip: If you want to steam a number of vegetables at the same time, steam vegetables with the same density together. For example, cauliflower and broccoli steam well together, but broccoli and asparagus don't because the broccoli takes longer to cook than the asparagus.

SWEET AND SPICY ROASTED SWEET POTATOES

PREP TIME: 20 MINUTES • COOK TIME 30 MINUTES

Yield: Makes 4 servings • *Portions*: 1 starchy vegetable, ½ fat

4 sweet potatoes, peeled and cut into 1" cubes

2 bell peppers, red, orange, yellow, or any combination, cut into 1½" cubes

1 red onion, cut into wedges

2 tablespoons coconut oil, melted

¼ teaspoon ground ginger

¼ teaspoon ground cumin

¼ teaspoon ground coriander

¼ teaspoon paprika

¼ teaspoon ground cinnamon

⅛ teaspoon ground nutmeg

½ teaspoon Celtic or pink Himalayan salt

¼ teaspoon ground black pepper

   Dash of cayenne

Preheat the oven to 425°F. Line 2 baking sheets with parchment.

In a large bowl or a resealable plastic bag, toss or shake the sweet potatoes, bell peppers, and onion with the oil, ginger, cumin, coriander, paprika, cinnamon, nutmeg, salt, pepper, and cayenne until the vegetables are coated with oil and spices.

Place the mixture in a single layer on the prepared baking sheets and roast for 25 to 30 minutes. Don't pile up the potatoes; you want them to roast, not steam.

> **NOTE:**
>
> *If you don't have all the spices, just use what you have on hand. The spice measurements don't need to be precise. Use what you like.*

SALAD DRESSINGS, DIPS, AND SAUCES

SPICY LIME VINAIGRETTE

PREP TIME: 5 MINUTES

Yield: *Makes eight 2-tablespoon servings (1 cup)* • **Portions:** *1 fat per serving*

½ cup extra-virgin olive oil

¼ cup + 2 tablespoons fresh lime juice

2 tablespoons water

½ teaspoon lime peel

½ teaspoon ground cumin

2 tablespoons coarsely chopped fresh cilantro

1 clove garlic, smashed

Dash cayenne

Dash of hot sauce (if you like spiciness, add more)

⅛ teaspoon Celtic or pink Himalayan salt

In a bowl or a jar with a tight-fitting lid, whisk or shake together the oil, lime juice, water, lime peel, cumin, cilantro, garlic, cayenne, hot sauce, and salt. Remove and discard the garlic before serving. Refrigerate.

NOTES:

This dressing has lots of Mexican and Southwest flavors. It makes a great spicy slaw, it's good on a salad with grilled chicken, and you can use it as a marinade. For chicken, fish, or shrimp, marinate for 2 hours; for beef, marinate as long as overnight.

The garlic is smashed to flavor the dressing without having minced garlic in it. Remove the garlic before serving the dressing.

This is best prepared ahead and refrigerated so the flavors can meld.

ROASTED CAULIFLOWER HUMMUS (NO BEANS!)

PREP TIME: 15 MINUTES • COOK TIME: 30 MINUTES

Yield: About 2½ cups or ten ¼-cup servings • *Portions:* ½ fat per serving

- 4 tablespoons extra-virgin olive oil
- 1 teaspoon Celtic or pink Himalayan salt
- ¼ teaspoon ground black pepper
- 1 teaspoon cumin
- Pinch of cayenne (optional)
- 1 large head cauliflower (about 2 pounds), cut into small florets
- 2–3 garlic cloves, unpeeled
- ⅓ cup tahini
- 2 tablespoons freshly squeezed lemon juice (½–1 lemon)

Preheat the oven to 400°F and place oven racks in the upper middle and lower middle positions. Line two baking sheets with parchment. In a small bowl, combine the oil, salt, pepper, cumin, and cayenne (if using). Place the cauliflower on the sheet pans, drizzle with the oil mixture, and toss. Roast for 15 minutes, then add the garlic to the pan and switch the position of the two pans for even baking. Roast for 15 to 20 minutes more, or until some of the florets have browned and are fork-tender. Remove from the oven and let cool for 5 to 10 minutes. Squeeze the garlic from its skin. In a food processor, combine the cauliflower, garlic, tahini, and lemon juice and blend until smooth. Taste and add more salt or pepper as desired. If you want a thinner consistency, add water, 1 tablespoon at a time, and blend until desired consistency is reached. Cover and refrigerate for up to 4 days.

NOTES:

Because cumin has such a distinctive flavor, feel free to adjust the amount to suit your personal tastes. Remember, you can always add more!

To serve, optionally drizzle with 1 teaspoon of olive oil and lightly sprinkle with paprika.

ROASTED RED PEPPER HUMMUS (NO BEANS!)

PREP TIME: 15 MINUTES • COOK TIME: 30 MINUTES

Yield: About 3 cups or twelve ¼-cup servings • *Portions:* ½ fat per serving

- 4 tablespoons extra-virgin olive oil
- 1 teaspoon Celtic or pink Himalayan salt
- ¼ teaspoon ground black pepper
- 1 teaspoon cumin
- Pinch cayenne (optional)
- 1 large head cauliflower, about 2 pounds, cut into small florets
- 8 ounces jarred roasted red peppers, drained
- ⅓ cup tahini
- 2 tablespoons freshly squeezed lemon juice (½ to 1 lemon)

Preheat the oven to 400°F and place the racks in the upper middle and lower middle positions. Line two baking sheets with parchment. In a small bowl, combine oil, salt, pepper, cumin, and cayenne (if using). Place the cauliflower on the sheet pans, drizzle with the oil mixture, and toss. Roast for 15 minutes, then switch the positions of the two pans for even baking. Roast for 15 to 20 minutes more, or until some of the florets have browned and are fork-tender. Remove from the oven and let cool for 5 to 10 minutes. In a food processor, combine the cauliflower, roasted peppers, tahini, and lemon juice and blend until smooth. Taste and add more salt or pepper as desired. If you want a thinner consistency, add water, 1 tablespoon at a time, and blend until desired consistency is reached. Cover and refrigerate for up to 4 days.

NOTES:

Because cumin has such a distinctive flavor, feel free to adjust the amount to suit your personal tastes. Remember, you can always add more!

One serving option is to drizzle with 1 teaspoon of olive oil and lightly sprinkle with paprika and/or toasted pumpkin seeds (pepitas).

THOUSAND ISLAND DRESSING

PREP TIME: 5 MINUTES

Yield: ⅔ cup • Portions: 1 fat per tablespoon

- ½ cup avocado oil mayonnaise
- 2 tablespoons avocado oil
- 2 tablespoons sugar-free ketchup or 1½ tablespoons tomato paste
- 2 tablespoons dill pickles or cornichons, cut into a small dice
- ⅛ teaspoon Celtic or pink Himalayan salt
- ⅛ teaspoon ground black pepper
- 1 teaspoon apple cider vinegar
- ⅛ teaspoon garlic powder
- Stevia or monk fruit sweetener to equal ½ teaspoon sugar (optional)

In a small bowl, combine all of the ingredients. Store covered in the refrigerator for up to 7 days.

> **NOTE:**
>
> *Cornichons are miniature gherkin cucumbers, only 1 to 2 inches in length, that are harvested before they are fully mature. Then they are fermented just as other pickles. They have a tart, acidic taste and a crunchy texture, and they really balance a mayonnaise-based dressing.*

TONNATO SAUCE

PREP TIME: 10 MINUTES

Yield: *ten 2-tablespoon servings* • *Portions*: *2 fats*

½ **cup olive oil**

½ **cup avocado mayonnaise**

4 **anchovies packed in olive oil, drained**

1 **(6–7 ounce) can tuna packed in olive oil, drained**

2 **tablespoons capers, rinsed and drained**

3 **tablespoons freshly squeezed lemon juice (about 1½ medium lemons)**

   Pinch Celtic or pink Himalayan salt

   Freshly ground black pepper

In a blender, combine all of the ingredients and puree until smooth and creamy. Store in a sealed container in the refrigerator for up to 4 days.

BALSAMIC VINAIGRETTE

PREP TIME: 5 MINUTES

Yield: Makes eight 2-tablespoon servings (1 cup) • Portions: 1 fat per serving

½ cup extra-virgin olive oil

½ cup balsamic vinegar

1 teaspoon mustard powder

½ teaspoon very finely chopped fresh thyme or ¾–1 teaspoon dried

1 clove garlic, smashed

⅛ teaspoon Celtic or pink Himalayan salt

In a bowl or a jar with a tight-fitting lid, whisk or shake together the oil, vinegar, mustard, thyme, garlic, and salt. Refrigerate. Remove the garlic from the dressing before serving.

NOTES:

The garlic is smashed to flavor the dressing without having minced garlic in it. Remove the garlic before serving the dressing.

This is best prepared ahead and refrigerated so the flavors can meld.

VARIATIONS:

I like fresh herbs in my salad dressings, so I use them liberally. You can substitute any herbs you prefer.

CREAMY AVOCADO SAUCE OR SALAD DRESSING AND 3 VARIATIONS

PREP TIME: 5 MINUTES

Yield: *Makes four ⅓-cup servings (about 1½ cups)* • **Portions**: *1 fat per serving*

2	avocados (6–7 ounces each)
1	small clove garlic
1½–2	tablespoons fresh lime or lemon juice
½–1	teaspoon Celtic or pink Himalayan salt
	Pinch of ground black pepper
⅓–¾	cup water

Slice each avocado in half, remove the pit, and scoop out the flesh with a spoon.

Place the avocado flesh, garlic, lime or lemon juice, salt, and pepper in a blender or food processor. Combine until smooth, stopping a few times to scrape down the sides. Thin as desired with the water, adding little by little until you reach the desired consistency.

Store in an airtight container in the refrigerator for up to 7 days. Use any of the variations below as a creamy salad dressing or as a sauce for vegetables, meat, poultry, or seafood.

VARIATIONS:

Avocado lime chipotle sauce or creamy dressing: Add about ¼ teaspoon chipotle powder, ¼ teaspoon ground cumin, and a pinch of cayenne. Optionally, add 1 to 2 teaspoons fresh cilantro and/or ½ teaspoon fresh lime peel.

Fresh herb avocado sauce or creamy dressing: Add a combination of your favorite chopped fresh herbs, such as thyme, basil, dill, chives, marjoram, parsley, or cilantro. Cilantro is by far my favorite with avocados.

Hot and smoky avocado sauce or creamy dressing: Use ½ teaspoon or more of chipotle chile pepper in adobo sauce. You can add smoked paprika for a smokier flavor.

CREAMY GINGER DRESSING

PREP TIME: 5 MINUTES

Yield: Makes five 3-tablespoon servings (1 cup) • *Portions: 1 fat per serving*

¾ cup full-fat coconut milk

1½ tablespoons coconut aminos

2 tablespoons white vinegar

2 teaspoons grated or minced fresh ginger

1–2 cloves garlic, minced

2 pinches of cayenne (just under ⅛ teaspoon)

In a bowl or a jar with a tight-fitting lid, whisk or shake together the milk, coconut aminos, vinegar, ginger, garlic, and cayenne. Refrigerate. Remove and discard the garlic before serving.

NOTES:

Only use fresh ginger.

The garlic is smashed to flavor the dressing without having minced garlic in it. Remove the garlic before serving the dressing.

This is best prepared ahead and refrigerated so the flavors can meld.

VARIATIONS:

If you can find kaffir lime leaves, add 1 or 2 to this dressing for a lovely Thai flavor. Remove and discard the leaves before serving.

This dressing is also excellent with poultry and fish, not just on your salad! Put it on shredded cabbage and you have an instant and delicious slaw salad. You'll find it on Napa Slaw with Creamy Ginger Dressing (page 227).

FRENCH VINAIGRETTE

PREP TIME: 5 MINUTES

Yield: Makes eight 2-tablespoon servings (1 cup) • *Portions:* 1 fat per serving

½ cup extra-virgin olive oil

⅓ cup red wine vinegar

2 tablespoons water

1½ teaspoons Dijon mustard

1 tablespoon finely minced shallots

⅛ teaspoon Celtic or pink Himalayan salt

In a bowl or a jar with a tight-fitting lid, whisk or shake together the oil, vinegar, water, mustard, shallots, and salt. Refrigerate.

> **NOTES:**
>
> *This is best prepared ahead and refrigerated so the flavors can meld.*
>
> *You can also add any herbs you like.*

LEMON VINAIGRETTE OR CREAMY LEMON DRESSING

PREP TIME: 5 MINUTES

Yield: Makes eight 2-tablespoon servings (1 cup) • *Portions: 1 fat per serving*

VINAIGRETTE

- ½ cup extra-virgin olive oil
- ¼ cup + 2 tablespoons fresh lemon juice
- 2 tablespoons water
- ½ teaspoon lemon peel
- ½ teaspoon finely chopped fresh thyme or ⅛ teaspoon dried (optional)
- 1 clove garlic, smashed
- ⅛ teaspoon Celtic or pink Himalayan salt

CREAMY DRESSING

- ½ cup Lemon Vinaigrette
- ½ cup full-fat coconut milk

To make the vinaigrette: In a bowl or a jar with a tight-fitting lid, whisk or shake together the oil, lemon juice, water, lemon peel, thyme (if using), garlic, and salt. Refrigerate. Remove and discard the garlic before serving.

To make the creamy dressing: Whisk together the vinaigrette and coconut milk or blend in a blender.

NOTES:

This vinaigrette is a fabulous marinade for chicken, fish, or shrimp; marinate for 2 hours before cooking.

This is best prepared ahead and refrigerated so the flavors can meld.

VARIATION:

You can substitute any herbs you like.

ORANGE VINAIGRETTE OR CREAMY ORANGE DRESSING

PREP TIME: 5 MINUTES

Yield: Makes eight 2-tablespoon servings (1 cup) • *Portions: 1 fat per serving*

VINAIGRETTE

- ½ cup extra-virgin olive oil
- ½ cup fresh orange juice
- 1 tablespoon red or white wine vinegar
- ½ teaspoon orange zest
- ½ teaspoon finely chopped fresh tarragon or rosemary or ⅛–¼ teaspoon dried
- 1 clove garlic, smashed
- ⅛ teaspoon Celtic or pink Himalayan salt

CREAMY DRESSING

- ½ cup Orange Vinaigrette
- ½ cup full-fat coconut milk

To make the vinaigrette: In a bowl or a jar with a tight-fitting lid, whisk or shake together the oil, orange juice, vinegar, orange zest, tarragon, garlic, and salt. Refrigerate. Remove and discard the garlic before serving.

To make the creamy dressing: Whisk together the vinaigrette and coconut milk or blend in a blender.

NOTES:

This is an excellent marinade for chicken, fish, or shrimp; marinate for 2 hours before cooking.

This is best prepared ahead and refrigerated so the flavors can meld.

VARIATION:

You can substitute any herbs you prefer.

COCKTAIL SAUCE

PREP TIME: 5 MINUTES • COOK TIME: 5–10 MINUTES

Yield: Makes eight 2-tablespoon servings (1 cup) • ***Portions:*** *No protein or fat*

½ cup tomato paste (sugar- and dextrose-free)

¼ cup apple cider vinegar

¼ cup apple juice, unsweetened

Pinch of onion powder

⅛ teaspoon ground cloves

2–3 tablespoons prepared horseradish

Dash of hot sauce

In a small saucepan, mix the tomato paste, vinegar, apple juice, onion powder, and cloves and heat over very low heat for about 5 minutes, continually stirring to prevent scorching.

If you want the sauce to thicken further, keep it at a very low simmer for a few more minutes.

Cool completely. Add the horseradish and hot sauce and stir. Adjust the horseradish and hot sauce to suit your tastes.

Store in the refrigerator in a jar with a tight-fitting lid. This dressing will keep refrigerated for about 2 weeks.

NOTES:

Heating this sauce encourages all the flavors to meld and will also slightly thicken it.

You can find prepared horseradish in the refrigerated case at the grocery store. Over time, horseradish loses its potency after it's been opened and refrigerated. If your horseradish isn't fresh, you'll need to use more.

This sauce is fabulous with shrimp!

MARINARA SAUCE

PREP TIME: 15 MINUTES • COOK TIME: 45 MINUTES

*Yield: Makes four 1-cup servings • **Portions**: ½ fat*

2 tablespoons ghee

1 large yellow onion, finely chopped

3 cloves garlic, minced

1 can (28 ounces) petite dice tomatoes

1 can (6 ounces) tomato paste

¼–½ cup water

1 tablespoon balsamic vinegar

¼ cup chopped fresh basil or 1½ tablespoons dried

2 tablespoons chopped fresh parsley

2 teaspoons chopped fresh thyme or ¾ teaspoon dried

1 teaspoon dried marjoram

1 teaspoon Celtic or pink Himalayan salt

¼ teaspoon ground black pepper

Heat the ghee in a saucepan over medium-high heat. Cook the onion until softened. Add the garlic and cook for 1 to 2 minutes. Add the tomatoes, tomato paste, water, vinegar, basil, parsley, thyme, marjoram, salt, and pepper and simmer uncovered for about 45 minutes. Adjust the salt and pepper to taste.

NOTE:

You can serve the marinara over Zucchini Wide-Cut Pasta (page 231). It's also great with Turkey or Chicken Italian Sausage (page 163). If you add the sausage, it makes a complete meal.

HOMEMADE MAYONNAISE
AND 6 VARIATIONS

PREP TIME: 15 MINUTES

Yield: Makes sixteen 1-tablespoon servings (1 cup) • *Portions: 1 fat per serving*

2 egg yolks

1 teaspoon Dijon mustard

1 tablespoon + 1 teaspoon fresh lemon juice

**1 cup macadamia nut oil or avocado oil (olive oil is not recommended—
see Notes)**

Celtic or pink Himalayan salt

Bring the ingredients to room temperature. Place the egg yolks in a food
processor. Add the mustard, lemon juice, and salt to taste and pulse until the
ingredients are completely combined. With the motor running, add the oil in a
very slow, steady stream until the mixture is thick and emulsified.

Refrigerate in an airtight container. Because this is a fresh egg product without
preservatives, use it within 5 days.

> **NOTES:**
>
> *Select very fresh, organic, free-range, properly refrigerated eggs with intact shells,
> and avoid contact between the yolks and the shell. If you feel more comfortable,
> use pasteurized eggs.*
>
> *I don't recommend olive oil because it has a strong flavor that can overpower the
> delicacy of mayonnaise.*

VARIATIONS:

You can add a lot of pizzazz to mayo by introducing additional ingredients.
There's no right or wrong way to add flavors to mayonnaise. Experiment, adjust
the seasonings to suit yourself, and taste as you create.

Roasted red pepper mayo: Add about ½ teaspoon minced roasted garlic and
about 2 tablespoons roasted red peppers to ½ cup mayo. This works well, but
remember, there are no rules. Trust your tastebuds! I like to leave bits of the
roasted red peppers, but you can completely puree them. I also suggest adding
about ⅛ teaspoon hot-pepper sauce (such as Tabasco) per ½ cup mayonnaise to
give it a little zing. A dash of cayenne will work, too.

Lime chipotle mayo: Substitute lime juice for the lemon juice when you make
the mayo. Add about ¼ teaspoon dried chipotle powder, ¼ teaspoon ground
cumin, ¼ teaspoon minced garlic, and a dash of cayenne per ½ cup of mayo.
Optionally, add 1 to 2 teaspoons fresh cilantro and/or ½ teaspoon fresh lime zest.

Herb mayo: Add a combination of your favorite chopped fresh herbs, such as thyme, basil, dill, chives, marjoram, parsley, and cilantro. Optionally, add ¼ teaspoon minced garlic per ½ cup mayo.

Aioli (garlic mayonnaise): Add a few cloves of very finely chopped garlic when you make the mayo. You can also use Roasted Garlic (page 263), which is milder and has a less pungent taste.

Hot and smoky mayo: Use about ½ teaspoon chipotle chile pepper in adobo sauce and ¼ teaspoon minced garlic per ½ cup mayo. Just as in the lime chipotle mayo, you can substitute lime juice for the lemon juice in the mayo recipe. You can also add ¼ teaspoon smoked paprika.

Horseradish mayo: Use ½ cup mayo and 1½ to 2 tablespoons prepared horseradish (from the refrigerated section of your grocery store) and a few twists of freshly ground black pepper. Optionally, you can add about ½ teaspoon finely chopped fresh rosemary. This is divine on beef.

KETCHUP

PREP TIME: 5 MINUTES • COOK TIME: 5–10 MINUTES

Yield: Makes eight 2-tablespoon servings (1 cup) • **Portions:** *No protein or fat*

½ cup tomato paste (sugar- and dextrose-free)

¼ cup apple cider vinegar

¼ cup apple juice, unsweetened

   Pinch of onion powder

⅛ teaspoon ground cloves

In a small saucepan, mix the tomato paste, vinegar, apple juice, onion powder, and cloves. Heat over very low heat for about 5 minutes, stirring continually to prevent scorching.

If you want the ketchup to thicken further, keep it at a very low simmer for a few more minutes.

Cool completely and store in the refrigerator in a jar with a tight-fitting lid. It will keep refrigerated for about 2 weeks.

NOTE:

Heating the ketchup encourages all the flavors to meld and will also slightly thicken it.

ROASTED GARLIC

PREP TIME: 2 MINUTES • COOK TIME: 40 MINUTES

Yield: *Makes multiple 1–2 clove servings* • *Portions*: *Negligible fat*

1 large head of garlic

1 teaspoon melted coconut oil or ghee

Move an oven rack to the center of the oven. Preheat the oven to 400°F.

Peel away the loose, papery outer layers around the garlic head. Leave the head intact with all the cloves connected. Trim about ¼" off the top of the head to expose the tops of the garlic cloves.

Drizzle with the melted coconut oil, allowing the oil to sink into the cloves. Wrap in foil and roast for 30 minutes. Remove from the oven and pierce the center clove with a knife. If the garlic is very soft and spreadable, it's done. If not, return it to the oven for 10 minutes, then check again. Even once it's soft, you can continue roasting, checking every 10 minutes, until the garlic becomes golden and caramelized. The roasting time will vary based on the size, variety, and age of the garlic.

Let cool slightly. To serve, press on the bottom of a clove to push it out of its paper. Roasted garlic can be refrigerated in a sealed container for 2 weeks or frozen for up to 3 months.

NOTES:

Talk about flavor! Roasting garlic transforms it from a hard, pungent flavor into an almost sweet, creamy, caramelized delight. Use it lavishly in cooking, salad dressings, sauces, or with meats or vegetables.

You can roast as many garlic heads as you like in 1 foil wrapper; use 1 teaspoon of fat per head.

FIESTA MARINADE

PREP TIME: 5 MINUTES

Yield: Makes 8 servings; enough for 2 pounds meat/poultry/seafood • **Portions:** 1 fruit

- ⅔–1 cup fresh orange juice
- ⅓ cup apple cider vinegar
- 2 cloves garlic, minced, or 1½ teaspoons garlic powder
- 1½–2 teaspoons dried oregano
- 1 teaspoon Celtic or pink Himalayan salt
- ¾ teaspoon ground cumin
- ½ teaspoon ground black pepper

In a bowl, whisk together the orange juice, vinegar, garlic, oregano, salt, cumin, and pepper. (Use a large, nonmetalic bowl if you will be marinating in the bowl.) Marinate poultry or seafood for 1 to 2 hours in the refrigerator. Marinate beef or pork as long as overnight in the refrigerator.

Because there's no fat in the marinade, brush or spray the marinated meat with coconut oil before grilling or sautéing.

> **NOTES:**
>
> *The cumin and oregano in this recipe give the meat a south-of-the-border flavor.*
>
> *This is a great marinade for chicken, beef, pork, or seafood. Be sure to try it for grilling! Serve any of the salsas (pages 267, 269, and 272) on the side.*

MY FAVORITE MARINADE

PREP TIME: 5 MINUTES

*Yield: Makes 8 servings; enough for 2 pounds meat/poultry/seafood •
Portions: Negligible fat*

2 tablespoons coconut oil, melted

3 tablespoons fresh lime juice

¼ cup coconut aminos

2 tablespoons finely chopped fresh ginger

2–3 cloves garlic, minced

1 teaspoon ground cumin

½ jalapeño, seeded and finely chopped (wear plastic gloves when handling)

¼ cup fresh cilantro, finely chopped

¼ teaspoon paprika

¼ teaspoon ground white pepper

In a bowl, whisk together the oil, lime juice, coconut aminos, ginger, garlic, cumin, jalapeño, cilantro, paprika, and white pepper. (Use a large, nonmetalic bowl if you will be marinating in the bowl.)

NOTES:

This is great on chicken, beef, pork, or seafood.

Be sure to try it for grilling!

When the meat comes off the grill or out of the skillet, serve it with Creamy Ginger Dressing (page 254) as a drizzle sauce. What a combo! Or serve leftover protein in a salad topped with Creamy Ginger Dressing.

CREAMY CHIMICHURRI

PREP TIME: 5 MINUTES

Yield: Makes sixteen 1-tablespoon servings (1 cup) • *Portions:* Negligible fat

- 1 avocado, pitted and peeled
- 1 tablespoon fresh lemon juice
- ½ teaspoon lemon peel
- 1½ tablespoons red wine vinegar
- 2 cloves garlic
- ½ teaspoon Celtic or pink Himalayan salt
- ⅛ teaspoon ground black pepper
- ⅛ teaspoon red-pepper flakes
- ¼ teaspoon ground cumin
- 1 cup fresh parsley leaves, tightly packed
- 1 cup fresh cilantro leaves, tightly packed

In a food processor or blender, combine the avocado, lemon juice, lemon peel, vinegar, garlic, salt, black pepper, red-pepper flakes, and cumin. Process or blend until smooth, stopping a few times to scrape down the sides. Add the parsley and cilantro and pulse to coarsely chop. Store in an airtight container in the refrigerator for up to 5 days.

NOTES:

If you're not a big fan of cilantro, you can use all parsley or a smaller amount of cilantro with parsley making up the difference. This sauce is fabulous on grilled beef, but you can use it on any meat—especially lamb.

Chimichurri is a flavorful Argentine herb sauce traditionally served with grilled beef and made with olive oil. When you substitute avocado for the oil, the flavors remain the same, but your portion is bigger to provide more flavor.

PESTO

PREP TIME: 5 MINUTES

Yield: Makes four ¼-cup servings (1 cup) • *Portions:* ½ fat

- 2 **cups fresh basil leaves, tightly packed**
- 1 **cup fresh baby spinach, tightly packed**
- 2 **cloves garlic**
- 1 **avocado, pitted and peeled**

- 2 **tablespoons pine nuts**
- 1 **tablespoon fresh lemon juice**
- ½ **teaspoon Celtic or pink Himalayan salt**

In a food processor or blender, combine the basil, spinach, garlic, avocado, pine nuts, lemon juice, and salt. Process or blend until smooth, stopping a few times to scrape down the sides. Store in an airtight container in the refrigerator for up to 3 days.

NOTE:

This sauce is fabulous on grilled or sautéed fish or chicken or tossed with zucchini or spaghetti squash "pasta."

PICO DE GALLO (SALSA FRESCA)

PREP TIME: 15 MINUTES

Yield: Makes eight ¼-cup servings (2 cups) • *Portions:* No protein or fat

- 8 **Roma tomatoes, seeded and diced**
- 1 **red onion, finely chopped**
- 1 **jalapeño, seeded and finely chopped (wear plastic gloves when handling)**

- ½ **cup coarsely chopped fresh cilantro**
- 1–2 **tablespoons fresh lime juice**

In a large bowl, mix the tomatoes, onion, jalapeño, cilantro, and lime juice. Refrigerate in a tightly sealed container for up to 5 days.

NOTES:

The usual serving size is ¼ cup, but you can have as much as you want because it's all vegetables and seasonings.

This can be prepared ahead and refrigerated.

Pico de Gallo adds a lot of flavor. It is excellent on any roasted, grilled, or sautéed meat, poultry, or seafood or on eggs.

ROASTED RED PEPPER SAUCE

PREP TIME: 5 MINUTES

Yield: Makes four ¼-cup servings (1 cup) • **Portions:** Negligible fat

- **2** jars (12 ounces each) roasted red peppers (sugar- and dextrose-free) or 1 pound peppers after draining (see Notes)
- **1** clove garlic
- **½** teaspoon fresh lemon juice
- **¼** teaspoon Hungarian paprika
- **¼** teaspoon Celtic or pink Himalayan salt
- **⅛** teaspoon ground black pepper
- **¼** cup full-fat coconut milk

Drain the roasted peppers well and blot with paper towels. In a food processor or blender, combine the roasted peppers, garlic, lemon juice, paprika, salt, black pepper, and coconut milk. Process or blend until smooth, stopping a few times to scrape down the sides. Store in an airtight container in the refrigerator for up to 7 days.

NOTES:

One 12-ounce jar will yield about 8 ounces peppers. If you use a different-size jar, about one-third of the weight in the jar will be water and two-thirds will be peppers. Labels often include the drained weight.

This sauce is fabulous on grilled or sautéed fish or chicken.

ROASTED SALSA VERDE (GREEN TOMATILLO SALSA)

PREP TIME: 5 MINUTES • COOK TIME: 10 MINUTES

Yield: Makes 1 cup • *Portions: No protein or fat*

- **8 ounces (5–6 medium) tomatillos, husked and rinsed**
- **½ serrano chile or jalapeño, seeded (wear plastic gloves when handling)**
- **1 teaspoon fresh lime juice**
- **3 tablespoons finely chopped onion**
- **3 tablespoons finely chopped fresh cilantro**
- **⅛ teaspoon Celtic or pink Himalayan salt (optional)**

Preheat the broiler. Broil the tomatillos and chile on a baking sheet for 4 to 5 minutes, or until darkly roasted and evenly blackened in spots. Turn them over and roast the other side for 3 to 4 minutes, or until the tomatillos and chile are blistered and blackened.

In a blender or food processor, combine the tomatillos and chile along with any juice left on the baking sheet and the lime juice. Add 2 to 3 tablespoons water and blend or process to a coarse puree. Stir in the onion and cilantro by hand and taste to see if you'd like more lime juice. Add the salt (if using) only after tasting.

Refrigerate in a tightly sealed container for up to 5 days.

> **NOTES:**
>
> *There's no limit on serving size; you can have as much as you want because it's all vegetables and seasonings.*
>
> *Roasted Salsa Verde adds a lot of flavor. It's excellent on any roasted, grilled, or sautéed meat, poultry, or seafood, or on eggs.*

SANTA FE SAUCE

PREP TIME: 5 MINUTES

Yield: Makes fifteen–sixteen ¼-cup servings (3¾–4 cups) • *Portions: Negligible fat*

- 1 teaspoon ghee
- 1 onion, chopped
- 1 green bell pepper, chopped
- 1 can (28 ounces) fire-roasted tomatoes (see Notes)
- 2 cloves garlic, minced
- 1 teaspoon adobo sauce from canned chipotle chile peppers in adobo sauce
- 2 teaspoons ground cumin
- 1 teaspoon Celtic or pink Himalayan salt
- Pinch of cayenne
- ¼ cup coarsely chopped fresh cilantro

Melt the ghee in a deep skillet on medium-high heat. Add the onion and cook for 5 to 7 minutes, or until translucent. Add the bell pepper and cook for 5 minutes. Add the tomatoes, garlic, adobo sauce, cumin, salt, and cayenne and bring to a simmer. Reduce the heat to low and simmer for about 20 minutes, stirring occasionally to break up the tomatoes. Taste, adjust seasoning if necessary, and stir in the cilantro. Refrigerate in a tightly sealed container for up to 5 days.

To use this as a simmer sauce, you may need to thin it with bone broth made with chicken or fish or with water. Adding about ½ cup broth or water to 2 cups Santa Fe Sauce should give you the right consistency.

NOTES:

Fire-roasted tomatoes are currently available in diced or crushed form in 28-ounce cans from Muir Glen Organics; they are excellent!

In contrast with Smoky Chipotle Salsa (page 272), Santa Fe Sauce is meant to be served warm and is excellent on any roasted, grilled, or sautéed meat, poultry, or seafood, or on eggs.

There's no limit on serving size; you can have as much as you want because it's all vegetables and seasonings.

VARIATIONS:

To use as a simmer sauce for chicken: In a large deep skillet, bring 2 cups Santa Fe Sauce to a simmer over medium-high heat. If the sauce seems too thick, add about ½ cup Chicken Bone Broth (page 98) or water. Reduce the heat to medium, add 4 pieces of chicken, and simmer for about 20 minutes, or until an instant-read thermometer inserted in the thickest portion of the chicken registers 165°F (for boneless) or 170°F (for bone-in) and the juices run clear. Excellent served over Cauliflower Rice (page 222).

To use as a simmer sauce for fish: In a large, deep skillet, bring 2 cups Santa Fe Sauce to a simmer over medium-high heat. If the sauce seems too thick, add about ½ cup Chicken Bone Broth or Fish Bone Broth (page 98 or 103) or water. Reduce the heat to medium, add 4 pieces of whitefish (such as cod, tilapia, and so on), and simmer for 7 to 12 minutes, depending on the size and thickness of the fish, or until the fish flakes easily (see the Note about perfectly cooked fish on page 185). Excellent served over Cauliflower Rice (page 222).

SMOKY CHIPOTLE SALSA

PREP TIME: 10 MINUTES

Yield: Makes ¾–1 cup • *Portions:* No protein or fat

- 3 Roma tomatoes, seeded and cut in quarters
- ½ onion, cut into wedges
- 2 cloves garlic
- ½ jalapeño, seeded (wear plastic gloves when handling)
- ½ cup fresh cilantro
- 1 can (14.5 ounces) fire-roasted tomatoes (see Notes)
- 1 teaspoon chipotle chile pepper in adobo sauce +
  2 teaspoons adobo sauce
- 1 teaspoon Celtic or pink Himalayan salt
- ½ teaspoon ground cumin
- 3 tablespoons fresh lime juice

In a food processor or high-powered blender, combine the Roma tomatoes, onion, garlic, jalapeño, and cilantro. Pulse until everything is evenly chopped. Add the canned tomatoes, chipotle pepper and adobo sauce, salt, cumin, and lime juice. Pulse 2 or 3 times to thoroughly blend. Taste and adjust the seasonings as needed. Add more chipotle peppers if you like extra spice. Refrigerate in a tightly sealed container for up to 5 days.

NOTES:

Fire-roasted tomatoes are available in diced or crushed form in 14.5-ounce cans from Muir Glen Organics; they are excellent!

There's no limit on serving size; you can have as much as you want because it's all vegetables and seasonings.

Smoky Chipotle Salsa is excellent on any roasted, grilled, or sautéed meat, poultry, or seafood, or on eggs.

DESSERTS

BAKED APPLES

PREP TIME: 5 MINUTES • COOK TIME: 30 MINUTES

Yield: *Makes 4 servings* • *Portions*: *1 fruit*

2 organic baking apples

1 or more teaspoons ground cinnamon

Pinch of ground nutmeg

Pinch of ground ginger

Move an oven rack to the center of the oven. Preheat the oven to 350°F.

Wash and core the apples. Place in a baking dish and sprinkle with the cinnamon, nutmeg, and ginger. Add about ½" water to the bottom of the dish. Cover and bake for 30 minutes, then check for doneness. The apples should be soft when pierced with a knife. If they aren't soft enough, cover and return to the oven, checking every 5 minutes. Baking time will vary based on the size and type of apple.

To serve, top with the baking juices.

POACHED PEARS

PREP TIME: 10 MINUTES • COOK TIME: 30 MINUTES

Yield: Makes 4 servings • *Portions: 1 fruit*

- **2 firm pears**
- **½ cup water**
- **1 teaspoon pure vanilla extract or almond extract**
- **Pinch of your favorite spice: ground nutmeg, ginger, or cinnamon (optional)**

Peel, halve, and core the pears. Put in a skillet, cut side up, with the water. Add the vanilla or almond extract. Add the spice(s), if using. Cover and heat over medium-high heat until the water begins to simmer. Reduce the heat to low and simmer for 10 to 15 minutes, or until the pears are tender.

To serve, top with the poaching juices.

NOTE:

Very firm pears are better for poaching. My all-time favorite is Bosc; Comice and Bartlett are too soft and tend to fall apart when poached.

STRAWBERRIES WITH A BALSAMIC REDUCTION

PREP TIME: 5 MINUTES • COOK TIME: 10 MINUTES

Yield: Makes 4 servings • *Portions: 1 fruit*

- **¼ cup balsamic vinegar**
- **1 pound fresh strawberries (about 1 quart)**
- **Dash of ground black pepper (optional)**

In a small saucepan, simmer the vinegar over medium-low heat until it is reduced to half. Meanwhile, remove the strawberry caps and cut the berries in half. Place in a medium bowl. When the vinegar has reduced, let it cool for about 5 minutes, then pour over the berries. Add the black pepper (if using).

SHAKES

BAKED APPLE SHAKE

PREP TIME: 5 MINUTES

Yield: Makes 1 serving • *Portions: 1 protein, 1 fat, 1 fruit*

1 small apple

¼ teaspoon ground cinnamon

Pinch of nutmeg

2 tablespoons water

1 scoop Dr. Kellyann's Vanilla Bone Broth Protein or a Dr. Kellyann–approved protein powder (see Note)

1 cup unsweetened almond milk

⅓ cup full-fat coconut milk

1 teaspoon pure vanilla extract

1 tablespoon ground flaxseeds (optional)

1 tablespoon chia seeds (optional)

Handful of ice (optional)

Slice the apple, remove the seeds, and place in a microwaveable bowl. Sprinkle with the cinnamon and nutmeg. Add the water and microwave for about 3 minutes on high.

In a blender, combine the apple mixture, protein powder, almond milk, coconut milk, and vanilla. If desired, add the flaxseeds, chia seeds, and ice. Blend until smooth and creamy. Sprinkle with additional cinnamon or nutmeg.

NOTE:

See Dr. Kellyann's list of approved protein powders on the Resources page at drkellyann.com/resources.

EASY DOES IT: SWAP OUT MEALS OR SHAKES!

Too busy to cook? You can use a collagen shake as a meal replacement for breakfast, lunch, or dinner on the Bone Broth Diet. Prep your ingredients ahead of time, and you'll have a meal in minutes.

You can substitute any shake on pages 275–278 for a meal. Limit the fruit to half an individual piece (half an apple, half an orange) or a closed fistful, about ½ a cup, of diced fruit or berries.

Want to invent your own shakes? Just follow this formula.

DO-IT-YOURSELF SHAKE

PREP TIME: 3 MINUTES • YIELD: 1 SERVING

- 1 cup water, coconut milk (not canned), or almond milk, unsweetened and carrageenan-free
- 1 scoop Dr. Kellyann's Bone Broth Protein Powder (flavor of your choice)
- 1 serving fat (page 68)
- 2 handfuls of leafy greens or nonstarchy veggies (pages 66–67; optional)
- 1 portion of fruit, if desired.
- Stevia or monk fruit sweetener to taste (optional)
- Herbs and spices to taste (optional)

GREEN GODDESS SHAKE

PREP TIME: 2 MINUTES

Yield: Makes 1 serving • *Portions: 1 protein, 1 fat*

1 scoop Dr. Kellyann's Vanilla Bone Broth Protein or Dr. Kellyann-approved protein powder (see Note, page 275)

1 cup unsweetened almond milk

1 cup fresh spinach, tightly packed

½ avocado, pitted and peeled

¼ teaspoon pure vanilla extract

1 tablespoon ground flaxseeds (optional)

1 tablespoon chia seeds (optional)

   Handful of ice (optional)

In a blender, combine the protein powder, almond milk, spinach, avocado, and vanilla. If desired, add the flaxseeds, chia seeds, and ice. Blend until smooth and creamy.

STRAWBERRY SHAKE

PREP TIME: 3 MINUTES

Yield: Makes 1 serving • *Portions: 1 protein, 1 fruit*

1 scoop Dr. Kellyann's Vanilla Bone Broth Protein or Dr. Kellyann-approved protein powder (see Note, page 275)

1 cup unsweetened almond milk

   Handful of fresh or frozen strawberries (about ½ cup)

½–1 teaspoon pure vanilla extract

1 tablespoon ground flaxseeds (optional)

1 tablespoon chia seeds (optional)

   Handful of ice (optional)

In a blender, combine the protein powder, almond milk, strawberries, and vanilla. If desired, add the flaxseeds, chia seeds, and ice. Blend until smooth and creamy.

BLUE AND GREEN SHAKE

PREP TIME: 3 MINUTES

Yield: Makes 1 serving • *Portions: 1 protein, 1 fat, 1 fruit*

- **1 scoop Dr. Kellyann's Vanilla Bone Broth Protein or Dr. Kellyann-approved protein powder (see Note, page 275)**
- **1 cup unsweetened almond milk**
- **Handful of blueberries (about ½ cup)**
- **1 cup fresh spinach, packed**
- **½ avocado, pitted and peeled**
- **½–1 teaspoon pure vanilla extract**
- **1 tablespoon ground flaxseeds (optional)**
- **1 tablespoon chia seeds (optional)**
- **Handful of ice (optional)**

In a blender, combine the protein powder, almond milk, blueberries, spinach, avocado, and vanilla. If desired, add the flaxseeds, chia seeds, and ice. Blend until smooth and creamy.

MOCKTAILS

BLUEBERRY MOJITO MOCKTAIL

PREP TIME: 5 MINUTES

Yield: 4 servings • *Portions: No protein, fat, or fruit*

2½ limes, sliced into 20 wedges

¼ cup fresh mint leaves + more for garnish

1 cup blueberries, fresh or frozen (thawed)

1 quart club soda, seltzer, or sparkling water (8 ounces per serving)

Stevia or monk fruit sweetener to taste (optional)

Place 16 of the lime wedges into an unbreakable bowl. Add the mint leaves and blueberries. Using a cocktail muddler or meat tenderizing mallet, mash the limes, mint, and blueberries to extract the juices and oils. Pour the mixture into a glass jar with a lid, add ¼ cup water, and shake to combine. Strain a quarter of the mixture through a fine-mesh sieve into a glass filled with ice and top with 8 ounces of the club soda. Add sweetener, if desired. Garnish with one of the remaining lime wedges. Repeat with the remaining mojito mixture or store leftovers in the lidded jar in the refrigerator for up to 3 days.

NOTES:

By adding the club soda when you are ready to enjoy the mocktail, it won't lose its effervescence.

If you don't like carbonated water, use flat water.

For a collagen boost, add a serving of plain, unflavored collagen protein or hydrolyzed collagen.

CUCUMBER GIMLET MOCKTAIL

PREP TIME: 10 MINUTES

Yield: 4 *servings* • *Portions:* No protein, fat, or fruit

2 cucumbers

4 limes + 4 lime wedges

1 quart club soda, seltzer, or sparkling water (8 ounces per serving)

Stevia or monk fruit sweetener to taste (optional)

Slice 4 wheels from one of the cucumbers to use for garnish, then peel, seed, and coarsely chop the remainder of the cucumbers. Place in a blender or a food processer and puree until smooth. Strain the pureed cucumber through a fine-mesh sieve, pressing to get as much liquid as possible. Discard the solids and pour the cucumber juice into a glass jar with a lid. Juice 4 of the limes. Add the lime juice and ¼ cup water to the cucumber juice and shake to combine.

Pour a quarter of the mixture into a tall glass filled with ice and top with 8 ounces of the club soda. Add sweetener, if desired. Garnish with a cucumber wheel and a lime wedge. Repeat with the remaining gimlet mixture or store leftovers in the lidded jar in the refrigerator for up to 2 days.

> **NOTES:**
>
> *By adding the club soda when you are ready to enjoy the mocktail, it won't lose its effervescence.*
>
> *If you don't like carbonated water, use flat water.*
>
> *For a collagen boost, add a serving of plain, unflavored collagen protein or hydro-lyzed collagen.*

LEMON-BASIL SPRITZER

PREP TIME: 5 MINUTES

Yield: 4 servings • Portions: No protein, fat, or fruit

¼ cup packed basil leaves + 4 more for garnish

4½ lemons, sliced into 20 wedges

1 quart club soda, seltzer, or sparkling water (8 ounces per serving)

Stevia or monk fruit sweetener to taste (optional)

Place 16 of the lemon wedges and the basil leaves into a unbreakable bowl. Using a cocktail muddler or meat tenderizing mallet, mash the lemons and basil to extract the juices and oils. Pour the mixture into a glass jar with a lid, add ¼ cup water, and shake to combine. Strain a quarter of the mixture through a fine-mesh sieve into a glass filled with ice and top with 8 ounces of the club soda. Add sweetener, if desired. Garnish with one of the remaining lemon wedges and a basil leaf. Repeat with remaining spritzer mixture or store in the lidded jar in the refrigerator for up to 3 days.

NOTES:

By adding the club soda when you are ready to enjoy the spritzer, it won't lose its effervescence.

If you don't like carbonated water, use flat water.

For a collagen boost, add a serving of plain, unflavored collagen protein or hydrolyzed collagen.

SALTED THYME AND MEYER LEMON MOCKTAIL

PREP TIME: 5 MINUTES

Yield: 4 servings • *Portions:* No protein, fat, or fruit

2½ **Meyer lemons, sliced in 20 wedges**

  6 **sprigs of fresh thyme**

    Pinch Celtic or pink Himalayan salt

  1 **quart club soda, seltzer, or sparkling water**

    Stevia or monk fruit sweetener to taste (optional)

Place 16 of the lemon wedges and 4 of the thyme sprigs in an unbreakable bowl. Using a cocktail muddler or meat tenderizing mallet, mash the lemons and thyme to extract the juices and oils. Pour the mixture into a glass jar with a lid, add ¼ cup water and the salt, and shake to combine. Strain a quarter of the mixture through a fine-mesh sieve into a glass filled with ice and top with 8 ounces of the club soda. Add sweetener, if desired. Garnish with one of the remaining lemon wedges and a thyme sprig. Repeat with remaining lemon-thyme mixture or store leftovers in the lidded jar in the refrigerator for up to 3 days.

NOTES:

By adding the club soda when you are ready to enjoy the mocktail, it won't lose its effervescence.

If you don't like carbonated water, use flat water.

For a collagen boost, add a serving of plain, unflavored collagen protein or hydro-lyzed collagen.

You can experiment using other herbs. Mint and lavender are great combinations with lemon.

RECIPES CONTAINING GELATIN

Remember the amazing gut-healing and wrinkle-blasting effects of gelatin I talked about in Chapter 3? In addition to obtaining gelatin from bone broth, you can obtain it from store-bought gelatin. It's such a powerful slimming, healing, and beautifying food that I'm including a special section of gelatin-based recipes here.

SWEET BLACK CHERRY GUMMIES

PREP TIME: 5 MINUTES • COOK TIME: 3 MINUTES

Yield: Makes ten 2½-piece servings • Portions: 1 fruit

- ¼–½ teaspoon coconut oil or coconut oil spray
- ¾ cup cold water
- 4 tablespoons unflavored pasture-raised beef gelatin, such as Great Lakes Gelatin
- ½ cup unsweetened apple juice
- 1 cup Chicken Bone Broth (page 98)
- 2 cups fresh or frozen black cherries, pitted and pureed

Brush or spray 24 cups of a mini muffin pan lightly with the oil.

Put the water in a small bowl. Pour the gelatin into the water and let stand for about 1 minute to soften.

Heat the apple juice and broth in a medium saucepan over medium-high heat. When the juice simmers, add the gelatin mixture and stir until completely dissolved. Remove from the heat and combine with the pureed cherries. Pour into the prepared muffin pan cups and refrigerate for 3 or more hours, or until firmly set.

To serve, run a knife around the edge of each muffin cup and gently coax out each gummie.

PANNA COTTA WITH
BALSAMIC-SOAKED STRAWBERRIES

PREP TIME: 5 MINUTES • COOK TIME: 3 MINUTES

Yield: Makes 10 servings • Portions: ½ fat, 1 fruit

PANNA COTTA

- ½ cup cold water
- 2 tablespoons unflavored pasture-raised beef gelatin, such as Great Lakes Gelatin
- ¼ cup unsweetened apple juice
- 2 cans (14 ounces each) full-fat coconut milk
- 2 or more teaspoons pure vanilla extract

STRAWBERRIES

- 4 cups fresh strawberries
- 2–3 tablespoons balsamic vinegar

To make the panna cotta: Put the water in a small bowl. Pour the gelatin into the water and let stand for about 1 minute to soften.

Heat the apple juice in a medium saucepan over medium-high heat. When the juice simmers, add the gelatin mixture and stir until completely dissolved. Remove from the heat and stir in the coconut milk and vanilla. Pour into 10 ramekins or custard cups and refrigerate for 3 or more hours, or until firmly set.

To make the strawberries: Wash the strawberries, cut off the caps, slice the berries, and place in a medium bowl. Pour the vinegar over the berries, stir, and let stand for 5 minutes. Refrigerate if not serving immediately.

To serve, run a knife around the edge of a ramekin and tip the panna cotta onto a small plate. Top with the berry mixture.

SALMON MOUSSE

PREP TIME: 15 MINUTES • COOK TIME: 5 MINUTES

Yield: Makes 9 servings • Portions: ¼ protein, ½ fat

1¼ cups Chicken Bone Broth (page 98) or Fish Bone Broth (page 103), divided

1 tablespoon unflavored pasture-raised beef gelatin, such as Great Lakes Gelatin

1 cup coconut milk

2 tablespoons Homemade Mayonnaise (page 262)

1 tablespoon finely chopped celery

1 tablespoon finely chopped onion

1 tablespoon fresh lemon juice

1 teaspoon finely chopped fresh dill

1 teaspoon lemon peel

1 teaspoon smoked paprika

Pinch of cayenne

½ teaspoon Celtic or pink Himalayan salt

¼ teaspoon ground black pepper

1 can (7½ ounces) red salmon, drained and finely flaked

Put ¼ cup of the broth in a small bowl. Sprinkle the gelatin over the broth and let stand for 1 minute to soften. In a medium saucepan, bring another ½ cup broth to a boil and add the gelatin mixture. Stir until the gelatin is completely dissolved. Remove from the heat and allow to cool to room temperature.

Add the coconut milk, mayonnaise, celery, onion, lemon juice, dill, lemon peel, paprika, cayenne, salt, black pepper, and the remaining ½ cup broth to the gelatin mixture. Gently fold in the salmon and transfer to a 1-quart mold or small loaf pan. Refrigerate for about 3 hours, or until set.

Serve as a spread with celery, carrots, jicama slices, zucchini sticks, etc., or on a bed of lettuce.

VARIATION:

You can substitute crab or shrimp for the salmon.

GAZPACHO MOLDED SALAD

PREP TIME: 10 MINUTES • COOK TIME: 3 MINUTES

Yield: Makes 8 servings • *Portions: Negligible fat*

¼–½ teaspoon coconut oil or coconut oil spray

2½ cups Chicken Bone Broth (page 98), divided

2 tablespoons unflavored pasture-raised beef gelatin, such as Great Lakes Gelatin

1 cup Roma tomatoes, seeded and diced

1 cup finely chopped avocado (about 1 medium)

½ cup finely chopped English cucumber

½ cup finely chopped red onion

¼ cup finely chopped red bell pepper

1 small jalapeño, seeded and finely chopped (wear plastic gloves when handling)

1 clove garlic

¼ cup chopped fresh cilantro

1 tablespoon lime juice

1 teaspoon ground cumin

1 teaspoon Celtic or pink Himalayan salt

Brush or spray a 1-quart mold or loaf pan with the oil.

Put ½ cup of the broth in a small bowl. Pour the gelatin into the broth and let stand for about 1 minute to soften. In a medium saucepan, heat the remaining 2 cups broth until it simmers. Add the gelatin mixture and stir until it completely dissolves. Let cool to room temperature.

Add the tomatoes, avocado, cucumber, onion, bell pepper, jalapeño, garlic, cilantro, lime juice, cumin, and salt to the gelatin mixture. Pour into the prepared mold or pan and chill for about 3 hours, or until firm. Remove the salad from the mold or pan and turn out onto a platter. If it doesn't unmold easily, put the pan in a hot water bath for 1 minute or less.

NOTE:

Serve on a bed of lettuce.

CHICKEN PÂTÉ

PREP TIME: 10 MINUTES • COOK TIME: 3 MINUTES

Yield: Makes 8 servings • *Portions: Negligible fat*

¼–½ teaspoon coconut oil or coconut oil spray

1 cup Chicken Bone Broth (page 98), divided

2 tablespoons unflavored pasture-raised beef gelatin, such as Great Lakes Gelatin

1 cup full-fat coconut milk

1 tablespoon white vinegar

2 cups white and dark meat chicken, shredded or very finely chopped (see Notes)

6 spears asparagus, blanched and finely sliced

2 tablespoons finely chopped red onion

¼ cup roasted red peppers, cut into very small pieces

¼ cup Spanish olives, thinly sliced

1 small clove garlic, minced

1 tablespoon finely chopped fresh tarragon or 1 teaspoon dried

Brush or spray a 1-quart mold or loaf pan with the oil.

Put ½ cup of the broth in a small bowl. Pour the gelatin into the broth and let stand for about 1 minute to soften. In a medium saucepan, heat the coconut milk and the remaining ½ cup broth until they simmer. Add the gelatin mixture and stir until it completely dissolves. Let cool to room temperature.

Add the vinegar, chicken, asparagus, onion, peppers, olives, garlic, and tarragon to the gelatin mixture. Pour into the prepared mold or pan and chill for about 3 hours, or until firm. Remove the salad from the mold or pan and turn out onto a platter. If it doesn't unmold easily, put the pan in a hot water bath for 1 minute or less.

NOTES:

This is a great place to use the soft chicken meat from your Chicken Bone Broth (page 98). Poached chicken also works well. If you shred the chicken, it will be more difficult to slice than if it's finely chopped, but I prefer bigger pieces. Use a serrated knife to slice.

Serve on a bed of lettuce.

Making Deposits in the "Good Health Bank"

Melissa Joulwan is the author of the cookbooks *Well Fed: Paleo Recipes for People Who Love to Eat* and *Well Fed 2: More Paleo Recipes for People Who Love to Eat* and the driving force behind the blog *MelJoulwan.com*. You can also find her on Twitter and Instagram at @meljoulwan.

Melissa, who's also a coauthor of the recipes in the *New York Times* best-selling book *It Starts with Food,* by Melissa Hartwig and Dallas Hartwig, struggled for decades with weight and health problems. She turned that life around. Here's how she keeps balanced now.

"I have excellent habits 95 percent of the time. I sleep 8 to 9 hours per night to recover from and prepare for heavy barbell lifting, occasional sprints, and plenty of yoga and walking. I stock the house with healthy foods and cook nutrient-dense meals so my husband and I can eat real food every day.

"Then, on rare occasions, I indulge. I become a temporary slug and give in to the temptation of grass-fed ice cream, buttered popcorn, or an icy-cold glass of Prosecco. I should also mention that I have a known whipped cream problem.

"These minor nutritional off-road excursions are possible because I make deposits in the good health bank the rest of the time. Every workout, every good night's sleep, every cup of bone broth, every healthy meal is a deposit, so that once in a while, I can make withdrawals for a food treat."

Eating Well on a Budget

Gunnar Lovelace, CEO, Thrive Market

thrivemarket.com

Here's what my friend Gunnar, CEO of Thrive Market, says about eating healthy on a budget.

"For far too many people, healthy food is just out of reach. Why? Because it's so expensive. I grew up with a single mom and saw this struggle firsthand. She worked so hard to make healthy choices. She later remarried a man who ran a health-food buying club from an organic farm where we lived in Ojai, California. I realized that healthy living can be accessed at much lower prices when people work together. For years, I've been interested in creating the 21st-century version of a health-food co-op online. That's why I started Thrive Market.

"Thrive Market is an online shopping club offering organic, non-GMO foods and healthy products at wholesale prices. Like a co-op, Thrive Market uses the power of group buying to dramatically drop the prices on the highest-quality natural foods and supplements, nontoxic cleaners and home goods, and environmentally safe bath and beauty products. For the first time ever, more than 3,000 healthy, natural foods and products are available at the same price (if not lower!) as conventional, highly processed options.

"I keep my kitchen stocked with healthy foods by shopping at just two places: Thrive Market for nonperishable staples and pantry essentials and my local farmers' market for fresh produce. A community supported agriculture (CSA) box is another great way to get fresh, local fruits and vegetables. I know I'm more likely to cook myself a healthy meal if I have a pantry brimming with spices, oils, vinegars, and other cooking supplies."

MUSHROOM PÂTÉ

PREP TIME: 10 MINUTES • COOK TIME: 3 MINUTES

Yield: Makes 8 servings • *Portions:* Negligible fat

- ¼–½ teaspoon coconut oil or coconut oil spray
- 2 tablespoons unflavored pasture-raised beef gelatin, such as Great Lakes Gelatin
- 1 cup Beef Bone Broth (page 100), divided
- 1 cup full-fat coconut milk
- 2 teaspoons fresh tarragon or 1 teaspoon dried
- 2 cups finely chopped cremini mushrooms or a combination of your favorite mushrooms (see Note)
- 2 tablespoons finely chopped onion
- 1 small clove garlic, minced
- 1 teaspoon Celtic or pink Himalayan salt
- ¼ teaspoon ground black pepper

Brush or spray a 1-quart mold or loaf pan with the oil.

Put ½ cup of the broth in a small bowl. Pour the gelatin into the broth and let stand for about 1 minute to soften. In a medium saucepan, heat the coconut milk, tarragon, and the remaining ½ cup broth to a simmer. Add the gelatin mixture and stir until it completely dissolves. Let cool to room temperature.

Add the mushrooms, onion, garlic, salt, and pepper to the gelatin mixture. Pour into the prepared mold or pan and chill for about 3 hours, or until firm. Remove from the mold or pan and turn out onto a platter. If it doesn't unmold easily, put the pan in a hot water bath for 1 minute or less.

NOTE:

White button mushrooms are the least flavorful. It's better to use cremini.

CHAPTER 9

Making It Easy

Meal Plans and Tips for Batch Cooking

I'LL ADMIT IT UP front: This diet isn't as simple as those programs that deliver tasteless, premade frozen-food packets to your doorstep. But wouldn't you rather eat real food than something from a plastic container? I thought so!

And here's good news: There are ways to make this diet really, really simple. In Chapters 7 and 8, I outlined supereasy meals that take just minutes to make—and even no-cook meals you can grab at the grocery store. If you do want to cook, this chapter provides you with meal plans that will take the work out of deciding what's for dinner (or lunch or breakfast). In addition, you'll find a shopping list that includes the ingredients you'll need—and best of all, I'll give you advice on how to use your time efficiently in the kitchen by doing batch cooking.

3 WEEKS OF MEAL PLANS

In addition to making your meals fun, I want your meal planning to be easy as possible. That's because I know that like me, you already have way too much to do every day.

So to simplify things for you, I've developed complete meal plans for each week of your diet. These plans allow you to cut down on cooking time and make great use of your leftovers. Here they are. Note that each week includes 5 days of meals, because you'll be doing your bone broth intermittent fasts on the other 2 days.

Meal Plan 1 (see also, "Assembling the Perfect Plate" on page 120 and suggestions for fat portions on page 122)

WEEK 1

	DAY 1	DAY 2	DAY 3	DAY 4	DAY 5
Breakfast	Baked Scotch Eggs (page 126)— 1 protein, ½ fat (double recipe; serve leftovers for day 3 breakfast) Handful of berries—1 fruit	Baked Egg Cups with Spinach (page 125)— 1 protein, ½ fat (double recipe; serve leftovers for day 4 breakfast) Handful of berries—1 fruit	Baked Scotch Eggs (leftovers from day 1 breakfast)— 1 protein, ½ fat Handful of berries—1 fruit	Baked Egg Cups with Spinach (leftovers from day 2 breakfast)— 1 protein, ½ fat Handful of berries—1 fruit	Southwest Breakfast Scramble (page 139)— 1 protein, ½ fat Handful of berries—1 fruit
Lunch	Turkey Meatloaf Loaded with Vegetables (page 169) with Ketchup (page 262)— 1 protein (double recipe; serve leftovers for day 4 lunch) Large garden salad with any Bone Broth Diet salad dressing (see Chapter 8)— 2 vegetables, 1 fat	Easy Roast Chicken Breasts (leftovers from day 1 dinner)— 1 protein Large garden salad with any Bone Broth Diet salad dressing— 2 vegetables, 1 fat	Turkey Taco Salad (page 171; use leftover turkey chili from day 2 dinner)— 1 protein, 2 vegetables, 1 fat	Turkey Meatloaf (leftovers from day 1 lunch) with Ketchup— 1 protein Mediterranean Peasant Salad (leftovers from day 3 dinner) served over 2 handfuls lettuce topped with a handful of olives— 2 vegetables, 1½ fat	Orange Chicken Salad (use leftover chicken from day 4 dinner)— 1 protein, 2 vegetables, 1 fat
Dinner	Easy Roast Chicken Breasts (page 149)— 1 protein (make enough for 2 meals by roasting a chicken with a raw weight of 4+ lbs or 2 smaller chickens of approx. 2½ lbs; serve leftovers for day 2 lunch) Steamed vegetables— 1 vegetable Garden salad with any Bone Broth Diet salad dressing—1 fat vegetable, 1 fat	Rich and Hearty Turkey Chili (page 168)— 1 protein (serve leftovers for day 3 lunch) Cauliflower Rice (page 222)— 1 vegetable (double recipe; serve leftovers for day 4 dinner) Garden salad with any Bone Broth Diet salad dressing— 1 vegetable, 1 fat	Greek-Style Beef or Bison Burger (page 182) served on a roasted portobello mushroom— 1 protein, 1 vegetable Mediterranean Peasant Salad (page 232)— 1 vegetable, ½ fat (double recipe; serve leftovers for day 4 lunch) Top each burger with 1 tablespoon of Homemade Mayonnaise (page 258)— 1 fat	Chicken with Orange-Rosemary Sauce (page 155)— 1 protein (serve leftovers for day 5 lunch) Cauliflower Rice (leftovers from day 2 dinner)— 1 vegetable Garden salad with ½ any Bone Broth Diet dressing— 1 vegetable, 1 fat	Roasted Salmon Gremolata (page 185)— 1 protein, 1 fat Steamed asparagus— 1 vegetable Garlic Mashed Cauliflower "Potatoes" (page 223)— 1 vegetable Poached Pear (page 274; Friday-night dessert)—1 fruit

Meal Plan
WEEK 2

	DAY 1	DAY 2	DAY 3	DAY 4	DAY 5
Breakfast	Mediterranean Scramble (page 132)— 1 protein, ½ fat Handful of berries—1 fruit	Pork and Eggs (page 133; use leftover pork loin from day 1 dinner)— 1 protein, ½ fat, 1 fruit	Vegetable Frittata (page 141)— 1 protein, ½ fat (serve leftovers for day 5 breakfast) Handful of berries—1 fruit	Smoked Salmon and Eggs (page 138)— 1 protein Handful of berries—1 fruit	Vegetable Frittata (leftovers from day 3)— 1 protein, ½ fat Handful of berries—1 fruit
Lunch	Kale Salad with Turkey (page 170)— 1 protein, 2 vegetables, 1 fat	Tuna-Stuffed Tomato (page 195) topped with ¼ of an avocado, sliced— 1 protein, 2 vegetables, 1 fat	Chopped Balsamic Chicken Salad (page 156)— 1 protein, 2 vegetables, 1 fat	Stir-Fry, your choice of beef, chicken, or shrimp (leftovers from day 3 dinner)— 1 protein, 2 vegetables, 1 fat	Fiesta Beef Fajitas (leftovers from day 4 dinner) topped with ¼ of avocado (sliced)— 1 protein, 1 vegetable, 1 fat Cauliflower Rice (leftovers from day 4 dinner)— 1 vegetable
Dinner	Balsamic Roast Pork Loin (page 184)— 1 protein (use leftovers in day 2 breakfast) Large serving roasted vegetables— 2 vegetables	Sliced turkey breast— 1 protein Large garden salad with any Bone Broth Diet salad dressing— 2 vegetables, 1 fat	Stir-fry with your choice of beef, chicken, or shrimp (page 157)— 1 protein, 2 vegetables, 1 fat (double recipe; serve leftovers for day 4 lunch) Cauliflower Rice (page 222)— 1 vegetable (double recipe; serve leftovers for day 5 lunch)	Fiesta Beef Fajitas (page 181) topped with ¼ of avocado (sliced)— 1 protein, 1 vegetable, 1 fat (serve leftovers for day 5 lunch)	One-Skillet Zucchini Pasta with Sausage (page 162) topped with a handful of sliced olives— 1 protein, 2 vegetables, 1½ fat Baked Apple (page 273; Friday-night dessert)— 1 fruit

Meal Plan
WEEK 3

	DAY 1	DAY 2	DAY 3	DAY 4	DAY 5
Breakfast	Sausage-and-Apple Frittata (page 136)— 1 protein, ½ fat, 1 fruit (double recipe; serve leftovers for day 3 breakfast)	Zucchini Breakfast Cakes (page 142)— 1 protein, ½ fat (double recipe; serve leftovers for day 4 breakfast) Handful of berries—1 fruit	Sausage-and-Apple Frittata (leftovers from day 1 breakfast)—1 protein, ½ fat, 1 fruit	Zucchini Breakfast cakes (leftovers from day 2 breakfast)— 1 protein, ½ fat Handful of berries—1 fruit	Beef, Egg, and Mushroom Breakfast (page 127)— 1 protein, ½ fat Handful of berries—1 fruit
Lunch	One-Skillet Zucchini Pasta with Sausage (page 162) topped with a handful of sliced olives— 1 protein, 2 vegetables, 1½ fat	Chicken Salad with Crunch (page 160)— 1 protein, 2 vegetables, 1 fat	Curried Chicken (leftovers from day 2 dinner)— 1 protein, 1 vegetables Cauliflower Rice (leftovers from day 2 dinner)— 1 vegetable with 1 Tbsp ghee— 1 vegetable, 1 fat	Asian Turkey Burger (leftovers from day 3 dinner)— 1 protein Napa Slaw with Creamy Ginger Dressing (leftovers from day 3 dinner)— 2 vegetables, 1 fat	1 roasted or grilled chicken breast (sliced and served on salad)— 1 protein Large garden salad with any Bone Broth Diet salad dressing— 2 vegetables, 1 fat
Dinner	Braised Chicken with Leeks and Mushrooms (page 159)— 1 protein, ½ fat Steamed asparagus— 2 vegetables Drizzle 1 tablespoon melted ghee over steamed asparagus— 1 fat	Creamy Chicken Curry (page 145)— 1 protein, 1 vegetable (double recipe; serve leftovers for day 3 lunch) Cauliflower Rice (page 222) with 1 Tbsp ghee— 1 vegetable, 1 fat (double recipe; serve leftovers for day 3 lunch)	Asian Turkey Burger (page 172)— 1 protein (double recipe; serve leftovers for day 4 lunch) Napa Slaw with Creamy Ginger Dressing (page 227)— 2 vegetables, 1 fat (double recipe; serve leftovers for day 4 lunch)	Salmon Gremolata— 1 protein, ½ fat Steamed Brussels sprouts— 1 vegetable Steamed green beans— 1 vegetable Drizzle 1 tablespoon melted ghee over steamed vegetables— 1 fat	Easy Beef or Bison Burger (page 173)— 1 protein Sautéed mushrooms and spinach with 1 Tbsp ghee or coconut oil— 2 vegetables, 1 fat Strawberries with a Balsamic Reduction (page 274; Friday-night dessert)—1 fruit

REMINDER

If you want to create your own recipes, you'll find a handy At-a-Glance Meal Plan on page 74. This plan makes it easy for you to calculate your servings for each meal.

Things to stock for your diet

The best way to succeed on this diet is to ensure you have everything you need on hand. Here's a list of all the ingredients you'll require for the 3 weeks of meals in the meal plans.

Proteins

Fresh eggs

Hard-cooked eggs

Chicken breasts (in the freezer)

Ground turkey or chicken (in the freezer)

Ground lean beef/bison (in the freezer)

Deli-sliced turkey—sugar-, dextrose-, nitrate-, and gluten-free (Applegate brand)

Canned tuna

Canned salmon

Smoked salmon—sugar-, dextrose-, nitrate, and gluten-free and wild, not farm-raised if possible

1 whole chicken, several legs and/or thighs, necks and backs, and at least 6 chicken feet or a pig's foot for Chicken Bone Broth (in the freezer)

5 pounds or more of beef bones such as knuckles, joints, feet, and marrow bones, as well as 2 to 3 pounds meaty bones such as oxtail, short ribs, and shank for Beef Bone Broth (in the freezer)

Fats

Olive oil

Coconut oil

Ghee

Fresh avocados—3 or 4 per week

2 cans olives, sliced or whole

Seeds or nuts (optional)

Bone Broth Diet salad dressings (see Chapter 8)—make at least 2 kinds

Vegetables

Several boxes/bags prewashed salad greens—for instance, baby kale, spring mix, romaine hearts, spinach, or arugula

Any of your favorite precut and prewashed vegetables on the Bone Broth Diet list

Celery

Carrots

Sweet potatoes or yams—4 or more

Cauliflower

Roma tomatoes for cooking—4 or more

Cucumber

Any of your favorite green vegetables, such as broccoli, asparagus, cabbage, Brussels sprouts, chard, or kale

Onions

Garlic

Fresh ginger—1 knob

Any of your favorite fresh herbs, such as parsley, cilantro, basil, or thyme

Fruits

Fresh berries—blueberries, strawberries, blackberries, and/or raspberries

Frozen berries—keep 2 bags in the freezer

Lemons—2 or 3

Limes—2 or 3

Tomatoes for salads—cherry, grape, heirloom, etc.

Seasonings and Spices

Celtic or pink Himalayan salt

Black pepper

Coconut aminos

Hot sauce

Bay leaves

Italian seasoning

Bell's Seasoning

Dried thyme

Dried basil

Ancho chili powder

Chili powder

Cinnamon

Cumin

Nutmeg

Hungarian or sweet paprika

Cayenne (ground red pepper)

Garlic powder

Red wine vinegar

Balsamic vinegar

Cider vinegar

Any of your favorite fresh herbs, such as parsley, cilantro, basil, thyme, etc. (also noted under Vegetables)

Canned, Jarred, or Bottled Goods

Large cans (28 ounces) diced tomatoes, sugar-, dextrose-, and gluten-free— 2 or 3

Small cans (6 ounces) tomato paste—2

Tuna (also listed under Proteins)

Salmon (also listed under Proteins)

Chipotle chile peppers in adobo sauce

Roasted red peppers

Coconut aminos (also listed under Seasonings and Spices)

Hot sauce (also listed under Seasonings and Spices)

Full-fat coconut milk—several cans

Here's a tip: It's a good idea to stock your kitchen as thoroughly as possible before you start the diet. That way, you can avoid those grocery aisles filled with candy, chips, and cookies. When you do need to make trips to the store to restock your fridge or pantry during your diet, here are some pointers for temptation-free shopping.

- Stick to your shopping list! Plan your meals ahead of time, and write down exactly what you'll need to have on hand. Decide that you will buy only food items that are on your list. Period.

- Eat well and drink plenty of water before you shop. When you're hungry, your willpower drops like a rock, and a chocolate doughnut can go from mildly tempting to irresistible.

- Shop the perimeter of the store. I know you've heard this rule before, but it's truly one of the easiest ways to shop smart. The perimeter is where you'll find nearly all of your core foods: meat, eggs, fish, fruits, and vegetables. Make side trips into the inner rows only for specific items.

- Read labels. Food manufacturers sneak additives, colorings, sugar, and other garbage into nearly every product you can imagine. So when you depart from the store perimeter and venture into the danger zone, read labels carefully. Remember to look for those "danger words" I listed back in Chapter 4.

Shopping Smart

Vani Hari, creator of FoodBabe.com and *New York Times* **bestselling author of** *The Food Babe Way*

foodbabe.com

Vani likes to say, "The only person who decides what you put in your body is you." Here's her advice for making your decisions.

"Every bite of food that passes through our lips—and every glass of water we drink—is a potential source of toxic chemicals, including pesticide residue, preservatives, artificial flavors and colorings, addicting sugars and fats, genetically modified organisms, and more. These toxins can travel to and settle into all the organs of your body, particularly the liver, kidneys, gastrointestinal tract, and lungs, and do great damage. Scientists are now blaming chemical-ridden food for the dramatic rise in obesity, heart disease, chronic fatigue syndrome, infertility, dementia, mental illness, and more. Our food system is in dire shape, and so are we.

"So what are we supposed to do? While some additives may be safe in small quantities, the FDA cannot regulate cumulative consumption when particular additives are being added to an insurmountable number of foods without any postmarket oversight. For instance, even if you think you're eating healthy, you could easily be eating small doses of several controversial ingredients over and over again in every meal of that day. Michael Taylor, the FDA's deputy commissioner for food, even admitted recently: 'We do not know the volume of particular chemicals that are going into the food supply so we can diagnose trends. We do not know what is going on postmarket.'[1]

"This is why you must read ingredient lists. If you don't know why a particular ingredient is there for health reasons, put the product back down. The majority of food additives and chemicals that have been invented in the last 50 years are there for only one reason: to improve the bottom line of the food industry. If they are not there to improve your health, why take the risk?"

TIPS FOR BATCH COOKING

Does this ever happen to you? You start a diet—but a week or so into it, you have a crazy day. Maybe you need to work late, or you have a family crisis.

When you get home, you're stressed, exhausted, and hungry. You have tons of healthy food in the fridge and the freezer, but you don't have the energy to thaw, chop, and cook it. And as the minutes on the clock tick by, that delivery menu from the Chinese restaurant or the pizza place starts to look better and better.

I totally understand this feeling. I've fallen for the takeout route plenty of times myself, when I've come home weary and faced two ravenous boys. I know from experience that this is the easiest time of the day to pick up the phone and order the same foods that put those extra pounds on in the first place.

Luckily, I've discovered a simple way to avoid this diet downfall. And better yet, it's fun. It's batch cooking. I also refer to this concept as food management. In any successful restaurant or organized home, there has to be some kind of management system. Think of this as an assembly line, an easy way to maximize results.

Here's the secret: You can make lots of food in a very short amount of time if you're organized. For instance, you can brown enough hamburger, sauté enough chicken, or chop enough onions for three or four recipes. And you can make double or triple batches of chili, stew, or soup. Smart planning like this can get you in and out of the kitchen in record time, with your fridge and freezer filled with ready-to-go ingredients and meals.

Now, I'll grant you that "batch-cooking day" is a bit of a project. However, it's also a fun time to share with kids (even the littlest ones can help stir or mix) or with a partner. And you'll thank yourself for it later.

That's because one day, not too long from now, you're going to come home exhausted and starving, and you'll realize that you don't need to cook dinner. So instead of panicking and blowing your diet, you're going to put your feet up, put on a movie, and relax—and say a big thank-you to yourself.

How to batch-cook your proteins for the week

Look through the recipes and see what strikes your fancy. Be sure to check out the supereasy protein recipes for burgers, a beef roast, chicken, turkey, a pork roast, curry, chili, sausage, and tuna. Most of your breakfast proteins can also be made ahead and refrigerated or frozen. For instance, if you're making a frittata, make two instead of one.

Decide what you want to prepare for the week. Assuming that you're cooking for four people, here's a sample list that will give you three protein portions (breakfast, lunch, and dinner) per day for 5 days.

- Turkey or Chicken Italian Sausage (page 163): Make 3 or more pounds; cook it all and freeze 2 pounds in 1-pound portions or shape as patties and freeze.

- Easy Roast Chicken Breasts (page 149): Make eight or more; freeze in individual portions for a grab-and-go meal.

- Rich and Hearty Turkey Chili (page 168): It's a double recipe you can make in a slow cooker; enjoy a second meal later in the week.

- Easy Roast Chicken (page 150): Roast a whole bird. Have it for dinner and save the leftovers for lunches.

- Easy Beef or Bison Burgers (page 173): Make 3 or more pounds; freeze 2 pounds shaped as patties and refrigerate the others to cook for another meal.

- Hard-cook eight eggs.

- Make a dozen Baked Egg Cups with Spinach (page 125).

Now, here's an important tip: Before you start cooking, build your *mise en place*. That's the French term for setting up your ingredients ahead of cooking time. Trust me on this—before I started following this rule religiously, I can't tell you how many times I got halfway through a recipe before I discovered that I was missing an ingredient. When you follow the mise en place rule, this won't happen to you.

Next, look through the recipes you want to make and find the common elements. For instance, you may need a total of three chopped onions, six cloves of minced garlic, and salt, pepper, garlic powder, Bell's Seasoning, and Italian seasoning. Prepare all these ingredients first. Then just grab what you need for each recipe and put it together. Simple.

How to batch-prepare your vegetables for the week

The easiest way to always have what you need is to wash and prep a variety of vegetables and pack them in tightly sealed containers or resealable plastic bags on your batch-cooking day. Figure that over the week you'll be having some salads, several steamed vegetables, several roasted vegetable medleys, and plenty of crunchy vegetables to enjoy as crudités with one of the Bone Broth Diet dressings. Review the vegetable list in the book and make a list of what you're likely to want.

Once your refrigerator is stocked and ready for the week, here are some ways you can prep your veggies on your batch-cooking day.

BONE BROTH DIET DEVOTEES

Joanne Abbott

I've lost more than 14 pounds in 21 days. I'm thrilled with that. My skin is much better. It's clearer, and I'm hoping the rosacea will continue to subside. I've been feeling really good—no napping during the day. The kids are very proud of me, and my husband's very proud of me, and everyone notices it. People are like, "What are you eating?"

BEFORE   AFTER

- Wash and cut celery, carrots, radishes, and onions. Store them in water in individual containers (you don't want the carrots to taste like onions) with tight-fitting lids. The water will keep them crunchy.

- Wash and cut some of the other vegetables you'll be using during the week. If you aren't sure you'll be using veggies within a few days, don't cut them. They'll lose vitamins, and they may get mushy.

- Wash tomatoes and cucumbers so they're ready to grab and go.

- If you didn't buy prewashed greens, wash, spin, dry, and package them so they're ready for use. Store them in resealable plastic bags and squeeze out all the air.

- Make a double recipe of Cauliflower Rice (page 222). It's a great accompaniment to any protein.

- Make a roasted vegetable medley. When you have a roast in the oven, you can also make roasted vegetables. Select your favorites and follow the roasting directions on page 224.

- Select a few vegetables to lightly steam. Good choices include broccoli, carrots, Brussels sprouts, and green beans.

- Make two Bone Broth Diet salad dressings of your choice.
- Make one or more of the salsas or sauces to enjoy with vegetables or meats.

And don't forget the bone broth

Batch-cooking day is a great time to make one or two pots of bone broth. It takes only minutes to toss your bones, veggies, and seasonings in the pot, and you're done. Your broth can simmer away happily on its own while you do the rest of your cooking.

And here's a tip: If you add some meat to your stock along with the bones, you'll get a double bonus. The broth will be richer and more flavorful, and you'll have more proteins ready to use with no extra effort. Chicken, beef, and turkey simmered in broth are very tender. Use these meals to top salads, serve over Cauliflower Rice, or enjoy with one of the Bone Broth Diet sauces or salsas.

CHAPTER 10

Mouthwatering Meals for Your Bone Broth Lifestyle Plan

WHEN YOU CROSS THE finish line on your Bone Broth Diet, you'll be ready to start on my Bone Broth Lifestyle plan (see Chapter 5)—and that means it's time to start adding more fun foods to your meals. Congratulations . . . you've earned it!

On my Bone Broth Lifestyle plan, you can choose one of two options:

- **The 80/20 Option.** If you choose this option, for 80% of your meals, you're going to eat the same foods you ate on the Bone Broth Diet. Then, for the other 20% of your meals, you're going to live it up a little.

- **The Carb Control Option.** Here, you're going to do a little homework to find out what range of carbs works best for you. If you stick within that range nearly all the time, you can have a few "cheats" each week.

Now, I said back in Chapter 5 that as long as you watch your portion sizes, you can occasionally indulge in anything you want. If you're craving mac and cheese or chicken and waffles once or twice a week, go for it. I won't stop you.

However, I don't just want you to stay *slim* for life—I want you to stay *healthy* for life, too. And the more nutrients (and the less high-carb junk) you feed your body, the more it'll love you back. I'm hoping that even for your "cheat" meals, you'll frequently choose only *slightly* sinful foods.

That's why I've designed the recipes in this chapter to be a little bit wicked, but not too naughty. From Overnight Breakfast Parfait to Sheet Pan Chicken Dinner, they'll satisfy your cravings and still help you stay slim, young, and healthy.

CHECK OUT THE FUN NEW LOW-CARB FOODS!

When you're on your 80/20 plan, you'll discover there's a whole new world of food out there that are low in carbs, grain-free, and often dairy-free. Here are some of my favorites; you can find them on Amazon, at online stores like Thrive Market, and sometimes in your local health food stores.

Cauliflower everything! Cauliflower mash, cauliflower rice, cauliflower pizza crust, cauliflower wraps . . . you name it. (Just check labels to make sure your choices don't include other high-carb or unhealthy ingredients.)

Cashew cheese

Shirataki pasta and rice (made from the root of the konjac plant)

Low-carb cake, cookie, brownie, pancake, and waffle mixes

Low-carb wraps, breads, and bagels

Low-carb salad dressings and condiments (Primal Kitchen is a good brand.)

Chicken chips

Grain-free granola

Fermented salsa

Ready-to-cook "prepped" proteins (I love Cocofood for these—and their spices are amazing, too!)

GOING GRAIN-FREE HAS NEVER BEEN EASIER!

When I first went grain-free, it was tough to replace the foods I loved. Now, however, it's a piece of cake (no pun intended). Here are some of my favorite new treats. (Note: Some of these are low-carb and some not so much, so make sure the carb counts are within your range.)

Siete chips and taco shells

Lynn's Life baking mixes

From the Ground Up chips and crackers

Thrive Market coconut wraps and coconut flakes cereal

Simple Mills crackers

Purely Elizabeth grain-free granola

Cappello's grain-free pizza, pasta, and cookie dough

80/20 MAINTENANCE PLAN

BUTTERNUT SQUASH BREAKFAST HASH (80/20 MAINTENANCE PLAN)

PREP TIME: 15 MINUTES • COOK TIME: 12 MINS

Yield: 6 servings • *Portions: Negligible fat, 1 starchy vegetable, ⅓ fruit*

- 2 tablespoons coconut, avocado, or olive oil
- 1 medium butternut squash, about 1½ pounds, peeled and diced into ¼ to ½" pieces
- 1 small onion, diced
- 1 red bell pepper, diced
- 1 medium apple, diced
- ½ teaspoon Celtic or pink Himalayan salt
- ¼ teaspoon ground black pepper
- ½ teaspoon or more ground or rubbed sage
- ½ teaspoon chili powder
- ¼ teaspoon cinnamon
- ½ teaspoon paprika
- ⅛–¼ teaspoon cayenne
- ⅛ teaspoon garlic powder (optional)
- 6 fried eggs, for serving (optional)
- Hot sauce, for serving (optional)

In a large skillet, heat the oil on high heat until it shimmers. Add the squash and reduce the heat to medium. Sauté, stirring occasionally, for about 5 minutes. Add the onion, bell pepper, apple, salt, pepper, sage, chili powder, cinnamon, paprika, cayenne, and garlic powder (if using), and sauté for 5 to 7 minutes, until the vegetables are softened. Top each portion with a fried egg and serve with hot sauce, if desired.

NOTES:

There are a number of meats you can add to this dish for a heartier meal. Try pork or turkey sausage, diced bacon, ham, or Canadian bacon (all of which should be sugar- and nitrate-free). If you're adding meat, cook it fully first, remove it from the pan, and drain it on paper towels while you cook the hash. You can cook the hash in the pan drippings. When the hash is nearly done, add the meat and toss together. If you are adding meat, use about 4 to 5 ounces per serving to create an entrée.

Squash is difficult to cut, but you can often find it peeled, seeds removed, and diced in the grocery store. The chunks tend to be rather large, so cut them down into a smaller dice.

CREAMY CHICKEN AND MUSHROOMS (80/20 MAINTENANCE MEAL)

PREP TIME: 10 MINUTES • COOK TIME: 25 MINUTES

Yield: *4 servings* • Portions: *1 protein, 1 fat*

2 tablespoons ghee, divided

4 (4–6 ounces each) boneless, skinless chicken breasts

½ teaspoon Celtic or pink Himalayan salt

¼ teaspoon garlic powder

¼ teaspoon ground black pepper

12 ounces mushrooms, white, cremini, or a mix, sliced

⅓ cup white wine or chicken bone broth

½ teaspoon arrowroot

¾ cup full-fat coconut milk, reserve 1 tablespoon

¼ cup Pecorino Romano or other hard goat's or sheep's milk cheese, grated

In a large skillet, heat 1 tablespoon of ghee over medium heat until it shimmers. Season both sides of the chicken with the salt, garlic powder, and pepper and cook for 4 to 6 minutes, flip, and cook for 4 to 6 minutes more, until the chicken is golden and the internal temperature reaches 165°F on an instant-read thermometer. Transfer the chicken to a plate, cover, and set aside. In the same skillet, raise the temperature to medium-high, add the mushrooms, and cook for about 4 minutes, until tender. Transfer the mushrooms to the plate with the chicken.

Lower the heat to medium and add the wine and bring to a simmer, scraping up all the brown pieces to deglaze the pan. Cook for 2 more minutes to reduce the wine by half. Add the remaining 1 tablespoon ghee and the coconut milk and stir to combine. In a small bowl or cup, dissolve the arrowroot in the remaining 1 tablespoon chicken coconut milk and add to the skillet. Continue to simmer for 3 to 4 minutes and stir until the sauce begins to thicken. Stir in the grated cheese. Taste and adjust seasoning if needed. Add the mushrooms and chicken to the skillet and cook for 1 to 2 more minutes to warm through.

NOTES:

Sheep's milk contains almost twice the fat and protein of goat's milk, and fat adds more flavor to cheese. Cheese made with sheep's milk also has higher protein content (casein) and is less apt to crumble. Sheep's milk is also more digestible than cow's or goat's milk because of the type of casein (protein) it contains and because the fat globules are smaller, making them more digestible.

Deglazing a pan simply means adding a liquid to a pan in which other ingredients were cooked. It is done to loosen the little caramelized brown bits left in the pan, adding more flavor to the sauce. Use a wooden spoon to scrape up the brown bits as the liquid simmers.

If you can only find oversized chicken breasts, follow the instructions for how to slice large chicken breasts in the first note on page 147.

MEDITERRANEAN QUINOA SALAD (80/20 MAINTENANCE MEAL)

PREP TIME: 30 MINUTES

Yield: *6 servings* • **Portions:** *2 fats, 1 legume protein*

1 cup dry quinoa, red, white, or black

⅓ cup + 1 teaspoon olive oil

1¾ cup Chicken Bone Broth (page 98) or water

1 teaspoon Celtic or pink Himalayan salt + more for the dressing

1 clove garlic, minced

1 cup grape or cherry tomatoes, halved

1 (15-ounce) can chickpeas, rinsed and drained

½ cup roasted red or yellow peppers, cut into 2" strips

2 scallions (white and light green parts), sliced

¼ cup Kalamata olives, pitted and cut in half

¼ cup pine nuts, toasted (optional)

1 tablespoon balsamic or white balsamic vinegar

¼ cup fresh basil, julienned

3 cups arugula or baby spinach

¼ cup sheep's milk feta cheese, if you are not sensitive to dairy (optional)

¼ teaspoon black pepper + more to taste

Place the quinoa in a fine-mesh sieve and rinse thoroughly in cold water, moving it around with your hand or a wooden spoon for about 1 minute. Drain well. Preheat a large skillet on medium-high heat and add 1 teaspoon of the oil. Add the quinoa and cook, stirring constantly, for about 3 minutes, until the quinoa is dry and starting to get toasty. Add the broth, 1 teaspoon salt, and the garlic and bring to a boil. Once boiling, cover the skillet, reduce the heat to low, and simmer for about 15 minutes. Remove from the heat and keep covered for 5 or more minutes. Uncover and allow the quinoa to cool to room temperature. To speed the cooling process, place the quinoa in a fine-mesh sieve and run cold water over it.

Meanwhile, in a large bowl, combine the tomatoes, chickpeas, roasted peppers, scallions, olives, and pine nuts (if using).

In a small bowl or lidded jar, combine ¼ cup of the olive oil, the balsamic vinegar, and basil. Whisk or shake to combine. Add the quinoa, arugula, feta (if using), and black pepper to the bowl with the vegetables. Pour the dressing over the salad. Season with more salt and pepper, if desired. If the salad seems too dry, add the remaining olive oil. Serve chilled or at room temperature.

OVERNIGHT BREAKFAST PARFAIT (80/20 MAINTENANCE MEAL)

PREP TIME: 10 MINUTES

Yield: *4 servings* • **Portions:** *1 protein, 1½ fat, 1 fruit*

- 2 cups unsweetened almond milk, another nut milk, or coconut milk (not canned)
- 4 scoops chocolate or vanilla protein powder
- ½ cup chia seeds
- 1 can full-fat coconut milk or coconut cream (sometimes called cream of coconut)
- Monk fruit or stevia equal 2–4 tablespoons sugar (optional; if the protein powder is sweetened, skip this ingredient)
- ½ teaspoon vanilla extract
- 2 cups fruit of your choice (berries work well here)

In a blender or a medium bowl, combine the almond milk and protein powder and blend or whisk until smooth. Add the chia seeds and pour into 4 tall glasses or jars, cover, and refrigerate overnight. Refrigerate the coconut milk and a mixing bowl so you will have a well-chilled bowl in the morning. If you are planning on using a stand mixer to whip the coconut milk, refrigerate the bowl that you use with the mixer.

The next morning, carefully open the can of coconut milk. The coconut cream will have hardened, separated from the coconut milk, and risen to the top of the can; the coconut water will remain in the bottom of the can. Scoop the hardened coconut cream into the chilled mixing bowl. Keep the coconut water to thin the coconut cream or save it for a smoothie. Using a hand or stand mixer, whip the coconut cream for about 30 seconds on high until creamy. Add sweetener (if using) and vanilla and whip for about 1 minute or more, until peaks form. If it seems too stiff, add some of the coconut water, 1 teaspoon at a time, to loosen the cream.

Top the chia pudding with fruit of your choice and the whipped coconut cream.

NOTES:

If you forgot to put the mixing bowl in the refrigerator, just put it in the freezer for about 20 minutes before whipping the coconut cream.

If you have leftover whipped coconut cream, it will keep for up to 2 weeks in the refrigerator. It will get firmer under refrigeration.

If you choose to sweeten the coconut cream, a powdered sweetener blends well with the cream; a granular sweetener could leave the cream with a gritty texture.

SHEET PAN CHICKEN DINNER (80/20 MAINTENANCE MEAL)

PREP TIME: 25 MINUTES • COOK TIME: 30 MINUTES

Yield: *4 servings* • Portions: *1 protein, 1 fat, 1 starchy vegetable, 1 vegetable*

¼ cup kosher salt

4 (4–5 ounces each) boneless, skinless chicken breasts

2 tablespoons avocado, coconut, or olive oil

1 pound acorn, butternut, or kabocha squash, seeded and cut into ½" to 1" cubes

1 medium head cauliflower, cut into florets

1 teaspoon Celtic or pink Himalayan salt, divided

½ teaspoon ground black pepper, divided

2 tablespoons pasture-raised butter or ghee, melted

¼ teaspoon garlic powder

¼ teaspoon cinnamon

¼ teaspoon ground nutmeg

¼ teaspoon ground cloves

¼ teaspoon allspice

Pour 4 cups of cold water into a large bowl and add the kosher salt. Immerse the chicken in the brine, cover, and refrigerate for 30 to 60 minutes. Thirty minutes is optimal, but even 10 minutes of brining will make a difference.

While the chicken is brining, preheat the oven to 400°F and place a rack in the center position. Line a baking sheet with parchment. In a large bowl, combine the oil, squash, and cauliflower and season with a ½ teaspoon salt and ¼ teaspoon pepper, tossing to coat. Scatter the vegetables on the prepared baking sheet and roast for 10 minutes.

In a small bowl, combine the butter, garlic powder, cinnamon, nutmeg, cloves, allspice, ½ teaspoon salt, and ¼ teaspoon pepper. Remove the chicken from the brine, rinse, and pat dry with paper towels. Brush both sides of each breast with the butter mixture and place them on the sheet pan with the squash and cauliflower. Flip the vegetables and return the pan to the oven for about 20 minutes.

Using an instant-read thermometer, test the chicken for doneness. It should be 165°F. If needed, continue to roast the chicken, testing it every 3 to 5 minutes. Let the chicken rest for about 5 minutes before serving.

NOTE:

If you've never had kabocha squash (also called Japanese pumpkin) you're in for a treat. The flesh is a dark, rich orange and denser than butternut or acorn squash and with a sweeter flavor. I discovered it years ago by accident, and I never went back to other winter squash varieties because this is, by far, my favorite.

SWEET POTATO LATKE WAFFLES (80/20 MAINTENANCE MEAL)

PREP TIME: 20 MINUTES • COOK TIME: 5 MINUTES/WAFFLE

Yield: *4 servings* • **Portions:** *½ protein, negligible fat, 1 starchy vegetable*

2 large or 3 medium sweet potatoes, about 1 pound, peeled

2 scallions (white and light green parts), finely chopped

½ cup almond flour

2 eggs, lightly beaten

1 teaspoon baking powder

1 teaspoon salt

½ teaspoon ground black pepper

Dash of cayenne

Avocado, coconut, or olive oil pan spray

Preheat a waffle iron to medium. Cut the sweet potatoes into 2" chunks and shred them in a food processor using the shredding/grating disk. Put the shredded sweet potatoes in a fine-mesh sieve and squeeze out as much water as you can, or wrap in a clean kitchen towel or paper towels and twist to dry the potatoes. (You will stain the towel, so don't use your best one.) In a large bowl, combine the sweet potatoes, scallions, almond flour, eggs, baking powder, salt, pepper, and cayenne and mix well.

When the waffle iron is hot, spray it with pan spray. Scoop a rounded ½ cup or less (depending on the size of your waffle iron) of the sweet potato mixture and pour it onto the center of the waffle iron. Cook for about 5 minutes, until browned. Repeat with the remaining sweet potato mixture. Serve the waffles warm.

NOTES:

The drier the sweet potatoes, the better the waffles.

Other add-ins you might like: cinnamon, nutmeg, or pumpkin pie spice.

If you don't have a food processor, use a box grater on the side with the round holes.

Every waffle iron is different. You may need to adjust the temperature or cook time a bit.

These refrigerate well if you have leftovers. You can reheat them in a microwave, but they retain their crispiness when reheated on the stovetop.

TZATZIKI (80/20 MAINTENANCE PLAN)

PREP TIME: 15 MINUTES

Yield: *about 2 cups, eight ¼ cup servings;* **Portions:** *fat, varies based on yogurt used*

- **1 medium cucumber**
- **1 cup unsweetened plain coconut yogurt**
- **1 or 2 garlic cloves, finely minced**
- **1 tablespoon freshly squeezed lemon juice (¼–½ lemon)**
- **1 tablespoon extra-virgin olive oil**
- **½ teaspoon Celtic or pink Himalayan salt**
- **⅛ teaspoon ground black pepper**
- **2 tablespoons fresh dill, large stems discarded, chopped**

Peel the cucumber, cut it in half lengthwise, and scoop out the seeds with a spoon. On the side of a box grater with the round holes, grate the seeded cucumber and then chop it so the pieces are small and not stringy. Place the cucumber pieces in a fine-mesh sieve over a bowl and press them down with your hand or a rubber spatula to squeeze out as much water as possible. Let the cucumber sit in the sieve for about 15 minutes, then wrap it in a clean kitchen towel and squeeze out any remaining moisture. Alternatively, pulse the cucumber pieces a few times in a food processor until finely diced and follow the steps above to squeeze out as much water as possible. Regardless of how you chop the cucumber, removing as much moisture as possible is important so the tzatziki doesn't get watery.

In a small bowl, combine the yogurt, garlic, lemon juice, oil, salt, and pepper. If you are serving immediately, add the cucumbers and dill to the yogurt, stir, and serve. If you are not serving immediately, refrigerate the yogurt mixture and cucumbers in separate containers. When ready to serve, mix the yogurt, cucumbers, and dill together.

NOTES:

If you don't have any digestive issues with dairy, you can also use goat, sheep, or cow yogurt.

You'll be surprised by how much water is in a cucumber! When it is well drained, you'll end up with ¼–⅓ cup of cucumber.

Refrigerating the yogurt before serving allows the garlic to mellow and lose some of its bite. It also allows for even more water to release from the cucumber.

MISSING RICE AND NOODLES?
TRY THESE FUN SWAPS!

One of the most important pieces of advice I give my patients is "Don't sacrifice—swap!" That's because there's a delicious and healthy alternative for every high-carb, unhealthy dish. All it takes is a little creativity and you can enjoy any food you like.

For instance, if you're pining for spaghetti and meatballs right now—or for fried rice or a cool Asian noodle salad—you can go right ahead and have it. It's just a matter of swapping out rice and grain-based noodles for yummy, low-carb alternatives.

Zucchini noodles. Everyone loves "zoodles," and they're easy to make with a spiralizer, julienne peeler, vegetable peeler, or mandoline. I like to make my zoodles with both zucchini and yellow squash, for more color. For extra flavor, gently sauté your zoodles with garlic in a little olive oil before adding them to your sauce. In addition to making zoodles in place of spaghetti, you can make pappardelle-style zoodles by using a vegetable peeler to slice one-inch-wide strips. Thinly sliced zucchini "coins" make a great substitute for lasagna noodles, too.

Cauliflower rice. This takes just minutes to make, and—like regular rice—it's incredibly versatile. Simply pulse cauliflower florets quickly in a food processor until the pieces are the size of rice grains and then mix them with your favorite flavorings.

Spaghetti squash noodles. These are packed with powerful nutrients, and they have a mild flavor that blends well with any sauce. They're especially fun to make with kids, who love scooping the strands out of the squash.

Shirataki noodles (konjac). These noodles—also called miracle noodles or konjac noodles—are made from the root of the konjac plant. They're loaded with fiber and have virtually no digestible carbs, and they come in different shapes and sizes so you can substitute them for long noodles, macaroni, or rice. And don't be put off by the funny smell when you open the package; simply rinse the noodles and heat them well in a dry pan. The aroma will disappear.

Hearts of palm noodles. These come in a variety of sizes, so you can use them for everything from Italian dishes to Asian food. They smell very strong at first, but drain them, soak them in milk for about 30 minutes, and drain them again, and they'll be fine.

Sweet potato noodles. Spiralize sweet potatoes, and you get a firm, slightly sweet noodle that holds up well in soups and broths. Save these for a day when you've worked out hard and can use the extra carbs.

Celeriac (celery root) noodles. Believe it or not, those ugly celery roots, which some people compare to the mandrakes in the Harry Potter series, can turn into beautiful noodles.

Broccoli noodles. The florets on broccoli always get the attention, but don't toss out those stems! Instead, spiralize them and use them as the base for a yummy salad.

Cucumber noodles. If you're a fan of cold, refreshing noodle salads, you'll love these—and all you need to make them is a spiralizer or julienne peeler.

Parsnip noodles. This is another great option if you're pining for Asian-style noodles. Parsnips add a nice little "bite" to a dish.

Peppers. If you want to transform meat and sauce into a one-pan meal, try replacing pasta or rice with either chile peppers or bell peppers. They'll give your dish a nice crunch and lots of extra flavor and nutrition.

One more tip:

You can buy lots of noodle and rice alternatives at the grocery store these days. Have fun trying them out, but read the package labels carefully before you buy. Sometimes manufacturers sneak wheat or starch into these products, so watch for suspicious ingredients or high carb counts.

FERMENTED FOODS: A QUICK PRIMER

Traditional foods are making a huge comeback these days, and one of the trends that makes me the happiest is the return to *fermented* foods.

From kimchi to sauerkraut to kombucha, these foods have been part of human history for centuries—and with good reason! While they may seem humble, they're superstars that supply us with the beneficial gut bugs we need to keep our metabolisms and immune systems operating at their best. Here's a quick introduction to these remarkable foods.

What are fermented foods?

Fermentation involves preserving foods in a way that fosters the growth of good bacteria while preventing the growth of bad bacteria. The end result is a tasty food that mainlines beneficial bugs to your gut. Here are some popular fermented foods you can add to your diet:

- Yogurt is cow's milk or coconut milk fermented with good bacteria. When you shop for yogurt, I recommend reaching for coconut milk–based yogurt rather than milk-based yogurt. (That's because dairy can cause bloating and other issues—see

Chapter 5 for more on this.) Also, select brands with no added sugar, sweeteners, or artificial ingredients.

- Kefir is made from cow's milk or coconut milk that's fermented with a combination of bacteria and yeasts. Again, I strongly recommend reaching for coconut kefir rather than dairy kefir.

- Pickles, kimchi, and sauerkraut are excellent sources of probiotics. Be sure to buy refrigerated versions, because pasteurized versions don't contain live bacteria. And read the labels carefully to make sure you're getting what you want. Fermented foods will be preserved in a salt brine, not in vinegar.

- Kombucha is a combination of tea and some form of sugar (honey, for instance) that's fermented to produce good bacteria. It's an excellent source of beneficial bugs, but one note of caution here: Save kombucha for your Bone Broth Lifestyle Plan, because some brands contain enough sugar to derail your diet.

How much, how often?

When you first start eating fermented foods, it may take a while for your body to adjust to them. (That's because you're changing your gut's ecosystem.) I recommend starting with a spoonful or so per day—or about a quarter-cup of kefir, kombucha, or coconut yogurt—and working up to a bigger serving.

Eventually, see if you can get into the habit of eating a good-size serving every day. For instance, have a cup of coconut kefir, or half a cup of sauer- kraut or kimchi, or a whole fermented pickle. If you're like most people, as your body realizes that they're good for you, you'll go from saying ugh to loving these foods.

If you have a sustained severe reaction to probiotic foods, you may be dealing with an issue like small intestinal bacterial overgrowth (SIBO). In this case, you may want to abstain from probiotic foods until you heal your gut with a healthy, natural, low- carbohydrate diet and daily bone broth.

Can you make your own probiotic foods?

Yes, you can! What's more, it's fun and fairly inexpensive to ferment your own foods. And it's amazing how many foods you can ferment, from green beans to carrots to okra.

If you want to get serious about it, I recommend books like *Nourishing Traditions* by Sally Fallon and Mary Enig; *The Art of Fermentation* by Sandor Ellix Katz (which won a James Beard Award); and *The Kimchi Diet* by Susanne Bennett.

Optimizing Your Results with EXERCISE, STRESS REDUCTION, and LIFESTYLE CHANGES . . . Plus My Top Ten Beauty Tips!

CHAPTER 11

Add More Fat-Burning Power with Exercise

IF I TOLD YOU I had a pill that could help keep you slender, combat the blues, and lower your risk of developing cancer, heart disease, and diabetes, would you take it? How about if I offered it to you for free? Of course you would.

That pill is *exercise*.

Adding exercise to your routine while you're on the Bone Broth Diet will help you lose weight faster—and after you finish your diet, exercising is going to be one of your best weapons when it comes to keeping those pounds off. That's because exercise powers up your metabolism, making your body burn more fat.

In addition, exercise helps ward off that blah feeling we're all prone to. No matter how good you look, if your energy is low and you're giving off "life sucks" vibes, you're not going to be the best *you* that you can be. Think of exercise as something like a good shot of tequila: a real attitude adjuster.

Want more? Exercise is one of your best defenses against the diseases associated with aging. A recent study found that people who simply walked often and briskly were far more likely to be alive 15 years later than people who hardly ever exercised.[1] (I'll talk a lot more about this in Chapter 12.)

And here's something else that studies like this tell us about exercise: It doesn't have to be hard. Even walking, the easiest exercise of all, can slim you down, shape you up, and keep you young.

In this chapter, I'm going to introduce you to a fat-blasting walking program designed specifically for the Bone Broth Diet by Kathy Smith, one of the world's most famous fitness icons. Kathy's program is simple and fun, but don't let that fool you—it's powerful medicine. Do it for even 3 or 4 days a week during your diet and you'll lose extra pounds and inches.

But before I tell you about Kathy's special program and two other exercise options, let's look more closely at why you'll want to make exercise part of your new slimmer, younger lifestyle.

HOW MOVING TRANSFORMS YOUR BODY AND MIND

I believe in primal rules, and one of my primal rules is that you need to move every day. Your body is made to move, not to sit. When you move the way nature intends, you get leaner—and you get stronger, healthier, and happier as well. Here's why.

First, exercise makes it easier for you to keep off extra pounds by helping you become a natural fat burner. It flips on your internal furnace and keeps it on, so even when you're sitting at your desk writing e-mails, you'll still be burning fat. It revs up your body so it plays at a higher level all day long.

Second, exercise protects against the blues (and helps treat severe depression[2]) because it changes your biochemistry. Exercise triggers the release of endorphins, which are "feel good" chemicals that make you happy and relaxed. It also helps your body break down kynurenine, a substance linked to depression.[3]

Third, even easy exercise makes you healthier all over. Here are some of the things that a simple activity like walking does for your body.

- It lowers your blood glucose levels, reducing your risk for obesity and diabetes. A recent study found that breaking up sitting with 2 minutes of light walking every 20 minutes reduces blood glucose levels significantly.[4]

- It reduces your belly fat. In one study, researchers found that office workers who took short walks and did other simple movements decreased their waist size compared with a control group.[5]

- It increases your circulation, nourishing your skin and making it glow.

- It helps prevent heart disease.

- It can reduce your risks of breast[6] and endometrial[7] cancer.

Now, it's true that you can get slim without exercising. (A number of people in our test groups easily lost 10 pounds or more on the Bone Broth Diet without exercising a single day.) However, you'll lose more weight if you work out. And if you want to be slim, healthy, and youthful looking for your entire life, exercise is a must.

This is why no matter how busy you are, I want you to schedule some regular exercise every week during your diet. But as you know, I believe in "personal play"—so I want you to pick an exercise program that works for *you*.

THREE EXERCISE OPTIONS

One thing I've learned from working with hundreds of patients is that a single exercise plan won't work for everyone. Some people want to reach the highest levels of fitness, and they're willing to put in a huge effort to achieve this goal. Some people want to get enough exercise to tone their bodies, stay healthy, and feel good. Some people hate workouts but love biking, swimming, or playing tennis. And some people are coping with medical problems or other big life issues that make getting any kind of exercise tough—especially on top of a major diet transformation.

So I'm not going to present a one-size-fits-all program. Instead, I'm going to give you a pick-what's-right-for-you program. Here's how it works.

First, no matter what level of exercise you choose, respect what your body tells you on your intermittent fasting days. If you don't feel up to exercising on these days or the days that immediately follow them, feel free to skip your workouts. Even if you're a high-level athlete, realize that you'll probably be less capable of exerting yourself on fasting days and the days right after them.

Second, pick an exercise routine that's right for you. Choose one of the options I list below, depending on which option suits your needs and fitness level.

Option 1: Easy does it

If you find even simple exercise very challenging, here's an option that will get you moving without stressing you out. Simply get an activity tracker (I like Fitbit, but any brand is okay) or even an old-fashioned inexpensive pedometer. Every nonfasting day, make sure you walk at least 10,000 steps. You can do this on intermittent fasting days as well, but only if you feel up to it.

Keep using your activity tracker after you finish your diet. If you decide that you're ready for more, see if you can move up to the next option.

Option 2: Kathy Smith's special workout—just for you

If you're like most of the world, you already know who Kathy Smith is. She's the creator of dozens of bestselling workout videos. She's a *New York Times* bestselling author who's written eight books on exercise, diet, and lifestyle, as well as

Asking the Right Questions

Robb Wolf, former research biochemist and *New York Times* bestselling author of *The Paleo Solution*

robbwolf.com

Robb, a former California state power-lifting champion, is a leading health and fitness expert who now coaches athletes at the highest levels of competition. Here's his take on ancestral wisdom and modern medicine.

"The ancestral health [AH] model is incredibly important in finding solutions, but in a perhaps counterintuitive way: The AH template allows us to start with the 'right' questions concerning sleep, food, exercise, and gut biome to help us formulate the outcomes that promote optimal health.

"The current reductionist medical model is fantastic for acute medical issues, particularly trauma, but has largely failed in providing substantive guidance on how to prevent or improve chronic disease states. This is due in large part to a framework that is not even asking the right questions—the biggest of which is 'What is our body naturally designed to eat or do?' So how can mainstream medicine possibly find the 'right' answers?"

the star of the public television special *Ageless Energy*. After 3 decades at the forefront of her field, she knows all there is to know about fitness.

Kathy is also a friend of mine—and when I told her about my Bone Broth Diet, she immediately offered to adapt her Lean Walk program specifically for the diet. (Now that's a friend!)

Kathy has designed this program to give you a great calorie burn without leaving you feeling wobbly, weak, or tired. While it looks easy, it'll accelerate your weight loss because it employs the principle of periodization.

If you aren't familiar with periodization, it's a trick that athletes use to "peak" before big events. Put simply, it means that you vary one of the three elements of your workout: length, activity, or intensity. When you do this, it forces your body to keep stepping up its game—and that means that you burn fat faster.

Each week on Kathy's walking program, you'll change either the duration or the intensity of your workout. As a result, you'll burn extra calories and take off more weight. Here's how it works.

Baseline

Before you start the program, figure out how long it takes you to walk 1 mile. This will give you a baseline so you can measure your progress and know when it's time to move up a level. Find a nice route, mark off a mile using your car's odometer or a distance-tracking app, and then walk the mile and record your time. Don't worry about how fast you're walking.

Week 1

This walk will get you going at a steady, comfortable pace. You'll be walking anywhere from 10 minutes to an hour at a speed that matches your fitness level.

You'll start off with an easy 5-minute warm-up, walking at a strolling pace. Then you'll increase your pace slightly to a "steady-state" pace. Using the chart below to gauge your exertion, try to stick close to the 4 to 5 level.

Here's a schedule for your first week. The length of time you spend walking at a steady-state pace will depend on your general fitness; you want to challenge yourself without overstressing your body.

WEEK 1	
Mini-Fast Days (And the Days That Immediately Follow Them) Exercise is optional.	**Nonfasting Days** 5 minutes: warm-up pace 10–50 minutes: steady-state pace (4 or 5 on the exertion scale) 5 minutes: cool-down pace

MEASURING YOUR EXERTION

To rate your exertion, think about how you feel as you're walking. Do your legs feel like they're hardly working, or do they hurt? Are you breathing easily or hard? Is your heart pounding? Are you sweating? Based on how you feel, rate your exertion using the system here.

1–2	Very, very light
3	Very light
4	Moderate
5	Somewhat hard
6	Hard
7–8	Very hard
9–10	Very, very hard

Note: Your warm-ups and cool-downs should be between 2 and 3.

As you start your walking program, work on developing good walking techniques. Here are some basics.

- **Posture.** Imagine that there's a string coming from the top of your head, pulling you up. Tilt your body slightly forward from your ankles (not your hips or waist). Pull in your abdominal muscles to keep your spine straight, and avoid arching your lower back or sticking your butt out. Focus your eyes straight ahead. Keep your shoulders down and back, opening your chest so you can breathe easily. Check periodically to make sure you're not slouching.

- **Arms.** Let your arms swing freely and purposefully. This will improve your balance and burn more calories.

- **Feet.** Contact the ground with your heel, letting your foot roll forward comfortably. At the end of each step, push off with your toes to propel your body forward. Use a stride that feels natural to you.

Week 2

If it takes you more than 20 minutes to complete a mile, stick with the week 1 walk. If you can walk a mile in under 20 minutes, lengthen your walk by 10 to 20 minutes. Here's a schedule you can follow. You should be hitting a 6 or 7 on the exertion scale.

WEEK 2	
Mini-Fast Days (And the Days That Immediately Follow Them) Exercise is optional.	**Nonfasting Days** 5 minutes: warm-up pace 20–70 minutes: steady-state pace 5 minutes: cool-down pace

Week 3

If the week 1 or week 2 walk pushes you to your limits, stick with the level that's comfortable for you. But if you want an extra challenge, it's time to kick things up a notch. This workout will increase your endurance and fitness and burn more calories because it uses interval training to push you a little harder for very short periods of time.

During your aerobic intervals, you should walk fast enough that it feels like a hard workout (but not so fast that you need to stop). You should be hitting between 7 and 9 on the exertion scale. During your recovery intervals, return to the steady-state pace you used in your earlier walks.

WEEK 3	
Mini-Fast Days (And the Days That Immediately Follow Them) Exercise is optional.	**Nonfasting Days** 5–10 minutes: warm-up pace 3 minutes: aerobic interval 3 minutes: recovery interval (steady-state pace) 3 minutes: aerobic interval 3 minutes: recovery interval (steady-state pace) 5–10 minutes: cool-down pace

Here are two tips for getting the most from your aerobic intervals.

- Pump your arms more quickly. Start by bending your elbows 90 degrees and holding your hands in loose fists. Swing forward, not side to side, and keep your elbows close to your body.

- Concentrate on actively pulling up your toes as your legs swing forward. (Otherwise you might trip yourself.)

Walking at this level will give you an extra calorie burn that will last for hours. If you keep walking after you finish your diet, work on increasing your pace during aerobic intervals so you achieve maximum fat-burning. Kathy has more advanced workouts if you want to take things to an even higher level. Here's a link to one of them: kathysmith.com/store/leanwalk.

Option 3: Keep up your typical workouts

If you regularly go to the gym or work out to exercise videos and you feel energetic while you're on the diet, keep following your normal routine—even on fasting days, if you want. In fact, you'll actually burn more fat if you exercise while you're fasting. In particular, if you're into HIIT (high-intensity interval training), consider doing a few workouts each week. HIIT, which involves short cycles of intense exercise alternated with cycles of gentle exercise, is a powerful belly-fat burner. For instance, one study of postmenopausal women with type 2 diabetes compared the effects of continuous moderate cycling to HIIT involving bursts of intense cycling followed by recovery periods. While both groups of women lost weight, the researchers found that "significant loss of total abdominal and visceral fat mass was observed only with HIIT."[8] Similarly, a 2019 study found that short bursts of intense activity are more effective for weight loss than longer, moderate-intensity workouts.[9]

However, don't force yourself to exercise at this level if you don't feel like it. You'll lose weight even if you don't—especially if you do Kathy Smith's program in option 2.

If you're a hard-core fitness buff who loves programs like WOD (workout of the day), metcon (metabolic conditioning), or CrossFit, do your regular workouts 3 or 4 days a week if it feels right to you (and do some light walking in between). But—and this is really, really important—if you choose to do intense workouts, be absolutely sure to follow your program's protocol for refueling after a workout. I can't stress this enough. You can easily satisfy this protocol and still stick to the approved foods on the Bone Broth Diet.

And again, listen to your body. On the days it's saying no to strenuous exercise, do Kathy's program in option 2 or just take a leisurely walk. I'm serious. No matter how strong you are, sometimes your body needs a little R&R.

One caution: If you haven't exercised at a strenuous level before and you're thinking about trying a program like CrossFit, metcon, or WOD, I strongly recommend choosing one of the other options during your 3-week diet. This will give your body a chance to recalibrate and reset so it'll be ready for a bigger challenge.

NOTES FOR EXTREME ATHLETES ONLY (WOD, METCON, CROSSFIT, ETC.)

After a very intense workout, you must refuel within a half hour because your body will start the recovery period faster and more effectively. Have a meal-size serving of easy-to-digest protein like egg whites, chicken breast, or salmon and a starchy carbohydrate such as winter squash, jicama, sweet potato, or pumpkin. After a strenuous workout, you need this "bonus meal." Right now, fat is less important. This is the only time you don't need to add it.

Eat your normal meal 60 to 90 minutes later. My personal favorite is scrambled eggs with diced sweet potatoes.

And here's a good preworkout tip: To signal to your body that activity is coming, eat a small amount of protein and fat 15 to 60 minutes before your workout. It's important, though, to skip the carbs here. Hard-cooked eggs and a handful of nuts work great—so do some jerky and a handful of coconut chips.

Above all, do what you love

There's an old cliché that the best form of exercise is the one you'll actually do. And here's why it's a cliché: It's true! So move in ways that make you happy—whether it's dancing, riding a bike, swimming, or playing hopscotch with your kids. Any form of exercise, as long as it's not unnatural or excessive, will help you stay slender, healthy, and fit. Just keep in mind that on your mini-fast days and the days that immediately follow them, you'll be less capable of intense exercise.

No matter which option you pick, stay flexible from day to day. For instance, if you're doing Kathy's program and you experience the carb flu I've talked about, step down to option 1 for a few days or even take those days off. Again, listen to your body and do what it tells you to do.

And remember the bottom line: Just move. And move at least a little every day, because it'll help keep you slim, healthy, and happy for life.

Live Long and Stay Healthy by Making Smart Choices

So far, I've focused mostly on the here and now, because I know your goal is to take off those extra pounds fast. However, in addition to getting slim, I know you want to stay healthy for a long, *long* time—because don't we all?

Well, guess what: They don't call me an anti-aging expert for nothing. I've spent two decades studying the most effective ways to stop the clock or even turn it back. I don't just want to help you get slim . . . I also want to set you up for a long, happy lifetime. My goal is to transport you into transformation. That's why right now I want to share some of my best tips for staying young, healthy, and vibrant *forever*.

TIP #1: KEEP YOUR GUT MICROBIOME HAPPY

Back in Chapter 3, I talked a little about your gut microbes—the trillions of "bugs" that call your gastrointestinal tract home. You'll remember that I told you how these bugs play a big role in fighting inflammation so your gut can stay strong and healthy.

That's the short story, but there's a lot more to it. Now I'd like to do a deep dive into this topic—because I'm not exaggerating when I say that you need to have a healthy gut to have a long, healthy life.

As we get older, our gut microbiome ages, too. Our gut bugs get less diverse, which is a very bad thing—and, worse yet, we have fewer "good" bugs. In fact, scientists can now tell how old you are, within about a four-year range, just by looking at your gut bugs.[1] And get this: The microbes in your gut can strongly predict whether you'll still be alive in 15 years.[2]

That's a little creepy, I know. But guess what: These facts aren't carved in stone. In reality, you can slow or even reverse your microbiome's slide into old age! And making your gut microbiome younger, in turn, can slow down aging in every part of your body, because a healthier gut enhances your antioxidant activity, improves your immune function, suppresses chronic inflammation, helps to regulate your metabolism, and aids in preventing insulin resistance.[3] Optimizing your gut microbiome may keep your brain healthy as you age, too (more about this later).

And here's another reason to keep your gut microbiome young and vibrant: It'll make it *way* easier to keep those extra pounds off for good.

How effective can those tiny gut bugs be when it comes to keeping you slim? Consider this: In an eye-opening study a few years ago, researchers enrolled sets of twins, with each twin pair including one obese and one slim twin. When the researchers transferred gut bacteria from the twins into mice, the mice with the bacteria from obese twins became fat, while the mice with the bacteria from slim twins stayed slim.[4]

So if you're blaming your weight issues on heredity, think again—because it turns out your gut bugs may have a much bigger say than your genes.

Happily, science shows that microbiome aging definitely *isn't* inevitable. In one study, for instance, researchers found that extremely healthy people in their 90s had gut microbiomes similar to those of people decades younger. One of the researchers commented, "The main conclusion is that if you are ridiculously healthy and 90 years old, your gut microbiota is not that different from a healthy 30-year-old in the same population."[5]

You're never too old to have a young gut. What's more, it's easy to "de-age" your gut microbiome. Here are some simple steps that will make your internal ecosystem thrive:

Eat probiotic foods several times each week. These are foods like kimchi, pickles, and coconut kefir that contain beneficial bugs that will settle into your gut.

Eat plenty of prebiotic foods. Prebiotics are foods that serve as "fertilizer" for your internal garden, helping your microbes to flourish. These foods include asparagus, onions, leeks, garlic, Jerusalem artichokes, and chicory.

Take prebiotic and probiotic supplements. Even if you work probiotic and prebiotic foods into your diet, I strongly recommend taking a high-quality supplement containing both. As a general rule, the more strains of probiotics and prebiotics your supplement contains, the better. (A big bonus here: probiotics are also awesome for your skin! See page 362.)

Avoid antibiotics as much as possible. Yes, sometimes antibiotic drugs can be lifesavers. But often—for instance, if you have a viral rather than a bacterial infection—they're worthless. And they *massacre* good bugs, frequently allowing bad bugs to gain a foothold. According to scientists, it can take up to a full year for your gut to recover from a single round of antibiotics.[6] You don't want your microbiome to suffer needlessly, so take antibiotic drugs only when they're really necessary.

Watch out for other drugs as well. NSAIDs, proton pump inhibitors, and many other drugs can mess with your gut microbiome. Use these drugs if you need them but be as sparing as you can.

Above all, keep drinking bone broth and using collagen! These foods fight inflammation and build a strong, solid gut wall, giving your gut bugs a safe, secure place to live.

When you're rebuilding your gut, be patient. You're likely to see some benefits early on, but it may take many months for that gut to really glow. Also, there may be a few bumps along the way, in the form of gas or diarrhea, as you sweep the bad bugs out and invite the good ones in. Stick with it, and your gut will thank you.

TIP #2: MAKE FASTING A PART OF YOUR LIFESTYLE

One of the biggest bonuses of doing my Bone Broth Diet is that you'll discover how *easy* fasting is. It's one of those things that sounds scary but isn't. When you do my bone broth fasts, it's *comfortable* fasting. In fact, many people who finish the diet choose to keep up the intermittent fasting habit.

This is a very smart idea, because fasting is one of the most powerful tools we have for promoting a long, healthy life. In fact, as I said back in Chapter 3, our bodies are genetically engineered to fast, because our ancestors didn't have a steady supply of food at their fingertips. Some days they ate like kings and queens, but other days they didn't eat at all—and their bodies used that food-free time to clean house and make repairs.

Today, however, it's eat-eat-eat for most of us. Frequently, we grab our first meal when it's still dark and keep snacking all the way through the late-night shows. As a result, our bodies never get the rest they desperately need. Picture a never-empty gut as a dorm room that never, ever gets cleaned. (Ick.)

Luckily, fasting—like bone broth—is another piece of ancient wisdom we're rediscovering. We now know that fasting isn't just an old tradition; it's potent modern medicine.

Every year, scientists are uncovering new benefits of doing intermittent fasts. I've already told you how fasting hikes your levels of human growth hormone, an anti-aging hormone that sculpts your muscles. On your Bone Broth Diet, you'll also see how fasting makes those extra pounds melt away quickly. In an article in the *New York Times*, health reporter Jane Brody recently summarized still more big fasting benefits: "Human studies of intermittent fasting found that it improved such disease indicators as insulin resistance, blood fat abnormalities, high blood pressure and inflammation, even independently of weight loss."[7]

And—as they say on TV—there's more! Here are some of the additional things intermittent fasting does for you:

It benefits your brain. I talked earlier about how fasting stimulates the production of brain-derived neurotrophic factor (BDNF). This promotes the growth of new brain cells and helps your existing brain cells work better. Animal research indicates that boosting your levels of BDNF can even help to protect against Alzheimer's disease.[8]

It increases your endurance. In a recent study of mice, researchers found that mice deprived of food every other day developed more efficient energy metabolism and improved running endurance.[9]

If you've had breast cancer, it can lower the risk of it recurring. Researchers investigating the effects of fasting for breast cancer survivors reported that fasting 13 or more hours a day (that includes sleeping hours) lowered the chances of recurrence significantly. The researchers say, "Prolonging the length of the nightly fasting interval may be a simple, nonpharmacologic strategy for reducing the risk of breast cancer recurrence."[10]

So once you've finished your diet, and you know that bone broth fasting isn't hard at all, I hope you'll do it on a regular basis. It's truly one of the best gifts you can give yourself.

(Need a little more motivation? It'll do wonders for your food bill . . . and you'll save hours and hours in the kitchen!)

My Bone Broth Diet involves doing two 24-hour fasts each week, which happens to be my favorite way of fasting. However, as you know by now, I'm all about personal play. Once your diet is done, pick any style of fasting that suits your needs. The best type of fast is the one you'll stick with.

For instance, if you find 24-hour fasts a little bit tough, try doing *time-restricted eating*. In this approach, you simply shorten your eating window. Research shows that by limiting your meals to a 10-hour period each day—for instance, eating only between 8 a.m. and 6 p.m.—you can lose weight, reduce your belly fat, lower your blood pressure and cholesterol, and more efficiently stabilize your blood sugar and insulin levels.[11]

There are all sorts of other fasts you can try, so experiment a little and see what works best for you. Any type of intermittent fasting will do your body good.

TIP #3: STAY LOW-CARB . . . AND CONSIDER DOING "KINDA KETO"

By the time you're done with my Bone Broth Diet, your body will be a fine-tuned fat-burning machine—and this means you will be able to stay satisfied, energetic, and craving-free without all those carbs you used to scarf down.

My hope is that once you reach this point, you'll keep your carb count low. That's because a low-carbohydrate diet has benefits that extend well beyond weight loss. There's growing evidence that the lower you go, carb-wise, the more benefits you may reap. That's why many people are adopting a ketogenic diet, in which you limit carbs to 20 to 25 net carbs or fewer per day.

Now, I want to say up-front that this diet works beautifully for some people but not others. Here's my suggestion: First, try doing moderate keto—what I call "kinda keto"—and see if this agrees with you. On a moderate keto plan, you can eat up to 50 carbs each day. (See my advice on counting carbs on pages 84–85.) Just make sure your carbs are coming from good natural sources such as fruits and vegetables as often as possible and not from packaged or processed foods. You can always go more hard-core if you want, but moderate keto lets you get virtually all of the benefits or keto without white-knuckling it. And those benefits are pretty remarkable.

For example, a 2020 study found that our brain pathways start to deteriorate in the late forties, which is scary news. However, the same study found a solution: teach the brain to burn ketones (those fats I talked about earlier) instead of glucose, by keeping carbs to a minimum. The researchers found that burning glucose decreased the stability of the brain's networks, while burning ketones stabilized these networks.[12] Similarly, a pilot study involving 14 older adults with mild cognitive symptoms suggestive of early Alzheimer's disease found that slashing carbs and loading up on fat improved brain function and memory.[13]

In addition, going keto may reduce your risk for cancer. A 2019 study found that feeding mice with squamous cell lung cancer a ketogenic diet inhibited tumor growth significantly. Earlier, a study of humans with cancer found "a robust correlation" between higher blood glucose concentrations and worse survival in the patients with squamous cell cancer. (It had no effect on adenocarcinoma, another form of cancer.[14])

More recently, a review of the research concluded that going keto can enhance the results of cancer treatments. The researchers stated, "The majority of preclinical and several clinical studies argue for the use of the ketogenic diet in combination with standard therapies based on its potential to enhance the antitumor effects of classic chemo- and radiotherapy, its overall good safety and tolerability and increase in quality of life."[15]

And if you're a migraine sufferer, here's some exciting news: Going keto might help to reduce those agonizing headaches that interfere so cruelly with your life. One group of researchers has reported, "Clinical data on the ketogenic diet in migraine—obtained from 150 patients investigated in case reports and prospective studies—suggest that [it] may be a rapid onset effective prophylaxis for episodic and chronic migraine."[16] Another group of scientists concluded that a keto diet helps to protect against migraines by improving the function of the mitochondria (the "power plants" in our cells), compensating for fluctuating levels of the brain chemical serotonin, decreasing levels of CGRP (an inflammatory protein), and suppressing neuroinflammation.[17]

Again, not everyone can or should do full-on keto. I know people who thrive on it and people who crash and burn. Give moderate keto a try first and then experiment with full-on keto and see if it's right for you. You're good either way, as long as you kiss most carbs good-bye.

TIP #4: MOVE!

I've already talked a little about the importance of exercise back in Chapter 11, but now I'd like to take a closer look at the benefits you get from it. Here are four big reasons why movement is medicine:

It lowers your risk of disease. Exercise is one of your strongest defenses against the diseases of aging. For instance, women have a 12% to 21% lower risk of breast cancer[18] when they exercise, and physical activity lowers the risk of colon cancer by 19%.[19] Exercise also lowers your risk of everything from obesity to diabetes to Alzheimer's disease to stroke.

It helps you sleep better. Sleep is crucial if you want to stay young and healthy (more on this shortly), and I think you'll be surprised at how much your sleep improves when you exercise. This is especially true if you're near or at menopause, when getting a good night's sleep can be particularly tricky. One recent study,[20] for instance, found that both aerobic and resistance exercises helped postmenopausal women with insomnia find relief.

It makes you happier. Think of exercise as a "happiness pill." In one recent large-scale study,[21] researchers found that all types of exercise—from team sports to cycling to gym workouts—can reduce mental health problems. In particular, exercise can help to reduce anger, depression, or anxiety, which is why growing numbers of psychologists and psychiatrists now "prescribe" workouts.[22]

It keeps you young. As I said back in Chapter 11, exercise is one of your best defenses against aging. That's because it turns back the clock at the cellular level.

In one study, researchers analyzed the telomeres of nearly 6,000 people. Telomeres are the caps on the ends of your chromosomes—kind of like the plastic tips, or aglets, on the ends of your shoelaces—and as you age, they get shorter and shorter, leading to DNA damage.

Remarkably, the researchers found that the most physically active people had much longer telomeres than the most sedentary people. In fact, the difference amounted to about *nine years* of cellular aging! That's a big payoff for simply working out.[23]

In addition to keeping you young physically, exercise can help to keep you young mentally. In a 2020 study, researchers asked 206 older adults to exercise four times a week, increasing over time from 20 to 40 minutes a day. At the end of six months, the participants had better scores on verbal fluency, word recall, and "executive function" (which includes planning, focusing on a goal, and multi-tasking). The blood flow to their brains also increased.[24]

And for more good news on exercise and aging, let's circle back to that all-important gut microbiome—because there's a strong correlation between exercise, the microbiome, and staying young.

In a recent study, scientists found that a sick gut microbiome can predict both cognitive problems and physical frailty. That's no surprise, of course, given what we already know about the influence of our gut bugs. But there was more: They also found that *exercise had a big impact on the health of the gut*. Their conclusion: Exercise can help to heal your microbiome, and a healthy microbiome in turn can make you stronger and smarter as you age.[25]

Remember: Each time you exercise, your gut bugs stand up and cheer. You're not just doing it for yourself . . . you're doing it for them, too!

One tip, however. If you're burned out, feel free to relax and sip on bone broth instead of doing heavy workouts. Just take easy walks, do simple yoga moves, and let your body heal.

TIP #5: GET ENOUGH SLEEP

It's a myth that staying awake into the wee hours of the night will burn off more calories and help you stay slim. In reality, the opposite is true; in fact, research indicates that sleeping one extra hour a night can burn off an extra 14 pounds over the course of a year, largely because it cuts down on night-time snacking.[26] Conversely, here's what sleeping too little does to you:

- It increases the fine lines on your face and reduces your skin's elasticity. (That's why you look so old when you burn the candle at both ends for a few nights.)

- It lowers your levels of human growth hormone—that youth-promoting hormone that sculpts lean muscle.

- It makes your metabolism sluggish.

- It causes you to crave sugar and carbs.

- It jacks up your level of the stress hormone cortisol, making you anxious and jittery.

Now, I know firsthand that getting enough sleep can be trickier than it sounds. However, practicing good "sleep hygiene," as the sleep experts call it, may help you fall asleep more easily and sleep more soundly. If you have trouble dozing off or staying asleep, try these tricks:

Set a bedtime and do your best to stick to it. Seriously . . . bedtime is not just for kids! Our biological clocks regulate everything from healing to digestion, and when you keep changing your bedtime, you'll constantly be out of sync with these clocks. This can pack pounds on your belly and increase your risk for depression. There's even a name for it—"social jet lag"—and it's as bad for you as travel-related jet lag. So try to get to bed around the same time each night.

Step away from your devices. The blue light from your phone, computer, or tablet messes with your sleep, telling your brain that it's daytime and keeping you alert. So end your screen time at least an hour before bedtime, or at least wear blue light–blocking glasses when you use your devices.

Treat yourself to nice bedding. If you can afford it, get a good mattress, a comfy pillow, and high-quality sheets.

Keep it dark. Even a small amount of light can make it harder for you to fall asleep. Worse yet, research shows that exposure to light at night is "a significant risk factor for overweight and obesity."[27] Keep your room as dark as possible and use blackout curtains to block outside light.

Turn down the thermostat. Like our ancient ancestors, we sleep best when our "cave"—or in this case, our bedroom—is nice and cool. If you can, keep the temperature in the mid-sixties.

Mellow out. Before bedtime, take an Epsom salt bath. The magnesium in the salt will soothe your skin and make you sleepy. In addition, rub a little lavender oil on your bedposts.

De-stress before you sleep. It's hard to get to sleep if your mind is spinning, so get in the habit of doing the stress-busting strategies I'll describe in Chapter 13. Do a little gentle stretching or yoga, but avoid doing vigorous workouts in the evening. A strenuous workout can rev you up instead of calm you down.

TIP #6: MINIMIZE YOUR BODY BURDEN OF TOXINS

It's a dirty world out there, and you can't avoid all of the toxins in it. However, you can dramatically reduce your exposure to these toxins by taking a few simple steps:

Drink filtered water. Get the best water filtration system you can afford, whether it's a water-filtering pitcher, filters on your faucets, or a whole-house system.

Eat organic when you can. I know that going all-organic may be too hard on your budget. If so, check the Environmental Working Group's "dirty dozen" and "clean fifteen" lists to find out which produce is fine to buy in nonorganic form and which isn't.

Buy "green" cleaners and beauty products. The Environmental Working Group is a handy resource here, too. Search under "EWGT Verified," and you'll find a database of nontoxic products you can trust.

TIP #7: DO A REGULAR CLEANSE

Let's face it: No matter how faithfully you try to take care of yourself, you're just human. And sometimes you're going to work too hard, sleep too little, grab junk food meals, and start skipping workouts. Add in the regular wear-and-tear of life—job stress, family crises, toxins you can't always avoid, and toxic *people* you can't always avoid—and you're on the path to burnout.

Stay on this path too long, and you're going to crash and burn. And believe me—you don't want that to happen.

What's the answer?

Simple: When you start to see the signs of burnout—aging skin, extra belly fat, fatigue, "brain fog," and a lack of joy in your life—*take charge* by doing a quick cleanse to push nutrients into your body and push toxins out. When you do this, you'll stop burnout in its tracks.

Remember: It all starts with food. Once you're restored and re-energized, you can tackle the other causes of your burnout—whether it's difficult people, a stressful job, or money problems. That's because you'll be back in fighting shape, and you'll be able to handle anything life throws at you.

Now, I'm very proud of my own plan, Dr. Kellyann's Cleanse and Reset. It healed me when I hit burnout, and now it has healed thousands of other people. However—I'll say it yet again—I'm a great believer in personal play, so choose any cleanse that works best for you. Just make sure you follow these guidelines:

■ Pick a cleanse that's rich in tissue-repairing foods like collagen and bone broth. These will renew, refresh, and revitalize you.

■ Avoid all-juice cleanses that leave you feeling stringy and weak. You want to pamper yourself, not punish yourself.

■ Include a variety of nonstarchy veggies in your cleanse, to help banish the bloat and flood you with nutrients. Also, add a little fruit—berries are best— but don't overdo it or you'll overload your body with sugar.

Doing regular cleanses is one of the most effective strategies you can employ to avoid "hitting the wall." In fact, I'm a big believer in doing a cleanse at the beginning of every season. Get in this habit yourself, and you'll enter each new season all shiny and new and crush that burnout before it even has a chance to rear its ugly head. That's what I call preventive medicine!

THE KEY TO SUCCESS: TAKE ONE STEP AT A TIME

I know I gave you a long "to-do list" in this chapter. But don't panic, you don't have to tackle everything at once! Just pick the step that's easiest for you to do and make that your starting point. Then, once that step becomes habit, pick the next one.

And don't worry if you backslide sometimes. (You can always undo the damage with a few bone broth fasts or a cleanse.) We're all perfectly imperfect, and that's just fine. If you practice *most* of these strategies *most* of the time, you'll get all of the benefit.

So pick your first step and get started on a long, healthy, happy, wonderful life!

REACH FOR THESE SUPER-CLEANSERS!

In between cleanses, you can help keep your body squeaky-clean by incorporating powerful detoxifying foods into your daily diet. Here are the top super-cleansers:

- **Bone broth.** Yep, I have to give my favorite food one more plug. As I've mentioned, bone broth is loaded with the amino acid *glycine*. Your liver needs glycine to do its job of detoxification, and its ability to cleanse your body is limited by the amount of glycine available. So drink up!

- **Onions.** That distinctive smell of onions comes from sulfur-containing compounds that are potent detoxifiers. That's one reason why eating onions can reduce your risk for liver and colon cancer.

- **Seaweed.** The alginate in seaweed absorbs toxins from your digestive tract so your body can get rid of them. (Want another plus? Research suggests that alginate might help you lose weight.) Seaweed is also loaded with minerals that help to whoosh toxins out of your system.

- **Cilantro and coriander.** *Cilantro* (also called Chinese parsley) refers to the leaves of the coriander plant, while *coriander* refers to its seeds. Research shows that cilantro can help reduce the amount of lead your body absorbs, and coriander can ramp up the power of your body's natural detoxifying agents.

- **Curcumin.** Is there anything this powerful detoxifying and anti-inflammatory spice can't do? It's linked to easier weight loss, a reduced risk of cancer, and has even improved memory in people with Alzheimer's disease.

- **Apples.** These yummy fruits are loaded with pectin, which can help remove heavy metals from your body.[28]

- **Raw cruciferous veggies.** Foods like broccoli, cabbage, kale, and Brussels sprouts contain *glucosinolates,* which break down to form cancer-fighting molecules including *indoles* and *isothiocyanates* (ITCs). These increase the detoxification of substances that otherwise could promote cancer. Cooking may reduce the bioavailability of ITCs, so regularly include raw or very lightly cooked cruciferous veggies in your diet.

- **Dandelions.** If you think dandelions are simply a lawn pest, you're missing out. Dandelions and other bitter greens can give a big boost to your liver's detox efforts. Toss a handful into salads or soups, take dandelion in capsule form, or try drinking dandelion tea.

■ **Milk thistle.** As your body's primary detoxifier, your liver takes a beating in today's polluted world. Milk thistle, which contains a powerful healing substance called *silymarin,* can help it bounce back from the damage that toxins do. In fact, milk thistle is used in many countries to help the liver recover from alcohol damage or even mushroom poisoning. You can use milk thistle in capsule or liquid form, or as a tea.

■ **Burdock root.** Eastern cultures prize burdock root as a blood purifier, and science shows that it has liver-protective and detoxifying properties. You can take burdock root in capsule form, as an extract, or as a tea.

■ **Beetroot, tea, garlic, citrus fruits, carrots, avocados, and coffee.** All of these are powerful liver cleansers.

Note: Avoid dandelion, milk thistle, and burdock root if you're allergic to ragweed, marigolds, chrysanthemums, and related plants. If you have any plant allergies at all, test a small amount first to make sure you do fine with it.

CHAPTER 13

Get Slimmer by Lowering Your Stress

THINK "WEIGHT LOSS" AND you automatically think about diet and exercise—and that's what we've talked about up to this point. But now I want you to consider a hidden culprit that nearly always plays a big role in weight gain: chronic stress.

I'm guessing that you're under a lot of stress. (Who isn't these days?) Maybe you wear your stress like a badge of honor: "Look at me, working full-time, raising a family, doing volunteer work, and . . . "

That's what I used to do, too. But here's what I learned the hard way. You can get away with this superhero act for a long time, maybe for years. But over time, if you don't take steps to counter the stress that your demanding routine is causing, it will wear you out—and I can guarantee that it will put an extra 10, 20, or 50 pounds on you.

If you want to stay slim and healthy for life, you've got to face down your stress. It's not an option—it's necessary.

In Chapter 14, I'll explain how to develop a mind-set that helps you stay "stress-resistant" forever. This is the most powerful thing I teach my own patients for keeping extra weight off. However, it'll take time for you to achieve that mind-set, and I want you to start taking control over your stress right away.

So in this chapter, I'll show you six ways to cut your stress levels immediately, no matter how crazy your life is right now. These techniques are easy and even fun, and they'll speed up your weight loss and de-age you, too.

But before we get to them, let's talk about all the bad stuff that chronic stress does to you.

STRESS MAKES YOU GAIN WEIGHT

When you're chronically stressed, your body craves relief. As a result, you're tempted to turn to food to "self-medicate." Research shows that many people eat more snacks when they're stressed and that they're likely to turn to candy, chips, and other junk foods.[1] That's because when we eat foods like these, we get a quick rush of feel-good chemicals—a food "high."

In fact, even thinking about something stressful that's coming up in your life can make you crave food. In one study, researchers divided college-age women into two groups. They told one group that they'd need to fill out a questionnaire about work (a low-stress activity). They told the other group that they'd need to give a speech about work to a panel of judges (a high-stress activity). Then the researchers took blood samples from the women. The result? The women who anticipated having to give a talk had higher levels of ghrelin, a hormone that makes you feel hungry.[2]

In short, stress makes you want to eat. And eating when you're stressed makes you feel good—temporarily.

Unfortunately, the relief that comes from that chocolate bar or carton of ice cream lasts for only a few seconds. When the rush fades, your stress comes right back—and worse yet, you'll probably add a layer of guilt on top of it. This guilt adds to your stress and tempts you to overeat once again in order to seek relief, creating a vicious cycle—a pattern I see all the time in my own practice.

STRESS MAKES YOU OLD AND WRINKLY

It's bad enough that stress can make you fat, but here's something else it does: It makes you age faster.

When you're stressed, your levels of a hormone called cortisol skyrocket. If your cortisol levels stay high month after month, your blood pressure and blood sugar levels will climb, and your levels of human growth hormone (which helps keep you young and lean) will drop.

High cortisol levels will cause you to put on fat around your belly. If anyone you know is thin but still has that "tire" around the waist, chances are it's a cortisol tire. Chronically elevated cortisol can give you a middle-aged gut no matter how young you are.

In addition, research shows that chronic stress weakens the integrity of your skin's collagen.[3] As a result, your skin gets saggy and wrinkly, adding years to your

HOW STRESS AGES YOU AT THE MOLECULAR LEVEL

To understand just how dangerous chronic stress is for your cells, you need to know a little more about telomeres—those caps on the ends of your chromosomes that keep them from unraveling.

Unfortunately, telomeres don't last. The cells that make up your organs, skin, bones, blood, and connective tissue typically divide 50 to 70 times. With each division, the telomere shortens, aging the cell until eventually it dies.

Psychological stress speeds up this process because it boosts inflammation as well as oxidative stress.[4] Both inflammation and oxidative stress cause your telomeres to get shorter, aging you and putting you at risk for diabetes, cancer, and other diseases of aging.

appearance. And worse yet, chronic stress wreaks havoc on your immune system. A weak immune system, in turn, makes you age more quickly.

Finally, when you're stressed, it's harder for you to take care of yourself. You're more likely to turn to alcohol or cigarettes, short yourself on sleep, or skip exercising—all of which will make you look and feel older.

SIX FAST WAYS TO LOWER YOUR STRESS

Clearly, chronic stress is bad for your body. And tackling that stress is essential if you want to be lean, energetic, sexy, and healthy.

But if you lead a busy life, I'm guessing that you're thinking, "OMG, Kellyann, I don't have time to add anything else to my day. Telling me to add stress reduction to my schedule will just stress me out more."

And I get that. I really do. My life is crazy, too, and I have days when I can't handle one more thing. But I promise you that I'm not asking the impossible. The good news about chronic stress is that if you give your mind and body a break from it for only a few minutes a day, you can begin to reverse its negative effects. So if you have 30, 15, or even 5 minutes to spare, you can start cutting your stress down to size.

What's more, the techniques I'm recommending are easy. In fact, they may sound far too simple to be effective. But trust me: When I recommend these strategies to my patients, they get healthier, happier, and more energetic. And I see clinical results in the form of lower blood pressure, lower blood sugar, and falling numbers on the scale.

So try these six natural strategies and see the results for yourself.

1. Meditate

As a kid, I remember thinking of meditation as something that only hippies or gurus did. But then I grew up and got interested in medicine—and, in particular, in how medical practitioners can heal the human body naturally. And I discovered that meditation is very, very powerful medicine. Here are some of its proven benefits.

- **It changes your brain in ways that protect you against stress.** One study of people participating in an 8-week meditation program found that the intervention actually altered their brain structure. Scans showed that their reductions in stress correlated with decreased gray-matter density in the amygdala,

Stress and Your Metabolism

Marc David, founder of the Institute for the Psychology of Eating and author of *Nourishing Wisdom* and *The Slow Down Diet*

psychologyofeating.com

Stress doesn't just influence how much you eat—it also influences how much benefit you get from your food, as my friend Marc explains below.

"One of the lesser-known nutritional principles that can be a metabolic game changer for so many people is that our frame of mind when we eat can be as important as the food itself. We could be eating the healthiest food in the universe, but if we aren't in the optimum state of digestion and assimilation—which happens to be relaxation—we won't be absorbing the full nutrient profile of our meal.

"Evolution has wired human beings to most fully metabolize any meal when we're in the state of parasympathetic nervous system dominance. This means stress free, eating slowly, savoring, enjoying, feeling nourished, and taking time for our meal. When we're in the extreme opposite state—sympathetic nervous system dominance—the brain automatically shuts down digestion. So when we eat under stress or in an anxious rush, or if we're thinking negative thoughts about ourselves when we eat, we literally diminish the nutritional value of our meal.

"So yes, take control of your health by eating good medicinal foods like nutrient-dense broths. But remember to put yourself in the best frame of heart and mind whenever you eat so your body can best receive the foods you offer it."

a region of the brain that plays a big role in anxiety and stress. At the same time, they exhibited increased gray-matter density in the hippocampus, which facilitates learning and memory, as well as in brain regions associated with self-awareness, compassion, and introspection.[5]

■ **It can help you get control over eating problems.** A research review found that meditation "effectively decreases binge eating and emotional eating" in people with these problems.[6] Another study involving obese participants participating in a six-month diet found that "mindful meditation enhanced weight loss by 2.8 kg (approximately 6 pounds) potentially through greater improvements in eating behaviors and dietary restraint.[7]

■ **It can slow your aging.** Remember how stress makes your telomeres shorter? A few years ago, researchers asked one group of breast cancer survivors—all experiencing high levels of distress—to participate in group sessions in which they learned how to perform meditation and gentle hatha yoga. Participants practiced meditation and yoga at home each day. They also participated in supportive group therapy.

The researchers found that telomere length stayed stable in the women who practiced meditation and yoga and participated in supportive therapy, while telomeres grew shorter in a control group of cancer survivors who merely participated in a 1-day stress management seminar.[8] This means that the group who meditated both slowed their aging and reduced their risk of getting cancer again.

In addition, meditation can lower your blood pressure,[9] improve your immune function,[10] and reduce anxiety and depression.[11] So isn't that worth 20 minutes of your life a few times each week? I think so.

What's more, meditation is simple, once you get in the habit of doing it. Here's how "mindful meditation," the most well-studied version of meditation, works.

■ Find a quiet place where no one will interrupt you. If necessary, lock yourself in the bathroom.

■ Get in a comfortable position in a chair or on the floor. Rest your hands lightly on your thighs.

■ Notice how you feel. Are you cool or warm? Are you experiencing tension or pain in any part of your body? How does your clothing feel against your skin? Are you hungry or full? Are you wide awake or tired?

■ Notice your surroundings. What do you see, hear, or smell?

- Let your mind wander where it will. At first it will probably be swirling with thoughts about work, money, or family issues. That's okay. Simply examine each thought without judging it, and then gently let it go.

- Focus on your breathing. Take deep breaths in, as if you're filling your abdomen with air. Then slowly let each breath out. Focusing on your breathing helps you stay anchored as you meditate. When your mind wanders, let it—and then return your attention to your breathing.

- Say a word or a sound as you breathe out, if it helps to relax you.

Be patient with yourself when you're just beginning to practice meditation, because it takes time to learn to be still. If you're like me and you're always on the move from one commitment to the next, simply sitting and *being* may make you crazy at first. But over time, you should be able to get in the zone more and more quickly—and when you do, you'll instantly feel the stress flowing from your body.

Here are a few tips for getting the most from your meditation.

- **Meditating for 10 minutes a day is infinitely better than meditating for 70 minutes once a week.** Try to meditate frequently (every day if possible), even if that just means sitting for a few minutes.

- **Start small.** If you try to meditate for 30 minutes right from the start, I can almost guarantee that you will get frustrated and discouraged. I recommend starting with 5 minutes and increasing that time only when you're comfortable. If you sit for 5 minutes and you find that your mind wanders the whole time, you will still receive incredible benefits from meditation.

- **Focus on your breathing.** When you do this, the rest will follow.

One note: If you're like some of my patients, there's a chance that even with practice, you won't fall easily into the meditation mind-set. If you try meditating for several weeks and still have trouble with it, here's another alternative you can try: moving meditation.

Tai chi is one popular form of moving meditation, but there are other, less structured options. Here are some of my favorites. If you try them, simply remember to focus on your breathing and let your thoughts flow in and out of your mind without judging them.

- **Take a walk.** As you're walking, observe what you're feeling, seeing, smelling, and hearing. Is there a breeze, or is the air still? Do you smell flowers or maybe the aroma of fresh-brewed coffee coming from a Starbucks? What colors are the homes or stores you're walking past? Do you hear the sounds of traffic or the murmur of neighbors conversing? Focus on the rhythm of your walking and the sensation of your feet hitting the ground.

■ **Cook.** Select a recipe that takes some time to prepare—for instance, a stew, soup, or chili. As you wash and chop each vegetable, consciously stop, feel the shape of it, and notice its color. Watch the water pouring over it as you wash it. Listen to the sharp sound as you chop and the sizzle as you cook. Notice the aromas of your food cooking and the flavors you taste. Really look at your pots, pans, plates, and glasses, noticing their colors, shapes, sizes, and even any chips or scratches on them.

■ **Weed the yard or rake the leaves.** As you're working, observe how your plants are changing with the season. Look for new leaves. Examine each weed as you pull it or each pile of leaves as you rake. Stop and really look at the sky and the clouds. Listen to birds, examine bugs, and notice airplanes flying overhead.

You can practice mindful meditation in other settings as well—for instance, if you're petting your cat, bathing a baby, or lying in bed first thing in the morning. You can do a quick "mini-meditation" when you're walking from the grocery store to your car. (Be creative!) The key is to try to meditate regularly so it becomes a habit.

2. Do breathing exercises

Stress makes your breathing shallower, and shallow breathing makes you feel more stressed. Over time, this becomes a downward spiral. When you break this pattern by learning to breathe correctly, you're likely to see a big difference almost immediately.

The first step in changing your breathing is to become aware of how you're breathing now. So take about 5 minutes to do this exercise.

1. Sit in a comfortable spot where you won't be distracted. Turn off your phone and the TV. If you have pets, put them in another room.

2. Close your eyes and focus on your breathing. Don't change anything at all; just become aware of the way in which you breathe in and out. Does your breathing feel rushed or shallow, or does it feel even, slow, and deep?

3. Next, notice where you feel your breath going as you breathe in. Do you feel it in your nose, your throat, or your chest? Does your abdomen move when you breathe? Do your ribs expand?

Now that you're aware of your typical breathing pattern, work on making it deeper, more even, and more relaxing. Here's an exercise that will train you to breathe correctly.

1. Lie on the floor. Put one hand on your stomach and the other on your chest, over your heart. As you inhale, feel your hands move. First, feel the hand on your belly rise up as you pull air into your body. Then feel the hand on your chest move up as your ribs expand. Feel your breath filling you from your abdomen to the top of your lungs, just under your collarbones.

2. Pause for a second, and then start to exhale. Feel the air leaving your belly, so your hand drops. Then feel the air leaving your chest and your hand dropping there.

3. Pause and practice this again until you feel comfortable with it. The key is to breathe deeply, feeling the breath from your abdomen up.

Once breathing this way starts to feel natural, try to make it a habit. Anytime you notice yourself becoming stressed during the day, check to make sure you're breathing slowly and evenly from your belly up.

If you're extremely stressed, try this 4-7-8 (Relaxing Breath) Exercise. You can do it anywhere. To begin, sit in a comfortable position with your back straight. Place the tip of your tongue against the ridge of tissue behind your top front teeth, and keep it there the entire time.

1. Exhale through your mouth, making a whooshing sound. If you find it tricky to breathe around your tongue, try pursing your lips.

2. Close your mouth and inhale silently through your nose to a count of four.

3. Hold your breath for a count of seven.

4. Exhale completely through your mouth, making a whooshing sound, to a count of eight.

5. Complete this entire cycle four times.

Remember to inhale quietly through your nose and exhale with a whoosh through your mouth. You can breathe at any speed that's comfortable for you; the ratio of 4:7:8 is what's crucial. The more you do this exercise, the better you'll get at breathing slowly and inhaling and exhaling more deeply.

3. Get a massage

Do you think of massage as a guilty pleasure? If so, stop viewing it as sinful and start thinking of it as smart, because a massage can dramatically lower your stress levels.

In one study, researchers at Cedars-Sinai Medical Center randomly assigned 53 volunteers to either deep-tissue Swedish massage or light massage.[12] The researchers took blood and saliva samples before and after the massages, and here's what they found.

- The people who received the Swedish massages exhibited marked decreases in their blood and saliva levels of cortisol—that stress hormone I've talked about—and in arginine vasopressin, another hormone that can cause increases in cortisol. In addition, they had high numbers of immune cells called lymphocytes, indicating that massage ramped up their immune systems.

Surrender to Self-Love

Kim D'Eramo, DO, author of *The Mind-Body Toolkit*
drkimderamo.com

My good friend Kim is no ordinary physician. In addition to her conventional medical training, she's studied mind-body medicine and learned about the body's ability to heal itself.

Kim has used the "mind-body connection" to free thousands of people from pain, anxiety, and depression, and she told me something wise about healing, de-stressing, and self-acceptance that I'd like to share with you.

"Your emotions are the root of all your actions and behaviors. The chemistry of your emotions either creates health or creates disease. When there are emotions you've not dealt with, like anger, fear, or loneliness, this sets up the inflammatory chemistry that makes you gain weight and get sick. The chemistry of your repressed emotions also creates food cravings and drives your eating behaviors. Depending on whether you're in a positive or a negative emotional state, the chemicals of your emotions create health or create disease. They drive healthy or self-sabotaging behaviors.

"What's the most powerful way to end cravings and the negative emotional states that destroy health and cause weight gain? Self-acceptance. It is counterintuitive, since society programs us to 'fight disease' and 'fight fat.' We're surrounded by reasons not to accept

■ The light massage group exhibited increases in the hormone oxytocin, which is associated with contentment and "warm fuzzy" feelings, along with a drop in adrenal corticotropin hormone, which promotes cortisol release.

So add massage to your repertoire of stress-reducing techniques. Don't think of it as a splurge; think of it as a medical treatment than can de-stress you, keep you younger, and help you keep extra weight off. (When you think of it that way, it makes that 60 dollars sound pretty cheap, doesn't it?)

4. Take saunas

If you're stressed, I strongly recommend getting into the habit of using a sauna. Saunas lower your levels of the stress hormone cortisol—that same hormone that can cause you to develop a "cortisol tire" around your belly even if you're not overweight overall.

ourselves until we're perfect. There can even be an underlying fear that if you were to accept yourself as you are, you would never get off the couch again or bother to eat healthy. However, the truth is, when you love and accept yourself fully, you are more motivated to care for and nurture yourself with the foods and activities that bring even more health and well-being.

"When you feel sluggish or have cravings, see if you can take three deep, slow, full breaths, and imagine bringing the idea of self-love and self-acceptance into your body. This ends the subconscious cycle of self-hatred that's making you sick and bringing your energy down. It takes courage to accept yourself when you've just done a self-defeating behavior like overeating or when you weigh 50 pounds over your ideal weight. However, when we love and accept ourselves fully, it changes our chemistry. We enter a higher emotional state that calms cravings, supports weight loss, and literally reverses disease.

"Do the Bone Broth Diet as a gesture of self-love. Nurture yourself with this powerfully enriching food. Instead of making this into one more thing you do to 'fight the fat' or 'beat the bulge,' simply accept your body and yourself and surrender to self-love."

If possible, use an infrared sauna. This type of sauna, which uses light to heat your body directly without heating the air, is easy to tolerate if you're not a fan of steam saunas. And while it's mellowing you out, it'll also rejuvenate your skin and even make you healthier on a cellular level.[13]

5. Get outside

Picture a lion on the savannah, a whale in the ocean, or a parrot flying in the Amazon. Then picture the lion in a cage at the zoo, the whale in a tank, and the parrot on a perch in somebody's living room. It doesn't seem natural, does it?

Now, picture *you* as you're genetically designed to be: outdoors, watching the sky for rain or the grasslands for prey to kill. Walking miles to get food. Standing still to admire a mountain range. Then picture your life now—dashing from your house to your car to your office, and then staying indoors for hours.

Don't get me wrong. Like you, I have no interest in living in a cave or walking miles to hunt meat for dinner. I love my house and my car and my job, and I'm glad that my local butcher hands me steak from an animal that I didn't have to stab to death with a spear.

But there's a trade-off for our modern lifestyle. It's true that we're rarely cold, wet, scared, or hungry, like our ancestors were—but like animals in cages or

"BIG BANG" THERAPY

Kate, a friend of mine, went through a bad time a while ago. She and her husband, Joe, had high-pressure jobs that left them tense and exhausted, and things got worse when Kate's mom became ill and needed lots of care. "At the end of the day, Joe and I were just wrecked," Kate told me. Too tired to cook and too burned out to exercise, they were putting on pounds and they felt miserable.

One night when she was doing the dishes, Kate turned on the TV in the background. Normally, she's a serious documentary-and-news kind of person, but that night she happened to land on an episode of *The Big Bang Theory*.

"I'd never watched it before," she told me, "and I just couldn't stop laughing. My husband wandered in, and pretty soon he couldn't stop laughing, either. We were actually laughing so hard that we were in tears."

At the end of the show, they were still chuckling. And Kate felt so energized that she got out her yoga mat for the first time in weeks.

The next day, Kate did something smart. "I went on Netflix," she told me, "and I rented a whole season of that show. I swear, it was better than Xanax."

tanks, we're not really living the life we're genetically engineered to live. We've almost completely divorced ourselves from our natural habitat—and on a cellular level, our bodies know that something is missing.

What's the solution? Schedule in Mother Nature on your calendar. As often as you can, get out of the house and into the park, the forest, or the garden. Research shows that spending a short time in a "green" environment can lower your stress, and sunshine is a potent natural de-stressor and mood elevator as well.[14]

Want more? Getting outdoors has major physical benefits as well. In Japan, where "forest bathing" (that is, walking in the forest) is a popular trend, researchers compared people who walked either through a city or through a forest. They reported that the forest bathers lowered their cortisol levels, their pulse rate, and their blood pressure.[15] In another study, also done in Japan, researchers found that forest bathing enhanced immune function and elevated the expression of anti-cancer proteins.[16]

6. Laugh

Laughing is fun—and it makes you feel good all over by easing your stress, increasing bloodflow to your organs, relieving pain, and strengthening your immune system. (Maybe this is why people love funny cat videos so much.) So find something every day that makes you laugh—whether it's a silly book, the Sunday funnies, or a comedy.

By the way, here's a bonus: In addition to easing stress, laughter burns calories. One study showed that hearty laughing causes a 10 to 20 percent increase in energy expenditure and heart rate.[17] So while you're reducing your stress, you'll also be reducing your waistline.

SMALL SACRIFICE, BIG RESULTS

I'll say it again: I know you're busy. Some days you're crazy, insane, beyond-belief busy. And adding anything new to your schedule is a challenge.

But here's the great thing: None of the stress-lowering strategies I've talked about will take more than a few minutes a day, and some of them will take hardly any time at all. Better yet, they'll boost your weight-loss results and help you sleep better, think better, feel better, and look better.

So promise me that you will pick at least one of these strategies, starting today (even if it's just watching a cat video or doing a mini-meditation while you're vacuuming). Then try adding one or two more during your 3-week diet—better yet, do all of them. I promise you: Your brain, your waistline, your skin, and your DNA will thank you.

CHAPTER 14

Develop a Positive Mind-Set to Keep Extra Pounds Off

WHEN YOU FOLLOW MY Bone Broth Diet and simple exercise plan, you'll be giving your body everything it needs to be slim, healthy, and energetic. Stick to my 80-20 maintenance plan and go back on the diet anytime you put on a few pounds, and you can easily stay slender for life.

But here is something you need to know. There's an emotional component to weight loss as well as a physical component, and you will stay slender and youthful only if you are in a healthy environment and have a peaceful state of mind. If you're chronically stressed, sad, or angry, you will put those pounds back on (and the wrinkles as well). I virtually guarantee it.

When new patients come to my office, they typically start out by saying, "I need to know how to eat right. Can you help me?" But often, when I dig a little deeper—which I nearly always do, because my philosophy is to help my patients heal both physically and emotionally—I find out that food isn't the only issue.

For instance, I'll hear something like this: "I know I need to eat better, but it's really hard right now. My mom has early stage Alzheimer's, and I have to juggle my job with her needs. My sister lives close by, but she just says, 'You're better with her than I am—and you don't have kids like I do.' So I'm on my own, and I know it's going to get worse as my mom gets sicker."

Or a patient will say something like this: "I used to look good, but now I just keep gaining more and more weight. I don't know why I can't control my eating. Things are stressful at home because my husband and I are going through a bad time. He hates how I look, and I'm afraid that if I don't lose weight, he's going to leave me."

Or I'll hear this: "I lost my sister to cancer last year, and I can't stop grieving. I feel so alone, because she was the only person I could really share things with."

When patients tell me things like these, I know that I can help them take their weight off by changing their diets and giving them an exercise plan—but I also know that to keep the weight off, they'll need to change their lives as well.

Because I'm a medical professional, my patients usually expect me to focus solely on their physical health. But here is what I know: We are much more than bodies. We are also spiritual and energetic beings. And our health and weight are directly related to the environment we are in.

If you are in an unhealthy environment, your body will adapt by creating illness. It will also adapt by causing you to crave fat and sugar—a natural response to stress. As a result, you'll wind up chronically unhealthy, old, and overweight. So in reality, your initial weight loss is just part of your transformation to a healthy, slim you.

The de-stressing tips I offered in Chapter 13 are part of that transformation. However, if you're under high, chronic stress, they aren't enough. You need to figure out what's causing that stress and address it.

I know that right now, you're primarily interested in taking off pounds fast. But if you're tempted to skip this chapter, please do me a favor and read it. Because trust me on this: If you want to have "forever" weight loss and vibrant physical health, you need to focus on your emotional needs as well as your physical needs. And I have some powerful tools you can use to satisfy those emotional needs.

Here are the most important of your emotional needs. Here they are.

1. Choose your inner circle wisely.

To stay physically and emotionally healthy, you need to surround yourself with people who will be "carriers of your vision." These are people who understand you and your life goals and will support you and believe in you. These people serve as a shield, protecting you and lifting you. They will not sabotage you, they will stop other people from sabotaging you, and they won't let you sabotage yourself. If you lose weight and get healthier and happier, they will celebrate—not feel jealous or insecure and secretly work to undermine you.

These people may be your family members, your coworkers, your neighbors, or even your gym buddies. They can even be friends you meet online. You just need to identify them. Here's how you'll know them.

- They leave you feeling energized.
- They leave you feeling better about yourself, not worse.
- They really listen to you.
- They don't let you make excuses. (This is a big one.) When you're hurting, they won't encourage you to do unhealthy things like overeating. Instead, they'll steer you straight—firmly, if need be.

One of my favorite people, Daymond John of *Shark Tank*, was kind enough to share with me his insights on creating a strong inner circle. The strategy he uses is what he calls the 10 people closest to you. These are the people, he says, who determine who you are and how far you will go—so you need to pick them carefully. That doesn't mean other people aren't important. But it means that when you're parceling out your time and energy, these are the people you'll always put first. That's because you know they will put you first.

So . . . who are *your* 10 people? Don't decide right away. Instead, think about it. Who are the people who always come through for you? Who have your best interests at heart? Who understand your purpose and work to help you achieve it? Who will motivate you to stay slender and healthy, rather than secretly hope that you'll gain your weight back?

Keep these people close to you—or seek them out if you don't know them yet. When you surround yourself with them, they will help you talk your way out of tough times instead of eating your way through them.

2. Have an inner doorman.

This rule goes hand in hand with the previous one. While you're creating an inner circle of people who will carry your vision, you also need to get very tough-minded about whom you let into your circle.

While some people will carry your vision, others will sap your strength. Give yourself freely to the people who matter the most to you, instead of squandering your time and energy on everyone.

And definitely tell your inner doorman to keep certain people out. These include people who don't share your values, people who encourage you to give up rather than stay strong when you're going through tough times, and people who just want to use you to achieve their own goals. These people won't just waste your time. They'll make you tired, unhappy, and stressed . . . and that leads to extra pounds.

3. Strategize your yeses.

So far I've talked about inviting good people into your inner circle and kicking toxic people out. But now I'm going to switch gears and ask you a question: Are you a good friend to yourself—or are you your own worst enemy?

To answer that question, ask yourself this one as well. Do you say yes to everything because you don't want to miss out on an opportunity or let someone down? If so, here's the problem: When you say yes to everything, you eventually exhaust yourself and sabotage your health and weight-loss goals.

I found this out the hard way myself. It started when I wrote my first book. That one book turned into five. At the same time, I was raising two young boys while working full-time at my clinic.

I was running from dawn until midnight every day. Then the books came out, and I felt that I had to say yes to every TV show, every radio show, and every book signing. I had to get my message out to people who needed it, in every way I could. Plus, I had to help my kids with their math homework, get them to eat their veggies, drive them to baseball games, and make sure their socks matched.

As you can guess, I finally crashed and burned.

I spent my days telling people how to eat well, and then skipped meals and gorged on starchy comfort foods. I told my patients to lead value-centered lives, and then said yes to every offer that came along—even if it meant shorting myself and sometimes my kids. While I preached about the importance of movement, I was sitting at my desk for 16 hours a day getting "flat butt."

My life was spiraling out of control. Luckily, I realized it—and I realized that I needed to become strategic about my time. So here's what I started doing. When new opportunities opened up, I didn't automatically say yes. Instead, I stopped and asked myself these questions.

- If I say yes, what am I really agreeing to? How much work will this entail? Is it worth that much work?
- If I say yes, what effect will my decision have on my family, my own life, and my work?
- If I say yes, will I be violating any of my core values—for instance, my belief that I need to eat well and keep my body strong?

These days I no longer promiscuously accept every offer that comes my way. Instead, I measure out my yeses. And I'm not just happier and saner, I'm also healthier and thinner.

Why? Because the stress that stems from overcommitment makes you sick. It lowers your immune function, making you easy prey for illness. It sucks nutrients out of your body, leaving your skin dry and wrinkly and your hair thin and brittle. It makes you short-tempered and depressed. And it makes your body churn out huge amounts of cortisol and other stress hormones, causing those cravings for sugar and fat that I talked about earlier. In short, it makes you "fat, bitchy, and bald."

If you're heading in that direction right now, let me repeat the advice that I learned the hard way: *No is as powerful as yes.* When you start saying no to the things that aren't crucial—whether it's baking three dozen cupcakes for the PTA or taking work projects home on the weekends—you give yourself time to relax, reenergize, and destress. As a result, you can turn "fat, bitchy, and bald" into slim, happy, relaxed, and sexy.

Remember, too, that saying no may mean being assertive and insisting that other people say yes. For instance, if you're trying to care for an aging parent alone, it may mean putting your foot down and demanding that your other relatives help you out. I see far too many patients (especially women) who are overweight and unhealthy because they're trying to shoulder heavy burdens that other people are shirking.

4. Break free from bad relationships.

Are you currently in an unhappy relationship, and are you trying to decide if it's worth the effort you're putting into it?

The answer is simple: Look at yourself in the mirror. Are you washed out? Is your hair limp and thin? Are you putting on weight? Are there "sad lines" instead of laugh lines around your eyes? If so, this is your body's way of telling you that you need to escape.

Here's the deal. You're not meant to be under stress every day—not even low levels of stress. You are supposed to be stressed if a big dog is chasing you or a car is about to hit you. But the chronic stress you experience in a bad relationship ages you and makes you sick in ways that range from high blood sugar to weight gain to depression. And you can't live that way.

It's especially unhealthy for you to remain in a relationship if you and your partner don't share common values. For instance, if one of you has strong spiritual values and the other is all about accumulating money—or if one of you values fidelity in a relationship and the other doesn't—you are headed for grief.

So ask yourself: Do you feel stressed nearly every day? Is it your relationship that's causing that stress? Are your values miles apart? If so, there are only two ways you can get well: Go to counseling if you think the relationship is salvage-able, or get out if it isn't. Don't wait until you get sicker and gain even more weight—make the choice.

....

When Carly came to my office, she needed to get rid of 50 pounds. But she also needed to get rid of her boyfriend.

I'm really good at reading my patients' body language, and I could tell when I first saw Carly that she had emotional issues that went beyond her weight. So I gently steered the conversation around to her life. And while I'm not a psychiatrist, even the little bit of information she shared with me had me concerned.

Carly told me that her weight made her insecure, and that her boyfriend, John, was the first man who'd loved her for who she was. But as our conversation contin-ued, I started to sense that it wasn't love at all. It sounded more like manipulation.

Carly casually mentioned that John didn't work, but she said that was okay because she could pay the bills. She also confessed that he drank a lot, but she said, "I accept that because he totally accepts my weight." And more warning bells went off when she said that John had strongly discouraged her from coming to see me because "he knows I'll just get hurt by another failure."

Carly lost her extra weight, but it was a harder journey than it should have been because John tried to sabotage it. At our appointments, she'd tell me things like, "John gave me chocolates for Valentine's Day, and I knew he'd be upset if I didn't eat some of them." Or she'd say that she didn't have time to exercise because she had to work overtime to pay the couple's bills.

Clearly, a sexy, healthy, confident Carly wasn't part of John's game plan. Instead, he wanted an overweight, insecure partner he could take advantage of. And here's my guess: If Carly stays with him, she'll regain the 50 pounds she lost . . . and then some.

Conversely, here's a look at two of my superstar patients, Pam and Drew, the couple I introduced you to in Chapter 2. They'd both gained weight because they were eating high-carb diets, but they lost it—250 pounds between the two of them— because they supported each other every step of the way. And that's why I know they'll keep the pounds off.

Together, Pam and Drew went through the pain of recognizing that they were unhealthy. They went through the initial discomfort of taking action and changing their lifestyle. They shopped together, supported each other, and loved and cared for each other as a team.

When Pam and Drew appeared on The Doctors with me a while ago, I got to enjoy their company for hours. I heard them laugh continually. I saw them look in each other's eyes with true love and adoration. I saw them support each other, trust each other, and have each other's back in a way that was deeply touching. After 34 years of marriage, they could still let themselves fall in love over and over again—and they could elevate each other to achieve great things.

This is the kind of relationship you deserve to have yourself. If you do have it, hang on to it, because it will motivate you to be the best you that you can be. But if you're in a destructive relationship like Carly's, recognize that it is dragging you down, making you sick, and putting extra pounds on you. And if you can, get out.

....

Remember: Getting out of a bad relationship won't just make you happier—it'll make you healthier. One recent study,[1] for instance, found that 50 percent of female smokers succeeded in quitting if their partners gave up the habit, compared with only 8 percent of women whose partners didn't. When it came to weight loss, both men and women were more than twice as likely to lose weight if their partners signed on to the effort. Think about it.

5. Live in your truth.

We all lie, and women in particular tend to lie all the time.

Are you guilty of this? You're lying if you write happy Facebook posts while you're actually crying because your life sucks right now. You're lying if you tell your family that you're doing great when you're actually sad, scared, or lonely. And you're lying if you're a "people pleaser" who goes along with your friends' opinions and hides your own because you're afraid that people won't like you otherwise.

All of this lying takes an enormous toll. As I said earlier, we are not just physical beings but also energetic ones. When you use up so much of your energy maintaining lies, it makes you weak and ill. Moreover, when you bottle up your feelings instead of expressing them to people who can support and comfort you, you turn to food for comfort instead.

So if you want to stay happy, healthy, and slim, here is my advice: Be transparent. Tell the truth. If it's not true, don't post it, don't tweet it, and don't say it. Be authentic, and let your friends know that it is absolutely safe for them to be authentic around you. You'll all be better off as a result.

6. Learn to say "next."

Life is a big adventure. But you know what? It's also incredibly scary. That's because at any moment, it can wound you deeply. And sometimes it can take you from the highest high to the lowest low in a heartbeat.

DR. KELLYANN'S PATIENT PROOF

Cheryl

Cheryl, a patient of mine, had plenty of reasons to feel sorry for herself. A decade earlier, she'd been attacked and savagely beaten at work. As a result, she suffered head injuries, needed surgery, developed seizures, and had to take steroid drugs that caused her to gain nearly 80 pounds. That would be enough to break many people.

But Cheryl is a strong woman, and she decided to take her life back rather than staying stuck in her trauma. Her driving force? "To just be able to live and not feel sick." Before the attack, Cheryl loved life, loved shopping, and loved being with crowds of people. And she wanted all that back.

Now that she's following my protocol of real foods, Cheryl is losing weight, sleeping more deeply, healing physically in many ways, and loving life again. She tells the story of Henri Charrière, a famous prisoner who escaped from the brutal and "inescapable" penal colony of Devil's Island when he realized that each seventh wave in the ocean below the penal colony carried objects farther out to sea and could carry him far enough away to escape. For her, Cheryl says, my program "is that seventh wave."

While Cheryl is grateful for my program, I'm grateful to her because she is such an inspiration. That's because she had the courage to say *next* when so many people in her situation would simply surrender.

Maybe your partner asks for a divorce. Maybe you lose a job you loved. Or maybe someone you trust deeply betrays you. And it rips your heart out.

For many of my patients, this is when the weight starts piling on. As months, years, or even decades go by, they stay stuck in their hurt, unable to move forward. And unless they address that pain, they're never going to keep their excess weight off permanently.

Even in the short run, a heartache or big disappointment can derail health and weight-loss goals. That's why so many people succeed at a diet for a few days or weeks and then crash and burn after a bad date, a terrible day at work, or a financial setback.

Here's what I've learned through my own experience. To avoid getting stuck in a disappointment, a betrayal, or a heartache, you need a way to dismantle the pain quickly. And luckily, I've discovered that way. This is the best skill I have ever learned. Here's how to do it.

First, face the situation. Process it. Be angry. Be hurt. Be sad. Maybe even throw something.

Then do this. Literally say in your mind . . . *next.*

Picture the word: *next.*

Now, replace the pain with a mental image that brings you joy. Maybe it's a memory of your kids when they were babies. Maybe it's the feeling you get when you're hiking in the mountains or snuggling with your cat. Focus on something that floods you with joy. This will bathe your body in feel-good hormones, changing your mental state instantly and allowing you to move forward.

In the days and weeks that follow, learn to keep your pain in its place. Allow yourself to think about what pains you once a day—and only once a day—for 10 minutes. Then you are done. Again, think of something that fills you with joy, and then say *next.*

I can't overemphasize how crucial this skill is. If you can't move on when life hurts you, you will stay stuck in that hurt forever. And what will you do to ease that hurt? You'll overeat. I know—because I've done it, too. So remember: *next.*

7. Let someone else be "the rock."

It's easy to fall into the trap of trying to solve every problem on your own. But if you try to be "the rock" everywhere—at home, at work, with your friends—you're going to get overwhelmed. And when you get overwhelmed, you eat.

So here's my advice: If you're feeling stuck, don't go through it alone. If you are worrying, don't go through it alone. If you're sad or scared, don't go through it alone.

If you're like me and tend to feel that *strength* means that you need to deal with things yourself, try looking at this a different way. What I've learned is that it actually endears you to people when they see that you are beautifully imperfect, just as they are. And helping you feel safe, loved, important, and motivated helps them experience these same feelings themselves.

More important, reaching out for help is one of the most effective ways to stop

Believe!

Elizabeth Lombardo, PhD, bestselling author of *Better Than Perfect: 7 Strategies to Crush Your Inner Critic and Create a Life You Love*
elizabethlombardo.com

My wonderful friend Elizabeth Lombardo says, "A key and often overlooked ingredient to good physical health is your self-esteem. This includes your beliefs in yourself."

Here are three of her tips for developing a mind-set that will empower you to achieve your health and weight-loss goals.

"Believe that you are worth it. Sure, there may be obstacles to healthy living. And when you believe you are worth it, those obstacles are not as much concrete barriers as roadblocks that you can maneuver. Consider the benefits to being healthier (having more energy, feeling happier, being a great role model for your children, feeling proud of your new body). And focus on them over the obstacles.

"Believe you can make positive changes in your life. The ways you think, eat, and interact with others are all learned behaviors. You did not come out of your mother reaching for comfort food when you feel stressed or telling yourself what a loser you are. Those are learned. And anything learned can be unlearned and relearned, regardless of how long this has been part of your life. I have worked with people in their late eighties and nineties, and they could change—so can you!

"Believe in being better than perfect. Stop perfectionistic, all-or-nothing thinking, like 'I had one cookie and screwed up my diet—might as well eat the whole plate.' One deviation does not make you a failure. When you do not eat the way you wanted to, reframe 'failure' as 'data.' Why did you not do what you wanted to? Were you feeling overwhelmed? Did you not have healthy food options on hand? Then use the data to determine steps you want to take in order to prevent that slipup from happening again."

yourself from making seriously unhealthy choices. For instance, I know that when I get stuck, I start looking for comfort foods. There are reasons we seek out certain foods when we're feeling low. We're looking for a "change of state." We're looking to alter our chemistry in any way we can. Our bodies are smart, and what they're really looking for is feel-good hormones.

A healing conversation with a trusted person in your inner circle can generate these hormones. So if you're stuck and you feel the urge to reach for fattening foods, first make that call to someone you love and trust. Say, "I need help." And then let that person be your rock.

Always remember . . . it's not just about the food

While it's easy to focus on food when you need to lose weight, keep reminding yourself that what you eat is just part of the story. Your thoughts are as important as what's in your cupboard when it comes to having a beautiful body, looking young, and being energetic. You can't have it all without having your mind in the right place.

So while you're transforming your body, transform your mind-set at the same time. Say good-bye to toxic friends, and create an inner circle of people who will be the wind beneath your wings. Stop saying yes to everything, and stop trying to handle every life crisis on your own. Live in your truth rather than living a lie. And when life hands you lemons, learn to say *next*.

Put all of these rules into motion, and I promise that you will be happier and healthier. And when you create an environment where you can thrive, you will be able to kiss your extra weight good-bye . . . forever.

CHAPTER 15

Look Drop-Dead Gorgeous with My Top Ten Beauty Tips

By now, you know I'm very serious about slimming you down and making you healthy. But a girl can't be serious *all* the time, right? So in this final chapter, let's have a little fun.

Beauty tips aren't life or death, but I know that looking great is a big component of *feeling* great. It's all part of the package.

And you know what? Beauty doesn't start on the outside—it starts on the inside. That's why I'm not going to focus most of my attention on mascara, hair extensions, or nail polish in this chapter (although I love them all). Instead, I'm going to share my best tips for looking beautiful *from the inside out*.

And I'm not talking about that cookie-cutter, fashion-model kind of beautiful, either. I'm talking about being the most beautiful YOU that you can be. Because we're all beautiful in our own way—we just need to stop hiding our beauty and let it shine through.

Of course, we've already talked about some of the biggest steps you can take to look *and* feel good: Eat right. Get enough sleep. Take control over your stress. Cultivate peace of mind. But now I want to share some bonus tips I hope you'll love. Some of these are strategies you can use every day, while others will help you look fabulous on special occasions.

TIP #1: DO DRY BRUSHING

When I want to look my best before a TV appearance, this is one of my go-to tricks. It's a quick way to remove dry, dead skin cells, unclog pores, help your lymph system "take out the trash," and rev up your circulation so you look radiant all over.

Here's how you do dry brushing:

- Buy a bristle brush that's specially designed for dry brushing. You'll need a brush with a long handle so you can reach every part of your body. You might even want to buy a kit that includes several brushes, including a very gentle one for your face.

- Take off all your clothes and stand in the bathtub. Brush your entire body, starting with the soles of your feet and moving upward to your heart. Then brush your hands, arms, face, neck, and back, always brushing toward your heart. Cover every part of your body, being very gentle when you brush sensitive areas.

- When you've finished brushing, take a warm shower. Afterward, pat yourself dry and apply a good-quality skin cream or oil. Then slip into something sexy and see how you glow.

TIP #2: "PRELOAD" YOUR BODY WITH WATER EVERY MORNING—AND DRINK WATER ALL DAY LONG

As my friend Audrey Zona, who's a health coach, likes to say, "Drink water like it's your job." Remember: Dried-out skin cells are flabby and sad. Hydrated skin cells, in contrast, are plump and dewy—and that's what you want.

My rule is to drink about half your body weight in ounces of water each day, plus more if you've done a lot of sweating. If you're planning on eating low-carb for life (which I strongly recommend), you'll need a little extra water because low-carb diets are diuretic.

POWER UP YOUR WATER WITH PROBIOTICS!

I take a probiotic and a prebiotic supplement every day with my morning glass of lemon water, because it helps me build the beautiful gut that I need to have glowing skin. According to dermatologists, probiotics and prebiotics can help prevent acne and clear up rosacea. In addition, dermatologist Whitney Bowe at Mt. Sinai Medical Center says, "Increased numbers of good bacteria may also help to hydrate aging skin, reduce sun damage and improve the appearance of fine lines and wrinkles."[1]

I start every morning with a big glass of water with a lemon squeezed into it. This gives my skin a double dose of beautifying power—first from the water and second from the vitamin C, which helps build collagen.

In addition, I always keep detox waters on hand. These are infused waters—that is, waters flavored by submerging fruit, vegetables, herbs, and spices in them. Some of my favorite detox water combos are cantaloupe and strawberry; cucumber and mint; green tea and ginger; lemon and thyme; orange and blueberry; pineapple and mango; and watermelon and mint.

TIP #3: BEFORE A BIG DAY, FOREGO FOODS THAT MAKE YOU FART

I know I didn't put that very elegantly, but I mean it. For 24 to 48 hours before a big day—whether it's a hot date, a job interview, or your wedding day—I want you to stay away from beans, bubbly alcohol drinks, sparkling water, dairy, artificial sweeteners, soft drinks, sugar, and sugary fruits. Also, say no to gluten, which wrecks your gut. Better yet, take it to the next level by cutting out grains altogether.

What's more, steer clear of cruciferous veggies like cabbage, cauliflower, and broccoli. These vegetables are fantastic for you, but they can also bloat your belly big-time—so save them for those not-so-important days. And cut down on salt (more about that in tip #4).

Instead, treat yourself to bloat-fighting foods like asparagus, avocados, bone broth, cayenne, celery, cucumbers, ginger, green tea, lemon water, and fermented foods like kimchi. Your gut loves these foods, and it'll thank you by behaving instead of bullying you on your big day (or night).

Those are the basics of bloat fighting—but if you want to elevate your game to the "pro level," consider doing intermittent fasting for one or two days before a big day. Simply quit eating by 7 p.m. and try not to eat until 11 or so the next morning. This is the most effective bloat-buster I know.

TIP #4: BE SMART WITH THE SALT

I've had the good luck to meet some of the world's best makeup artists. And one message I've heard from them, over and over again, is that salt can dry out your skin and make you look saggy, baggy, and old.

But here's the deal: You don't need to give up salt; you just need to use the *right* salt. I like to say that salt can kill you or cure you—and it can also make you look old and tired or help you look young and vibrant. The secret to making salt your friend instead of your enemy is to toss out your table salt and replace it with unrefined Celtic sea salt or pink Himalayan salt. Here's why.

Refined salt is nothing but sodium and chloride, along with harsh and toxic chemicals, including bleaches and anti-caking agents. (Incredibly, manufacturers even add some chemicals to *remove* minerals your body craves—what they call "impurities.") Because there are no beneficial minerals left to balance out the sodium and chloride, you get an overdose of them. Your cells can't handle this, and the result is "puffy" skin—especially under your eyes.

Unrefined mineral salts, on the other hand, contain no toxic additives. They also contain smaller amounts of sodium and chloride than table salt. Better yet, they contain more than eighty minerals—silicon, potassium, magnesium, sulfur, calcium, and the list goes on—that energize your cells and help make you beautiful.

If you're worried about getting enough iodine if you give up table salt, it turns out—according to Dr. David Brownstein, an expert on iodine deficiency—that iodized salt actually isn't all that good a source of iodine. You're better off getting it from food sources like sea vegetables, turkey, cod, tuna, eggs, and Himalayan salt (which contains some natural iodine).

TIP #5: LIFT HEAVY THINGS

Back in Chapter 11, I told you that exercise can make you healthier. But here's another reason to do it: It makes your body sleek and sexy, so that little black dress hugs all the right curves.

As I've said, any form of exercise is good for you. However, *the only way you can sculpt muscle is to work it hard.* And the way to do that is with resistance exercise. So stick to walking, yoga, and light exercise during your diet—but afterward, add resistance training to your workouts.

I've known for years that resistance training is the biggest secret for getting the sexy shape you want. In fact—a little bit of trivia here—in my early days I was a body builder, and I once won the title of Miss St. Louis! I learned early on that to get truly sculpted, you need to lift weights and do resistance exercises like planks, pushups, and squats. However, I had to relearn this lesson just recently when the COVID-19 pandemic struck.

During the lockdown, I couldn't hit the gym, and I had no weights at home. At the time, I thought, *No problem. I'll just take a long, brisk walk every day.*

I did this religiously. And you know what happened? Within weeks, my waistline started to expand, my legs started to get flabby, and I started to get the dreaded "turkey wattles" under my arms. That's because walking simply wasn't enough to keep my muscles in shape.

I learned my lesson and bought myself a set of weights. It took weeks of weightlifting to get back to my pre-pandemic figure, but eventually I did.

The good news here is that it doesn't take a whole lot of resistance exercise to sculpt your muscles. In fact, you don't want to do it every day, because your body needs a day off to recuperate after a resistance workout. Schedule two or three workouts each week, aiming for 20 to 30 minutes each time. Gradually increase the number of repetitions you do, the size of your weights, or both. Keep this habit up for life, and you'll have the sculpted curves of a 30-year-old when you're 50. I kid you not.

TIP #6: PAMPER YOUR EYES

What's the first thing we notice about people we meet? Their eyes.

Our eyes truly are the windows to our souls, and they speak volumes about us. Audrey Hepburn once said, "The beauty of a woman is not in the clothes she wears, the figure that she carries, or the way she combs her hair. The beauty of a woman is seen in her eyes, because that is the doorway to her heart, the place where love resides."

Unfortunately, if your eyes take a daily beating from too much computer time, too little sleep, or pollutants in the air, they can be sending the wrong message about you: not that you're beautiful and loving, but that you're tired, old, out of energy.

Luckily, there are certain superfoods that help to make your eyes bright and beautiful, so your soul can shine through them. They include:

Berries. The anthocyanins in these fruits are nutritional powerhouses that help to keep your eyes clear and protect them from sun damage.

Omega-3 fatty acids. These nutrients, found in foods like fish and chia seeds, help to keep your eyes moist and minimize redness.

Kale and other leafy greens. These are rich in vitamin K, which helps to prevent those little blood vessels in your eyes from leaking. Translation—less "red eye" and more sparkle.

TIP #7: GET UPSIDE-DOWN

My good friend Kathy Smith, who contributed the fun and easy exercise plan in Chapter 11, also has a tip for making wrinkles vanish: Stand on your head! When you do this, you dramatically increase circulation to the skin of your face. This helps clean out the toxins that age your skin while bathing it in nutrients that make it young and healthy.

Try standing on your head for 1 to 3 minutes every day, if possible. If that sounds like too much of a challenge, here's an alternative: Lie on your bed with your head hanging over the edge. (For more of Kathy's beauty tips, check out her website: kathysmith.com.)

TIP #8: STAND UP STRAIGHT

I know I'm sounding like everyone's mom right now, but Mom was right! Good posture truly is a big deal. Here's why it matters:

- **Good posture makes you healthier.** When you slouch, you put extra stress on your back, your neck, and your shoulders. In addition, you prevent your lungs and digestive system from working at their best. When you stand up straight, all of your bones, joints, and organs are aligned correctly so they can function efficiently.

- **Good posture makes you happier.** In one study, researchers found that walking in a slouched posture made people feel "zombie-like" and increased feelings of sadness, loneliness, isolation, and sleepiness. In contrast, when participants stood upright while skipping and swinging their arms in opposition to their legs, they reported higher levels of energy and happiness.[2]

- **Good posture makes you look younger.** Try this experiment yourself. Stand in front of a full-length mirror and assume a slouched posture. Then stand upright and notice the difference. You'll look years younger and pounds lighter when your posture is good.

To improve your posture, try this exercise every day. Stand with your back against a bare wall, with your feet shoulder-width apart and your heels and butt touching the wall. If you can, touch the wall with your shoulders and the back of your head as well. (If you can't do this at first, no worries—just get as close as you can. Practice every day, and you'll make progress.) Hold this position as you breathe deeply in and out about ten times, keeping your head level. This exercise will teach your body to stand up straight.

TIP #9: BEFORE A ROMANTIC EVENING, EAT SOME "ENERGY FOODS"

This is one of those times when carbs come in handy. So indulge in a sweet potato, some winter squash, or a little extra fruit on the day of a special date. This will keep you going through the dinner, the dancing, and, well, whatever happens next!

TIP #10: HIT THE MALL (REALLY)

Finally, here's one more beauty tip, and I think you'll love it: *Go shopping.* I know this may not sound like making yourself beautiful from the inside out, but trust me—it is.

Here's the thing. If you've been battling weight problems for a while, you probably have a negative loop playing in your head that says, "I'm not beautiful." Even though you're going to be all shiny and new after your Bone Broth Diet, that same old script may keep playing over and over again. And if you don't erase it, you'll never be the most beautiful you that you can be.

That's why you need an attitude adjustment—and the ideal place to start is at the mall.

First, I want you to update your wardrobe. Right now, I'm betting you have a closet full of clothes designed to hide your figure. But now's the time to flaunt it instead, so stop aiming for "invisible" and start going for "look at me." Splurge a little—you've earned it—and buy some bold outfits that show off the new you. (Think slinky, sexy, and sassy.)

While you're at it, buy new undies. A well-fitted bra with a little push-up can take years off your figure, and panties that fit snugly without cutting into your butt can help to erase cellulite while eliminating those dreaded panty lines.

Next, take advantage of the smooth, glowing skin, strong nails, and silky hair you'll have as a result of loading yourself with bone broth and collagen. Treat yourself to some goodies at the makeup counter, and if you have any change left over, have your hair styled and get a manicure. If you're in your 30s or older, update your look by switching from black to brown mascara and minimizing foundation and blush; also, cut off long hair, because thinning hair looks fuller in a short cut.

Finally, take some selfies and send them to everyone you know. Show off your beautiful smile and your confidence, and the world see the new, radiant you. You're truly beautiful, inside and out—so it's time to stop hiding and start strutting!

SPREAD THE WORD!

I'VE GUIDED HUNDREDS OF patients to slimmer, healthier, happier lives, and I'm delighted and honored to be your guide as well. I wish you great success, and I'd love to hear from you about your results! I hope you'll share your stories and photos with me on my website.

Once you decide to start your Bone Broth Diet, tell someone!

Scientists studying change and habit say that if you share your commitment with friends and family, you're much more likely to stick to it. Knowing that others are going to ask you about your diet will give you added motivation to succeed.

Also, let me know how you're doing by going to:

drkellyann.com/resources

LET'S CONNECT ON SOCIALS

The Bone Broth Diet official hashtag is #BoneBrothDiet. If you add this hashtag to any posting you do, my social media team or others looking for bone broth inspiration will be able to view your photo and connect with you. You can search this hashtag for any social media platform and see what others are sharing about the program.

You can also follow me on social media for recipe inspirations and additional tips on staying slim, young, and healthy for life! You can find me on Instagram at @DrKellyannPetrucci, on YouTube at youtube.com/DrKellyannPetrucci, and on Facebook at facebook.com/drkellyann. While you're on Facebook be sure to check out my supportive Bone Broth Diet Facebook Group at facebook.com/groups/bonebrothdietrevolution for support and encouragement from others who are doing the Bone Broth Diet as well as members of my own team who are there answering your questions. You can also find me on Twitter at @DrKellyann and on TikTok @DrKellyann.

MEASUREMENT TRACKER AND CARB COUNTER

FILL OUT THIS FORM before and after your diet so you can quantify your results. I also suggest taking before-and-after photos of yourself from different angles.

BEGINNING OF THE DIET					COMPLETION OF THE DIET				
CURRENT WEIGHT					CURRENT WEIGHT				
CURRENT MEASUREMENTS					CURRENT MEASUREMENTS				
BICEPS	CHEST	WAIST	HIPS	THIGHS	BICEPS	CHEST	WAIST	HIPS	THIGHS
CURRENT BMI					CURRENT BMI				

To calculate your BMI (body mass index):

Measure your height in inches. To do this, stand against a wall and use a pencil to make a mark at the top of your head.

Take your height in inches and square the number. (Multiply the number of inches by itself.)

Divide your weight in pounds by your height in inches squared.

Multiply the answer by 703. This is your body mass index. While this number isn't infallible, it can give you a rough idea of the amount of body fat you have. Here's a guide you can use.

BMI	WEIGHT
Below 18.5	Underweight
18.5—24.9	Normal or healthy weight
25.0—29.9	Overweight
30.0 and Above	Obese

Before-and-After Medical Tests

If you're interested in how the diet affects your overall health, ask your doctor to do tests before and after the diet and record this information at each point.

- Your blood pressure
- Your blood sugar levels
- Your levels of C-reactive protein
- Your cholesterol and triglyceride levels
- Your pH (acid-base balance)

Carb Counter: Whether you want to stay moderately low-carb or go full-out keto, it's important to know the carb counts of the foods you choose. Here's a handy chart (originally published in my most recent book, *Dr. Kellyann's Cleanse and Reset*) that tells you how many carbs—and, more important, how many *net* carbs—there are in different fruits, veggies, nuts, and seeds.

NUTS AND SEEDS	SERVING SIZE	TOTAL CARBS (G)	FIBER (G)	NET CARBS (G)
Almonds	¼ cup	11	6.5	4.5
Brazil Nuts	¼ cup	6	3.75	2.25
Cashews	¼ cup	15	1.65	13.35
Chestnuts	¼ cup	17.5	0	17.5
Chia Seeds	2 Tbsps	10.5	8.5	2
Flaxseeds	2 Tbsps	7.25	6.75	2.5
Hazelnuts	¼ cup	8.5	4.85	3.65
Hemp Seeds	¼ cup	4.35	4	0.35
Macadamia Nuts	¼ cup	7	4.3	2.7
Peanuts	¼ cup	8	4.75	3.25
Pecans	¼ cup	7	4.8	2.2
Pine Nuts	¼ cup	6.5	1.85	4.65
Pistachios	¼ cup	13.5	5.5	8
Poppy Seeds	2 Tbsps	7	5	2
Pumpkin Seeds	¼ cup	5.5	3	2.5
Sesame Seeds	2 Tbsps	5.75	3	2.75
Sunflower Seeds	¼ cup	10	4.3	5.7
Walnuts	¼ cup	7	3.35	3.65

FRUITS	SERVING SIZE	TOTAL CARBS (G)	FIBER (G)	NET CARBS (G)
Apricots	½ cup	11	2	9
Bananas	½ cup	23	2.6	20.4
Blackberries	½ cup	9.6	5.3	4.3
Blueberries	½ cup	14	2.4	11.6
Boysenberries	½ cup	12	5.3	6.7
Cantaloupes	½ cup	8.2	0.9	7.3
Cherimoyas	½ cup	18	3	15
Cherries (sour)	½ cup	12	1.6	10.4
Cherries (sweet)	½ cup	16	2.1	13.9
Clementines	½ cup	12	1.7	9.3
Coconut	½ cup	15	9	6

FRUITS	SERVING SIZE	TOTAL CARBS (G)	FIBER (G)	NET CARBS (G)
Cranberries	½ cup	12	3.6	8.4
Currants	½ cup	14	4.3	97
Elderberries	½ cup	18	7	11
Figs	½ cup	19	2.9	16.1
Gooseberries	½ cup	10	4.3	5.7
Granny Smith Apple	½ cup	14	2.4	11.6
Grapes	½ cup	18	0.9	17.
Grapefruit	½ cup	8.2	0	8.2
Guava	½ cup	14	5.4	8.6
Honeydew	½ cup	9.1	0.8	8.3
Huckleberries	½ cup	8.7	0	8.7
Jackfruits	½ cup	23	1.5	21.5
Jujubes	½ cup	20	0	20
Kiwis	½ cup	15	3	12
Kumquats	½ cup	16	6.5	9.5
Lemons	½ cup	9.3	2.8	6.5
Limes	½ cup	11	2.8	8.2
Longans	½ cup	15	1.1	13.9
Loquats	½ cup	12	1.7	10.3
Mangoes	½ cup	15	1.6	13.4
Mulberries	½ cup	9.8	1.7	8.1
Nectarines	½ cup	11	1.7	9.3
Papayas	½ cup	11	1.7	9.3
Passionfruit	½ cup	23	10	13
Peaches	½ cup	14	0.6	13.4
Pears	½ cup	15	3.1	11.9
Pineapple	½ cup	13	1.4	11.6
Plantains	½ cup	32	2.3	29.7
Plums	½ cup	11	1.4	9.6
Pomegranate	½ cup	19	4	15
Pummelos	½ cup	9.6	1	8.6
Quinces	½ cup	15	1.9	13.1
Raspberries	½ cup	12	6.5	5.5
Rhubarb	½ cup	4.5	1.8	2.7
Star Fruit	½ cup	6.7	2.8	3.9
Strawberries	½ cup	7.7	2	5.7
Tangerines	½ cup	13	1.8	11.2
Watermelon	½ cup	7.6	0.4	7.2

VEGETABLES	SERVING SIZE	TOTAL CARBS (G)	FIBER (G)	NET CARBS (G)
Acorn Squash (raw)	1 cup	15	2.1	12.9
Arrowroot (raw)	1 cup	16	1.6	14.4
Artichoke Hearts (canned)	½ cup	11	5.4	5.6
Arugula (raw)	1 cup	0.8	0.4	0.4
Asparagus (raw)	1 cup	5.2	2.8	2.4
Avocados (raw)	1 cup	13	10	3
Beet Greens (raw)	1 cup	1.7	1.4	0.3
Beets (raw)	1 cup	13	3.8	9.2
Bell Peppers, Green (raw)	1 cup	4.3	1.6	2.7
Bell Peppers, Red (raw)	1 cup	5.6	1.9	3.7
Bell Peppers, Yellow (raw)	1 cup	6.3	0.9	5.4
Broccoli (raw)	1 cup	6	2.4	3.6
Broccoli Rabe (raw)	1 cup	1.1	1.1	0
Brussels Sprouts (raw)	1 cup	7.9	3.3	4.6
Butternut Squash (raw)	1 cup	16	2.8	13.2
Cabbage, Green (raw)	1 cup	4.1	1.8	2.3
Cabbage, Red (raw)	1 cup	5.2	1.5	3.7
Carrots (raw)	½ cup	9.6	2.8	6.8
Cassava (raw)	¼ cup	19.5	0.9	18.6
Cauliflower (raw)	1 cup	5.3	2.1	3.2
Celery (raw)	1 cup	3	1.6	1.4
Celery Root (raw)	1 cup	14	2.8	11.2
Chile Peppers (raw)	½ cup	8.8	1.5	7.3
Chinese Cabbage (raw)	1 cup	1.5	0.7	0.8
Chives (raw)	2 tbs	0.2	0.2	0
Collard Greens (raw)	1 cup	2	1.4	0.6
Cucumbers (raw) with peel	1 cup	3.8	0.6	3.2
Daikon Radish (raw)	1 cup	4.8	1.9	2.9
Eggplant (raw)	1 cup	4.8	2.5	2.3
Endive (raw)	1 cup	1.6	1.6	0
Fennel (raw bulb)	1 cup	6.4	2.7	3.7
Ginger Root (raw)	2 Tbsp	2.15	0.25	1.9
Green Beans (raw)	1 cup	7	2.7	4.3
Green Onions (raw)	1 cup	7	2.6	4.4
Jalapeño Peppers (raw)	1 cup	5.9	2.5	3.4
Jicama (raw)	1 cup	11	6.4	4.6
Kale (raw)	1 cup	1.4	0.6	0.8

VEGETABLES	SERVING SIZE	TOTAL CARBS (G)	FIBER (G)	NET CARBS (G)
Kohlrabies (raw)	1 cup	8.4	4.9	3.5
Leeks (raw)	1 cup	13	1.6	11.4
Lettuce, Green Leaf (raw)	1 cup	1	0.5	0.5
Lettuce, Romaine (raw)	1 cup	1.6	1	0.6
Mushrooms, Portobello (raw)	1 cup	3.3	1.1	2.2
Mushrooms, White (raw)	1 cup	2.3	0.7	1.6
Mustard Greens (raw)	1 cup	2.6	1.8	0.8
Napa Cabbage (raw)	1 cup	1.5	0.7	0.8
Okra (raw)	1 cup	7.5	3.2	4.3
Olives (canned)	10 olives	3	1	2
Onions, White (raw)	1 cup	15	2.7	12.3
Parsnips (raw)	½ cup	12	6.5	5.5
Peas, green (raw)	1 cup	21	8.3	12.7
Potatoes, Red (raw)	½ cup	12	1.3	10.7
Potatoes, White (raw)	½ cup	12	1.8	10.2
Potatoes, Yellow (raw)	½ cup	12	2	10
Pumpkin (raw)	1 cup	7.5	0.6	6.9
Radicchio (raw)	1 cup	1.8	0.4	1.4
Radishes (raw)	1 cup	3.9	1.9	2
Onions, red (raw)	1 cup	16	2	14
Rutabaga (raw)	1 cup	12	3.2	8.8
Shallots (raw)	¼ cup	6.8	1.2	5.6
Spaghetti Squash (raw)	1 cup	7	1.5	5.5
Spinach (raw)	1 cup	1.1	0.7	0.4
Summer Squash (raw)	½ cup	3.4	1.1	2.3
Sweet Potatoes (raw)	½ cup	13.5	2	11.5
Swiss Chard (raw)	1 cup	1.4	0.6	0.8
Tomatoes (raw)	1 cup	7	2.2	4.8
Turnip Greens (raw)	1 cup	3.9	1.8	2.1
Turnips (raw)	1 cup	8.4	2.3	6.1
Watercress (raw)	1 cup	0.4	0.2	0.2
Yams (raw)	½ cup	21	3.1	17.9
Zucchini (raw)	1 cup	3.5	1.1	2.4

NOTES

CHAPTER 3

1 B. O. Rennard et al., "Chicken Soup Inhibits Neutrophil Chemotaxis in Vitro," *Chest* 118, no. 4 (October 2000): 1150–57.

2 G. Samonina et al., "Protection of Gastric Mucosal Integrity by Gelatin and Simple Proline-Containing Peptides," *Pathophysiology* 7, no. 1 (April 1, 2000): 69–73.

3 D. F. McCole, "The Epithelial Glycine Transporter GLYT1: Protecting the Gut from Inflammation," *Journal of Physiology* 588, no. 7 (April 2010): 1033–34.

4 Z. Zhong et al., "L-Glycine: A Novel Antiinflammatory, Immunomodulatory, and Cytoprotective Agent," *Current Opinion in Clinical Nutrition and Metabolic Care* 6, no. 2 (March 2003): 229–40.

5 A. Howard and B. H. Hirst, "The Glycine Transporter GLYT1 in Human Intestine: Expression and Function," *Biological and Pharmaceutical Bulletin* 34, no. 6 (2011): 784–88.

6 M. C. Hochberg et al., "Combined Chondroitin Sulfate and Glucosamine for Painful Knee Osteoarthritis: A Multicentre, Randomised, Double-Blind, Non-Inferiority Trial versus Celecoxib," *Annals of the Rheumatic Diseases* (January 14, 2015), http://ard.bmj.com/content/early/2015/01/14/annrheumdis-2014-206792.long.

7 S. L. Navarro et al., "Randomized Trial of Glucosamine and Chondroitin Supplementation on Inflammation and Oxidative Stress Biomarkers and Plasma Proteomics Profiles in Healthy Humans," *PLOS ONE* 10, no. 2 (February 26, 2015): e0117534.

8 F. R. Nelson et al., "The Effects of an Oral Preparation Containing Hyaluronic Acid (Oralvisc) on Obese Knee Osteoarthritis Patients Determined by Pain, Function, Bradykinin, Leptin, Inflammatory Cytokines, and Heavy Water Analyses," *Rheumatology International* 35, no. 1 (January 2015): 43–52.

9 C. Kawada et al., "Ingested Hyaluronan Moisturizes Dry Skin," *Nutrition Journal* 13 (July 11, 2014): 70.

10 M. Díaz-Flores et al., "Oral Supplementation with Glycine Reduces Oxidative Stress in Patients with Metabolic Syndrome, Improving Their Systolic Blood Pressure," *Canadian Journal of Physiology and Pharmacology* 91, no. 10 (October 2013): 855–60.

11 M. González-Ortiz et al., "Effect of Glycine on Insulin Secretion and Action in Healthy First-Degree Relatives of Type 2 Diabetes Mellitus Patients," *Hormone and Metabolic Research* 33, no. 6 (June 2001): 358–60.

12 K. Kasai, M. Kobayashi, S. I. Shimoda, "Stimulatory Effect of Glycine on Human Growth Hormone Secretion," *Metabolism* 27, no. 2 (February 1978): 201–8.

13 M. Bannai and N. Kawai, "New Therapeutic Strategy for Amino Acid Medicine: Glycine Improves the Quality of Sleep," *Journal of Pharmacological Sciences* 118, no. 2 (2012): 145–48.

14 Mayo Clinic, "Arginine," mayoclinic.org/drugs-supplements/arginine/background/HRB-20058733.

15 Ibid.

16 "A New Potential Cause for Alzheimer's: Arginine Deprivation," *Duke Today*, Duke University, April 14, 2015.

17 Bonnie Prescott, "Glutamine Supplements Show Promise in Treating Stomach Ulcers," *Harvard Gazette*, May 15, 2009.

18 J. A. Monro, R. Leon R, and B. K. Puri, "The Risk of Lead Contamination in Bone Broth Diets," *Medical Hypotheses* 80, no. 4 (April 2013): 389–90.

19 Original report accessed from drkaayladaniel.com/boning-up-is-broth-contaminated-with -lead/.

20 M. J. I. Baxter et al., "Lead Contamination during Domestic Preparation and Cooking of Potatoes and Leaching of Bone-Derived Lead on Roasting, Marinading, and Boiling Beef," *Food Additives and Contaminants* 9, no. 3 (May–June 1992): 225–35.

21 Y. H. Youm et al., "The Ketone Metabolite b-Hydroxybutyrate Blocks NLRP3 Inflammasome-Mediated Inflammatory Disease," *Nature Medicine* 21, no. 3 (March 2015): 263–69.

22 N. Collins et al., "The Bone Marrow Protects and Optimizes Immunological Memory during Dietary Restriction," *Cell*, 178(5), 1088–1101, August 22, 2019, https://www.cell.com/cell /fulltext/S0092-8674(19)30849-9.

23 S. Jordan et al., "Dietary Intake Regulates the Circulating Inflammatory Monocyte Pool," *Cell*, 178(5), 1102–14, August 22, 2019, https://www.cell.com/cell/fulltext/S0092-8674(19) 30850-5.

24 A. Chen, "'Magic Soup': How Intermittent Fasting May Enhance the Immune System," WBUR, August 23, 2019, https://www.wbur.org/commonhealth/2019/08/23/intermittent -fasting-immune-system.

25 T. Kishi et al., "Calorie Restriction Improves Cognitive Decline via Up-Regulation of Brain-Derived Neurotrophic Factor," *International Heart Journal* 56, no. 1 (January 21, 2015): 110–15.

26 Intermountain Medical Center, "Study Finds Routine, Periodic Fasting Is Good for Your Health, and Your Heart," news release, April 3, 2011. Original research was presented April 3, 2011, at the scientific sessions of the American College of Cardiology conference in New Orleans.

27 " 'Fast-Mimicking Diet' May Promote Health and Longevity," *Medical News Today*, June 21, 2015.

28 C. Zauner et al., "Resting Energy Expenditure in Short-Term Starvation Is Increased as a Result of an Increase in Serum Norepinephrine," *American Journal of Nutrition* 71, no 6 (June 2000): 1511–15.

CHAPTER 4

1 "New Research Shows Obesity Is Inflammatory Disease," *Science Daily*, December 2, 2013.

2 K. Esposito et al., "Inflammatory Cytokine Concentrations Are Acutely Increased by Hyperglycemia in Humans: Role of Oxidative Stress," *Circulation* 106, no. 16 (October 15, 2002): 2067–72.

3 N. A. Melville, "Fructose Intolerance, Malabsorption a Common Culprit in Pediatric Abdominal Pain," *Medscape Multispecialty*, October 20, 2010.

4 "Sugary Foods Linked to Pancreatic Cancer Risk," Reuters, June 15, 2010.

5 I. Romieu et al., "Dietary Glycemic Index and Glycemic Load and Breast Cancer Risk in the European Prospective Investigation into Cancer and Nutrition (EPIC)," *American Journal of Clinical Nutrition* 96, no. 2 (August 2012): 345–55.

6 A. M. Port, M. R. Ruth, and N. W. Istfan, "Fructose Consumption and Cancer: Is There a Connection?" *Current Opinion in Endocrinology, Diabetes, and Obesity* 19, no. 5 (October 2012): 367–74.

7 A. Abbott, "Sugar Substitutes Linked to Obesity," *Nature*, September 17, 2014.

8 A. Aubrey, "Diet Soda May Alter Our Gut Microbes and Raise the Risk of Diabetes," National Public Radio, September 17, 2014.

9   L. Tran et al., "Soy Extracts Suppressed Iodine Uptake and Stimulated the Production of Autoimmunogen in Rat Thyrocytes," *Experimental Biology and Medicine* 238, no. 6 (June 2013): 623–30.

10 *Bulletin de l'Office Federal de la Santé Publique*, no. 28, July 20, 1992.

11 K. L. Watson et al., "High Levels of Dietary Soy Decrease Mammary Tumor Latency and Increase Incidence in MTB-IGFIR Transgenic Mice," *BMC Cancer* 15, no. 1 (February 6, 2015): 37.

12 X. Yang et al., "Dietary Soy Isoflavones Increase Metastasis to Lungs in an Experimental Model of Breast Cancer with Bone Microtumors," *Clinical and Experimental Metastasis* 32, no. 4 (April 2015): 323–33.

13 J. E. Chavarro et al., "Soy Food and Isoflavone Intake in Relation to Semen Quality Parameters among Men from an Infertility Clinic," *Human Reproduction*, 23, no. 11 (November 2008): 2584–90.

14 B. Chassaing et al., "Dietary Emulsifiers Impact the Mouse Gut Microbiota Promoting Colitis and Metabolic Syndrome," *Nature* 519, no. 7541 (March 5, 2015): 92–96.

15 K. He et al., INTERMAP Cooperative Research Group, "Association of Monosodium Glutamate Intake with Overweight in Chinese Adults: The INTERMAP Study," *Obesity* 16, no. 8 (August 2008): 1875–80.

16 "Caramel Coloring Chemical Linked to Cancer Found in 'Too High' Levels in Some Colas," NBC News, January 23, 2014.

17 H. Blankson et al., "Conjugated Linoleic Acid Reduces Body Fat Mass in Overweight and Obese Humans," *Journal of Nutrition* 130, no. 12 (December 2000): 2943–48.

18 K. H. Courage, "Fiber-Famished Gut Microbes Linked to Poor Health," *Scientific American*, March 23, 2015.

CHAPTER 7

1   Berta Buey et al. "Comparative Effect of Bovine Buttermilk, Whey, and Lactoferrin on the Innate Immunity Receptors and Oxidative Status of Intestinal Epithelial Cells," *Biochemistry and Cell Biology*, June 13, 2020 (online), https://pubmed.ncbi.nlm.nih.gov/32538128/.

2   Ágnes A. Fekete et al. "Whey Protein Lowers Blood Pressure and Improves Endothelial Function and Lipid Biomarkers in Adults with Prehypertension and Mild Hypertension: Results from the Chronic Whey2Go Randomized Controlled Trial," *American Journal of Clinical Nutrition* 104(6), December 2016, 1534–1544, https://pubmed.ncbi.nlm.nih.gov/27797709/.

3   Sebely Pal et al. "Effects of Whey Protein Isolate on Body Composition, Lipids, Insulin and Glucose in Overweight and Obese Individuals," *British Journal of Nutrition* 104(5), September 2010, 716–723, https://pubmed.ncbi.nlm.nih.gov/20377924/.

4   Jaya Benjamin et al. "Glutamine and Whey Protein Improve Intestinal Permeability and Morphology in Patients with Crohn's Disease: A Randomized Controlled Trial," *Digestive Diseases and Sciences* 57(4), April 2012, 1000–1002, https://pubmed.ncbi.nlm.nih.gov/22038507/.

5   A. E. Carroll, "Behind New Dietary Guidelines, Better Science," *New York Times*, February 23, 2015.

6   R. Chowhury et al., "Association of Dietary, Circulating, and Supplement Fatty Acids with Coronary Risk: A Systemic Review and Meta-Analysis," *Annals of Internal Medicine* 160, no. 6 (March 18, 2014): 398–406.

7   L. A. Bazzano et al., "Effects of Low-Carbohydrate and Low-Fat Diets: A Randomized Trial," *Annals of Internal Medicine* 161, no. 5 (September 2, 2014): 309–18. See also A. O'Connor, "A Call for a Low-Carb Diet That Embraces Fat," *New York Times*, September 1, 2014.

CHAPTER 9

1   K. Kindy, "Food Additives on the Rise as FDA Scrutiny Wanes," *Washington Post*, August 17, 2014.

CHAPTER 11

1   G. Reynolds, "How Exercise Can Help You Live Longer," *New York Times*, April 2, 2014.

2   G. Reynolds, "Prescribing Exercise to Treat Depression," *New York Times*, August 31, 2011.

3   G. Reynolds, "How Exercise May Protect Against Depression," *New York Times*, October 1, 2014.

4   D. P. Bailey and C. D. Locke, "Breaking Up Prolonged Sitting with Light-Intensity Walking Improves Postprandial Glycemia, But Breaking Up Sitting with Standing Does Not," *Journal of Science and Medicine in Sport* 18, no. 3 (May 2015): 294–98.

5   A. Puig-Ribera et al., "Patterns of Impact Resulting from a 'Sit Less, Move More' Web-Based Program in Sedentary Office Employees," *PLOS ONE* 10, no. 4 (April 1, 2015): e0122474.

6   X. Zhang et al., "Adult Body Size and Physical Activity in Relation to Risk of Breast Cancer According to Tumor Androgen Receptor Status," *Cancer Epidemiology, Biomarkers, and Prevention* 24, no. 6 (June 2015): 962–68.

7   D. Schmid et al., "A Systematic Review and Meta-Analysis of Physical Activity and Endometrial Cancer Risk," *European Journal of Epidemiology* 30, no. 5 (May 2015): 397–412.

8   F. Maillard et al., "High-Intensity Interval Training Reduces Abdominal Fat Mass in Postmenopausal Women with Type 2 Diabetes," *Diabetes & Metabolism*, August 24, 2016, 42(6): 433–42; https://www.sciencedirect.com/science/article/abs/pii/S1262363616304700.

9   "Short Bursts of Exercise 'Better for Weight Loss,'" Laurel Ives, BBC Health, February 16, 2019, https://www.bbc.com/news/health-47242940.

CHAPTER 12

1   E. Mullin. "The Bacteria in Your Gut May Reveal Your True Age," *Science Magazine*, January 11, 2019, https://www.sciencemag.org/news/2019/01/bacteria-your-gut-may-reveal-your-true-age.

2   R. P. Ortega. "The Microbes in Your Gut Could Predict Whether You're Likely to Die in the Next 15 Years," *Science Magazine*, January 22, 2020.

3   A. M. Vaiserman et al, "Gut Microbiota: A Player in Aging and a Target for Anti-Aging Intervention," *Ageing Research Reviews*, 35, May 2017, 36–45, https://www.sciencedirect.com/science/article/pii/S1568163716302653.

4   G. Kolata. "Gut Bacteria from Thin Humans Can Slim Mice Down," *New York Times*, September 5, 2013, https://www.nytimes.com/2013/09/06/health/gut-bacteria-from-thin-humans-can-slim-mice-down.html?_r=0.

5   G. Bian et al. "The Gut Microbiota of Healthy Aged Chinese Is Similar to That of the Healthy Young," *mSphere*, September 27, 2017 (online), https://msphere.asm.org/content/msph/2/5/e00327-17.full.pdf. See also: "'Ridiculously Healthy' Elderly Have the Same Gut Microbiome as Healthy 30-year-olds," news release, Western University, October 11, 2017, https://mediarelations.uwo.ca/2017/10/11/ridiculously-healthy-elderly-gut-microbiome-healthy-30-year-olds/.

6   Y. Brazier. "One Course of Antibiotics Disrupts Gut Microbiome for a Year," *Medical News Today*, November 15, 2015.

7   J. Brody. "The Benefits of Intermittent Fasting," *New York Times*, February 17, 2020, https://www.nytimes.com/2020/02/17/well/eat/the-benefits-of-intermittent-fasting.html.

8   "Growth Factor Protects Key Brain Cells in Alzheimer's Models," *Medical Xpress*, February 8, 2009.

9   K. Marosi et al. "Metabolic and Molecular Framework for the Enhancement of Endurance by Intermittent Food Deprivation," *FASEB Journal*, 32:7, July 2018, https://pubmed.ncbi.nlm.nih.gov/29485903/. See also: "Intermittent Dietary Restriction May Boost Physical Endurance," NIH Research Matters, March 6, 2018, https://www.nih.gov/news-events/nih-research-matters/intermittent-dietary-restriction-may-boost-physical-endurance.

10 C. Marinac et al. "Prolonged Nightly Fasting and Breast Cancer Prognosis," *JAMA Oncology*, 2(8), August 1, 2016, https://pubmed.ncbi.nlm.nih.gov/27032109/.

11 M. Brubaker. "Weight for It: Time-Restricted Eating Benefits Those at Risk for Diabetes, Heart Disease," UC San Diego Health, December 5,2019, https://health.ucsd.edu/news/releases/Pages/2019-12-05-time-restricted-eating-diabetes-and-heart-disease.aspx.

12 L. Mujica-Parodi et al. "Diet Modulates Brain Network Stability, a Biomarker for Brain Aging, in Young Adults," *Proceedings of the National Academy of Sciences*, March 17, 2020 (online), https://www.pnas.org/content/117/11/6170. See also: Amelia Hill. "Low-Carb Diet May Reverse Age-Related Brain Deterioration, Study Finds," *The Guardian*, March 6, 2020, https://www.theguardian.com/science/2020/mar/06/low-carb-diet-may-reverse-age-related-brain-deterioration-study-finds.

13 "Low-Carb 'Keto' Diet ('Atkins-Style') May Modestly Improve Cognition in Older Adults," Johns Hopkins Newsroom, June 27, 2019, https://www.hopkinsmedicine.org/news/newsroom/news-releases/low-carb-keto-diet-atkins-style-may-modestly-improve-cognition-in-older-adults.

14 K. Holland. "How the Keto Diet May Help Fight Certain Cancer Tumors," Healthline, August 16, 2019, https://www.healthline.com/health-news/what-to-know-about-keto-diet-and-cancer#A-secondary-finding-targets-sugar.

15 D. D. Weber et al. "Ketogenic Diet in the Treatment of Cancer—Where Do We Stand?" *Molecular Metabolism*, 33, 2020, 102–21, https://www.sciencedirect.com/science/article/pii/S2212877819304272.

16 P. Barbanti et al. "Ketogenic diet in migraine: rationale, findings and perspectives," *Neurological Sciences*, 38(Suppl 1), May 2017, 111–15, https://pubmed.ncbi.nlm.nih.gov/28527061/.

17 S. R. Jahromi et al. "Association of Diet and Headache," *Headache Pain*, 20(1), November 14, 2019, https://pubmed.ncbi.nlm.nih.gov/31726975/.

18 "Physical Activity and Cancer," NIH Cancer Institute, https://www.cancer.gov/about-cancer/causes-prevention/risk/obesity/physical-activity-fact-sheet.

19 Ibid.

20 G. Karandiker-Agashe and R. Agrawal. "Comparative Study of the Effect of Resistance Exercises Versus Aerobic Exercises in Postmenopausal Women Suffering from Insomnia," *Journal of Mid-Life Health*, 11(1), January-March 2020, https://pubmed.ncbi.nlm.nih.gov/32684719/.

21 S. R. Chekroud et al. "Association Between Physical Exercise and Mental Health in 1.2 Million Individuals in the USA Between 2011 and 2015: A Cross-Sectional Study," *The Lancet*, August 8, 2018 (online), https://www.thelancet.com/journals/lanpsy/article/PIIS2215-0366(18)30227-X/fulltext#seccestitle10.

22 "Exercise: Psych Patients' New Natural Prescription," *Science Daily*, May 21, 2019.

23 A. MacMillan. "Exercise Makes You Younger at the Cellular Level," *Time*, May 15, 2017.

24 B. DeAngelis. "How Aerobic Exercise Helps Us Keep Our Wits About Us as We Age," Hotchkiss Brain Institute, University of Calgary, May 19, 2020, https://cumming.ucalgary.ca/news/how-aerobic-exercise-helps-us-keep-our-wits-about-us-we-age-0.

25 H. Shin et al. "Exercise, the Gut Microbiome, and Frailty," *Annals of Geriatric Medicine and Research*, 23(3), September 23, 2019 (online), https://pubmed.ncbi.nlm.nih.gov/32743298/.

26 M. Sivak. "Sleeping More as a Way to Lose Weight," *Obesity Reviews*, 7(3), August 2006, 295–6, https://pubmed.ncbi.nlm.nih.gov/16866976/. See also: "Want to Lose Weight? Try Sleeping More," Medical Xpress, July 24, 2006, https://medicalxpress.com/news/2006–07 -weight.html.

27 K. Y. Lai et al. "Exposure to Light at Night (LAN) and Risk of Obesity: A Systematic Review and Meta-Analysis of Observational Studies," *Environmental Research*, 187, August 2020, https://pubmed.ncbi.nlm.nih.gov/32497902/.

28 Isaac Eliaz et al. "The Effect of Modified Citrus Pectin on Urinary Excretion of Toxic Elements," *Phytotherapy Research*, vol. 20, July 11, 2006, 859–64, https://schoolafm.com /wp-content/uploads/2013/09/Heavy-metals-and-Modified-Citrus-Pectin.pdf.

CHAPTER 13

1 G. Oliver and J. Wardle, "Perceived Effects of Stress on Food Choice," *Physiology & Behavior* 66, no. 3 (May 1999): 511–15.

2 K. Raspopow et al., "Anticipation of a Psychosocial Stressor Differentially Influences Ghrelin, Cortisol, and Food Intake among Emotional and Non-Emotional Eaters," *Appetite* 74 (March 2014): 35–43. See also A. Daly, "A Surprising Reason You May Be Eating More," *Women's Health*, December 4, 2013.

3 V. Kahan et al., "Stress, Immunity, and Skin Collagen Integrity: Evidence from Animal Models and Clinical Conditions," *Brain, Behavior, and Immunity* 23, no. 8 (November 2009): 1089–95.

4 J. K. Kiecolt-Glaser and R. Glaser, "Psychological Stress, Telomeres, and Telomerase," *Brain, Behavior, and Immunity* 24, no. 4 (May 1, 2001): 529–30.

5 "Mindfulness Meditation Training Changes Brain Structure in Eight Weeks," *Science Daily*, January 21, 2011.

6 S. N. Katterman et al., "Mindfulness Meditation as an Intervention for Binge Eating, Emotional Eating, and Weight Loss: A Systematic Review," *Eating Behaviors* 15, no. 2 (April 2014): 197–204.

7 K. C. Spadaro et al. "Effect of Mindfulness Meditation on Short-Term Weight Loss and Eating Behaviors in Overweight and Obese Adults: A Randomized Controlled Trial," *Journal of Complementary and Integrative Medicine*, 15(2), December 2017, https://www.degruyter.com /view/journals/jcim/15/2/article-20160048.xml.

8 L. E. Carlson et al., "Mindfulness-Based Cancer Recovery and Supportive-Expressive Therapy Maintain Telomere Length Relative to Controls in Distressed Breast Cancer Survivors," *Cancer* 121, no. 3 (February 1, 2015): 476–84.

9 M. K. Koike and R. Cardoso, "Meditation Can Produce Beneficial Effects to Prevent Cardiovascular Disease," *Hormone Molecular Biology and Clinical Investigation* 18, no. 3 (June 2014): 137–43.

10 C. Y. Fang et al., "Enhanced Psychosocial Well-Being Following Participation in a Mindfulness-Based Stress Reduction Program Is Associated with Increased Natural Killer Cell Activity," *Journal of Alternative and Complementary Medicine* 16, no. 5 (May 2010): 531–38.

11 A. Aubrey, "Mindfulness Meditation Can Help Relieve Anxiety and Depression," NPR, January 7, 2014, http://www.npr.org/blogs/health/2014/01/07/260470831/mindfulness -meditation-can-help-relieve-anxiety-and-depression.

12 R. C. Rabin, "Regimens: Massage Benefits Are More Than Skin Deep," *New York Times*, September 20, 2010.

13 Harry T. Whelan et al. "NASA Light-Emitting Diode Medical Applications from Deep Space to Deep Sea," CP552, *Space Technology and Applications International Forum*, 2001, edited by M. S. El-Genk.

14 L. Tyrväinen et al., "The Influence of Urban Green Environments on Stress Relief Measures: A Field Experiment," *Journal of Environmental Psychology* 38 (June 2014): 1–9.

15 B. J. Park et al. "The Physiological Effects of Shinrin-Yoku (taking in the forest atmosphere or forest bathing): Evidence from Field Experiments in 24 Forests across Japan," *Environmental Health and Preventive Medicine*, 15(1), January 2010, 18–26, https://www.ncbi.nlm.nih.gov /pubmed/19568835.

16 Q. Li et al. "Forest Bathing Enhances Human Natural Killer Activity and Expression of Anti-Cancer Proteins," *International Journal of Immunopathology and Pharmacology*, 20 (2), Supp 2, April–June 2007, 3–8, https://www.ncbi.nlm.nih.gov/pubmed/17903349.

17 M. S. Buchowski et al., "Energy Expenditure of Genuine Laughter," *International Journal of Obesity* 31, no. 1 (January 2007): 131–37.

CHAPTER 14

1 S. Jackson, A. Steptoe, and J. Wardle, "The Influence of Partner's Behavior on Health Behavior Change: The English Longitudinal Study of Ageing," *JAMA Internal Medicine* 175, no. 3 (March 2015): 385–92.

CHAPTER 15

1 Cari Nierenberg, "Probiotics Hold Promise for 4 Skin Conditions," *LiveScience*, June 24, 2014, https://www.livescience.com/46502-probiotics-hold-promise-skin-conditions.html.

2 Erik Peper and I-Mei Lin. "Increase or Decrease Depression: How Body Postures Influence Your Energy Level," *Biofeedback*, 40(3), Fall 2012, 125–30, https://doi.org/10.5298/1081-5937 -40.3.01.

INDEX

A

Abbott, Joanne, 300
Acute inflammation, 7
Adrenal fatigue, 40–41
Aioli (garlic mayonnaise) recipe, 261
Air fryer
    Air Fryer Fish and Zucchini "Fries,"
        186–188
    Breakfast Meatballs, 129
    Buffalo Cauliflower, 238
    Zucchini Fritters, 241–242
Air Fryer Fish and Zucchini "Fries" recipe,
    186–188
Alcohol, 60–62, 80
Allicin, 107
Amino acids, 36–37
Ancestral health (AH) model, 320
Apples
    Baked Apples, 273
    Baked Apple Shake, 275
    Pork Tenderloin with Apples and
        Onions, 183
    Sausage and Apple Frittata, 136
    as super-cleansers, 336
    Sweet and Savory Breakfast Hash, 140
Arginine, 36
Artificial ingredients, dangers of, 59–60
Artificial sweeteners, 47, 50–51
Asian Chicken Bone Broth recipe, 108
Asian Sesame Noodle Salad recipe, 234
Asian Turkey Burgers recipe, 172
Asparagus and Mushroom Crustless
    Quiche recipe, 124
Autoimmune disorders, 14
Avocado Egg Salad, Grab-and-Go, 196
Avocados
    Avocado Egg Salad, Grab-and-Go, 196
    benefits of, 218–219

carbohydrates within, 86
Chili Omelet, 130
Cool and Creamy Avocado-Pumpkin
    Soup, 215
Creamy Avocado Sauce or Salad
    Dressing, 253
Creamy Chimichurri, 266
Gazpacho Molded Salad, 286
Green Goddess Shake, 277
Pesto, 267

B

Baked Apple Shake recipe, 275
Baked Apples recipe, 273
Baked Egg Cups with Spinach recipe, 125
Baked or Mashed Sweet Potatoes recipe,
    243
Baked Scotch Eggs recipe, 126
Balsamic Roasted Brussels Sprouts recipe,
    235
Balsamic Roast Pork Loin recipe, 184
Balsamic Vinaigrette recipe, 252
Batch cooking, tips for, 297–301
Beans/legumes, 48, 59
Beauty tips, 361–367
Beef
    Beef, Egg, and Mushroom Breakfast,
        127
    Bolognese, 174–175
    Easy Beef or Bison Burgers, 173
    Easy Pot Roast, 179
    Fiesta Beef Fajitas, 181
    Greek-Style Beef or Bison Burgers, 182
    Hearty Beef and Vegetable Soup, 203
Beef, Egg, and Mushroom Breakfast recipe,
    127
Beef Bone Broth
    Easy Pot Roast, 179

Beef Bone Broth *(cont.)*
  Hearty Beef and Vegetable Soup, 203
  making of, 94
  Mushroom Pâté, 290
  recipe for, 100
  Rich and Hearty Turkey Chili, 168
Black pepper, 107
Blue and Green Shake recipe, 278
Blueberry Mojito Mocktail recipe, 279
Bolognese recipe, 174–175
Bone broth. *See also specific types*
  benefits of, 3–4, 6–7, 31, 37, 211, 219
  preparing, 31
  as super-cleanser, 336
Bone Broth Egg Drop Soup recipe, 207
Bone Broth Soup, Grab-and-Go, 197
Bone marrow, 35, 102
Brain, food and, 60
Brain-derived neurotrophic factor (BDNF),
    39–40
Braised Chicken with Leeks and
    Mushrooms recipe, 159
braising, 199
Breakfast Egg Muffins with Italian Sausage
    recipe, 128
Breakfast Meatballs recipe, 129
Breakfasts
  Asparagus and Mushroom Crustless
      Quiche, 124
  Baked Egg Cups with Spinach, 125
  Baked Scotch Eggs, 126
  Beef, Egg, and Mushroom Breakfast,
      127
  Breakfast Egg Muffins with Italian
      Sausage, 128
  Breakfast Meatballs, 129
  Butternut Squash Breakfast Hash, 304
  Chili Omelet, 130
  Egg and Tomato Skillet, 131
  Mediterranean Scramble, 132
  Overnight Breakfast Parfait, 308
  Pork and Eggs, 133
  Quick and Easy Lox, 134
  Roasted Red Pepper and Basil Egg Bites,
      135
  Sausage and Apple Frittata, 136
  Savory Vegetable Waffles, 137
  Smoked Salmon and Eggs, 138
  Southwest Breakfast Scramble, 139
  Sweet and Savory Breakfast Hash, 140
  Vegetable Frittata, 141
  Zucchini Breakfast Cakes, 142

Breathing exercises, 344–345
Broccoli noodles, 313
Broccoli Salad with Creamy Poppyseed
    Dressing recipe, 236
Brussels Sprouts Salad with a Sweet and
    Tangy Vinaigrette recipe, 237
Buffalo Cauliflower recipe, 238
Burdock root, 337
Burger, Grab-and-Go, 197
Butter, benefits of, 71
Butternut Squash Breakfast Hash recipe,
    304
Buttery Salmon and Asparagus recipe, 189

C

Calcium, 34
Calf's foot jelly, 37
Call-to-Action Soups
  Cool and Creamy Avocado-Pumpkin
      Soup, 215
  Mary's Hot-and-Sour Soup, 212
  Red Bell Pepper Soup, 214
  Salmon and Leek Chowder, 220
  Shiitake Mushroom Soup, 213
  Watercress Soup, 216
Calories, of intermittent fasting, 42–43
Capsaicin, 107
Carb Control System, 84–86, 302
Carb counter, 372–375
Carb flu, 20–23, 75
Carbohydrates, 62–63
Cardamom, 107
Carrots
  Beef Bone Broth, 100
  Bolognese, 174–175
  Chicken Bone Broth recipe, 98
  Chicken Salad with Crunch, 160
  Chopped Balsamic Chicken Salad, 156
  Easy Pot Roast, 179
  Fish Bone Broth, 103
  Greek-Style Lemony Chicken Soup, 202
  Hearty Beef and Vegetable Soup, 203
  Red Bell Pepper Soup, 214
  Rotisserie Chicken Bone Broth, 101
  Savory Vegetable Waffles, 137
  Spicy Chicken Soup, 208
  Tomato, Basil, and Italian Sausage
      Soup, 209
  Turkey Bone Broth, 99
  Turkey Meatloaf Loaded with
      Vegetables, 169

Tuscan Seafood Soup, 210
Zucchini Breakfast Cakes, 142
Cauliflower
    benefits of, 303
    Buffalo Cauliflower, 238
    Cauliflower Rice, 222, 312
    In-a-Hurry No-Prep Stir-Fry, 151–152
    Louisiana Creole Jambalaya, 153
    Roasted Cauliflower Hummus, 248
    Roasted Curry Cauliflower, 228
    Roasted Red Pepper Hummus, 249
    Sheet Pan Chicken Dinner, 309
Cauliflower Rice recipe, 222
Cayenne pepper (ground red pepper), 107
Celeriac (celery root) noodles, 313
Celery
    Beef Bone Broth, 100
    Bolognese, 174–175
    Chicken Bone Broth recipe, 98
    Chicken Salad with Crunch, 160
    Eastern European Beef Bone Broth, 108
    Easy Pot Roast, 179
    fish bone broth, 103
    Hearty Beef and Vegetable Soup, 203
    Herb-Infused Chicken Soup, 204
    Louisiana Creole Jambalaya, 153
    Red Bell Pepper Soup, 214
    Rotisserie Chicken Bone Broth, 101
    Spicy Chicken Soup, 208
    Thanksgiving Turkey Bone Broth, 106
    Turkey Bone Broth, 99
    Turkey Meatloaf Loaded with
        Vegetables, 169
    Vegetarian Potassium-Rich Broth, 105
Chicken
    Braised Chicken with Leeks and
        Mushrooms, 159
    Chicken à la Carte, Grab-and-Go, 196
    Chicken Cutlets with French Herbs and
        Creamy Roasted Red Pepper
        Sauce, 146–147
    Chicken Pâté, 287
    Chicken Shawarma, 148
    Chicken Stir-Fry, 157–158
    Chicken with Orange-Rosemary Sauce,
        155
    Chopped Balsamic Chicken Salad, 156
    Coconut Curried Chicken Soup, 200
    Creamy Chicken and Mushrooms,
        305–306
    Creamy Chicken Curry, 145
    Easy Roast Chicken, 150

    Easy Roast Chicken Breasts, 149
    Greek-Style Lemony Chicken Soup, 202
    Herb-Infused Chicken Soup, 204
    In-a-Hurry No-Prep Stir-Fry, 151–152
    Louisiana Creole Jambalaya, 153
    One-Skillet Zucchini Pasta with
        Sausage, 162
    Orange-Rosemary Chicken Salad, 161
    Portuguese Kale and Sweet Potato Soup,
        206
    Sheet Pan Chicken Dinner, 309
    Spicy Chicken Drumsticks or Thighs,
        154
    Spicy Chicken Soup, 208
    Tomato, Basil, and Italian Sausage
        Soup, 209
    Turkey or Chicken Chorizo, 164
    Turkey or Chicken Italian Sausage, 163
    Turkey or Chicken Savory Sausage, 163
Chicken à la Carte, Grab-and-Go, 196
Chicken Bone Broth
    Bone Broth Egg Drop Soup, 207
    Braised Chicken with Leeks and
        Mushrooms, 159
    Chicken Pâté, 287
    Coconut Curried Chicken Soup, 200
    Cool and Creamy Avocado-Pumpkin
        Soup, 215
    Cream of Wild Mushroom Soup, 201
    Creamy Chicken Curry, 145
    Gazpacho Molded Salad, 286
    Greek-Style Lemony Chicken Soup, 202
    Herb-Infused Chicken Soup, 204
    Italian Wedding Soup, 205
    Louisiana Creole Jambalaya, 153
    making of, 94
    Mary's Hot-and-Sour Soup, 212
    Mediterranean Quinoa Salad, 307
    Portuguese Kale and Sweet Potato Soup,
        206
    Quick Egg Drop Soup, Grab-and-Go,
        196
    recipe for, 98
    Red Bell Pepper Soup, 214
    Rich and Hearty Turkey Chili, 168
    rotisserie recipe for, 101–102
    Salmon and Leek Chowder, 220
    Salmon Mousse, 285
    Shiitake Mushroom Soup, 213
    Slow Cooker Southwest Pulled Pork, 180
    Spicy Chicken Soup, 208
    Sweet Black Cherry Gummies, 283

Chicken Bone Broth *(cont.)*
Tomato, Basil, and Italian Sausage
Soup, 209
Watercress Soup, 216
Chicken Cutlets with French Herbs and
Creamy Roasted Red Pepper
Sauce recipe, 146–147
Chicken Pâté recipe, 287
Chicken Salad with Crunch recipe, 160
Chicken Shawarma recipe, 148
Chicken Stir-Fry recipe, 157–158
Chicken with Orange-Rosemary Sauce
recipe, 155
Chili Omelet recipe, 130
Chondroitin, 35
Chopped Balsamic Chicken Salad recipe,
156
Chronic inflammation, 7
Cilantro, 336
Cleansing, 334–335
Cocktail Sauce recipe, 258
Coconut, benefits of, 144, 219
Coconut Curried Chicken Soup recipe,
200
Collagen, 6–7, 32–34, 111
community supported agriculture (CSA)
boxes, 289
Cool and Creamy Avocado-Pumpkin Soup
recipe, 215
Coriander, 336
Corn-based foods, elimination of, 47, 53–54
Cream of Wild Mushroom Soup recipe,
201
Creamy Avocado Sauce or Salad Dressing
recipe, 253
Creamy Chicken and Mushrooms recipe,
305–306
Creamy Chicken Curry recipe, 145
Creamy Chimichurri recipe, 266
Creamy Ginger Dressing recipe, 254
Creamy Lemon Dressing recipe, 256
Creamy Orange Dressing recipe, 257
Creamy Poppyseed Dressing recipe, 236
Cucumber Gimlet Mocktail recipe, 280
Cumin, 107
Curcumin, 107, 336

D

Dairy, 48, 54–55
Dairy-Free Creamy Ranch Dressing recipe,
239

Dandelions, 336
Deitch, Beverly, 28
Desserts
Baked Apples, 273
Poached Pears, 274
Strawberries with a Balsamic Reduction,
274
Diabesity, 52
Diabetes, 14
Diet soft drinks, dangers of, 51
Dips
Roasted Cauliflower Hummus, 248
Roasted Red Pepper Hummus, 249
Do-It-Yourself Shake recipe, 276
Dressings
Asian Sesame Noodle Salad, 234
Balsamic Vinaigrette, 252
Brussels Sprouts Salad with a Sweet and
Tangy Vinaigrette, 237
Creamy Avocado Sauce or Salad
Dressing, 253
Creamy Ginger Dressing, 254
Creamy Lemon Dressing, 256
Creamy Orange Dressing, 257
Creamy Poppyseed Dressing, 236
Dairy-Free Creamy Ranch Dressing,
239
French Vinaigrette, 255
Lemon Vinaigrette, 256
Orange Vinaigrette, 257
Spicy Lime Vinaigrette, 247
Thousand Island Dressing, 250
Dry-heat cooking methods, 198–199,
224–225

E

Eastern European Beef Bone Broth recipe,
108
Easy Beef or Bison Burgers recipe, 173
Easy Pot Roast recipe, 179
Easy Roast Chicken Breasts recipe, 149
Easy Roast Chicken recipe, 150
Easy Roast Turkey Breast recipe, 165
Easy Turkey Burgers recipe, 166
Eating disorders, 15
Egg and Tomato Skillet recipe, 131
Eggs
Asparagus and Mushroom Crustless
Quiche, 124
Avocado Egg Salad, Grab-and-Go, 196
Baked Egg Cups with Spinach, 125

Baked Scotch Eggs, 126
Beef, Egg, and Mushroom Breakfast, 127
benefits of, 9
Bone Broth Egg Drop Soup, 207
Breakfast Egg Muffins with Italian Sausage, 128
Chili Omelet, 130
Egg and Tomato Skillet, 131
Eggs and Salmon, Grab-and-Go, 196
Greek-Style Lemony Chicken Soup, 202
hard-cooked, 126
Homemade Mayonnaise, 260–261
Mediterranean Scramble, 132
myths regarding, 143
Pork and Eggs, 133
Quick Egg Drop Soup, Grab-and-Go, 196
Roasted Red Pepper and Basil Egg Bites, 135
Sausage and Apple Frittata, 136
Savory Vegetable Waffles, 137
Smoked Salmon and Eggs, 138
Southwest Breakfast Scramble, 139
Sweet Potato Latke Waffles, 310
Vegetable Frittata, 141
Zucchini Breakfast Cakes, 142
Eggs and Salmon, Grab-and-Go, 196
80/20 system
Butternut Squash Breakfast Hash, 304
Creamy Chicken and Mushrooms, 305–306
low-carb foods on, 303
Mediterranean Quinoa Salad, 307
Overnight Breakfast Parfait, 308
overview of, 80–84, 302
Sheet Pan Chicken Dinner, 309
Sweet Potato Latke Waffles, 310
Tzatziki, 311
Exercise
benefits of, 318–319, 331–332
breathing, 344–345
lifting, 364–365
options for, 319–325
overview of, 317–318

F

Fasting. *See also* Intermittent fasting
benefits of, 5–6, 37–42, 329
overview of, 328–329
process of, 37–42
schedule for, 18–19
Fats, 61, 143
Fats, healthy, 63, 71, 81
Fermented foods, 313–314
Fiesta Beef Fajita Lettuce Wraps, Grab-and-Go, 197
Fiesta Beef Fajitas recipe, 181
Fiesta Marinade recipe, 264
Fish Bone Broth
iodine in, 34–35
making of, 94
recipe for, 103
Salmon and Leek Chowder, 220
Tuscan Seafood Soup, 210
French Onion Beef Bone Broth recipe, 109
French Vinaigrette recipe, 255
Fructose, 49
Fruit
within the 80/20 system, 81
Baked Apples, 273
Blueberry Mojito Mocktail, 279
Creamy Lemon Dressing, 256
Creamy Orange Dressing, 257
Cucumber Gimlet Mocktail, 280
dangers of, 75
Fiesta Marinade, 264
Lemon Vinaigrette, 256
Orange Vinaigrette, 257
Panna Cotta with Balsamic-Soaked Strawberries, 284
Poached Pears, 274
portions of, 120
Strawberries with a Balsamic Reduction, 274
Strawberry Shake, 277
Sweet Black Cherry Gummies, 283
Fuller, Don and Cindy, 112

G

Garlic, 107, 263
Garlic Mashed Cauliflower "Potatoes" recipe, 223
Gazpacho Molded Salad recipe, 286
Gelatin
Chicken Pâté, 287
Gazpacho Molded Salad, 286
Mushroom Pâté, 290
overview of, 32–34
Panna Cotta with Balsamic-Soaked Strawberries, 284

Gelatin *(cont.)*
  Salmon Mousse, 285
  Sweet Black Cherry Gummies, 283
Ghee, 71, 119
Ginger, 107
Glucagon, 5–6, 39
Glucosamine, 35
Glucose, elimination of, 46
Glutamine, 36
Gluten, 53, 87
Glycine, 32, 36–37
Grab-and-Go Meals, 196–199
  Avocado Egg Salad, 196
  Bone Broth Soup, 197
  Burger, 197
  Chicken à la Carte, 196
  Eggs and Salmon, 196
  Fiesta Beef Fajita Lettuce Wraps, 197
  Instant Salad, 196–197
  Quick Egg Drop Soup, 196
  Rich and Hearty Turkey Chili, 196
  Roast Turkey Breast, 197
  Tuna or Salmon, 197
  Turkey Meatloaf, 196
  Zesty Salmon Patty, 196
Grain/grain-containing foods, dangers of,
  47, 52–54, 303
Greek-Style Beef or Bison Burgers recipe,
  182
Greek-Style Lemony Chicken Soup recipe,
  202
Green Goddess Shake recipe, 277
Griffin, Dolores, 44
Grilling, 199
Gut health, 33–34, 46–47, 326–328

H

Healthy fats, 63, 71, 81
Heart, healing of, 113
Hearts of palm noodles, 312
Hearty Beef and Vegetable Soup recipe,
  203
Herb-Infused Chicken Soup recipe, 204
Herb Mayo recipe, 261
HIIT workouts, 323
Homemade Mayonnaise recipe, 260–261
Hormones, 5–6, 40–41, 56–57, 63
Horseradish Mayo recipe, 261
Hot and Smoky Mayo recipe, 261
Human growth hormone (HGH), 6, 40

Hyaluronic acid, 36
Hydrolyzed collagen, 34

I

Immune system, 33, 39
In-a-Hurry No-Prep Stir-Fry recipe,
  151–152
Inflammation, 7, 32–33, 35, 36, 39, 46, 53,
  54, 63
Inner circle, choosing, 351–352
Instant Pot
  broth making within, 96–97
  Roasted Red Pepper and Basil Egg Bites,
    135
Instant Salad, Grab-and-Go, 196–197
Insulin, 9, 10, 36, 38, 49, 52
Intermittent fasting. *See also* Fasting
  benefits of, 329
  overview of, 30–31
  snacks for, 110–113
  why it works, 42–43
Iodine, 34–35
Italian Beef Bone Broth recipe, 109
Italian Wedding Soup recipe, 205

J

Joints, 35–36

K

Kale Salad with Turkey recipe, 170
Katzman, Sara, 55
Kefir, 314
Ketchup recipe, 262
Ketogenic diet, 330–331
Ketosis, 46
Kinda keto, 330–331
Kombucha, 314

L

Laughter, 349
Lead, myths regarding, 38
Leaky gut, 33–34
Lectins, 53
Legumes/beans, dangers of, 48, 59
Lemon-Basil Spritzer recipe, 281
Lemon-Roasted Asparagus recipe, 226
Lemon Vinaigrette recipe, 256
Lemony Cucumber Salad recipe, 226

Leonardi, Nadine, 25
Leptin, 9, 10, 52–53
Lime Chipotle Mayo recipe, 260
Lipotropic foods, 10, 63
Lobo, Rosita and Rohit, 104
Louisiana Creole Jambalaya recipe, 153
Low-Carb Veggies
  Asian Sesame Noodle Salad, 234
  Balsamic Roasted Brussels Sprouts, 235
  Broccoli Salad with Creamy Poppyseed
    Dressing, 236
  Brussels Sprouts Salad with a Sweet and
    Tangy Vinaigrette, 237
  Buffalo Cauliflower, 238
  Cauliflower Rice, 222
  Dairy-Free Creamy Ranch Dressing,
    239
  Garlic Mashed Cauliflower "Potatoes,"
    223
  Lemon-Roasted Asparagus, 226
  Lemony Cucumber Salad, 226
  Mac and Cheese, 233
  Mediterranean Peasant Salad, 232
  Napa Slaw with Creamy Ginger
    Dressing, 227
  Ratatouille, 230
  Roasted Curry Cauliflower, 228
  Roasted Kohlrabi, 240
  Roasted Portobello Burger "Buns," 229
  Roasted Sweet Onions, 229
  Zucchini Fritters, 241–242
  Zucchini Wide-Cut Pasta, 231
Lunch Entrées
  Air Fryer Fish and Zucchini "Fries,"
    186–188
  Asian Turkey Burgers, 172
  Balsamic Roast Pork Loin, 184
  Bolognese, 174–175
  Braised Chicken with Leeks and
    Mushrooms, 159
  Buttery Salmon and Asparagus, 189
  Chicken Cutlets with French Herbs and
    Creamy Roasted Red Pepper
    Sauce, 146–147
  Chicken Salad with Crunch, 160
  Chicken Shawarma, 148
  Chicken Stir-Fry, 157–158
  Chicken with Orange-Rosemary Sauce,
    155
  Chopped Balsamic Chicken Salad, 156
  Creamy Chicken Curry, 145

  Easy Beef or Bison Burgers, 173
  Easy Pot Roast, 179
  Easy Roast Chicken, 150
  Easy Roast Chicken Breasts, 149
  Easy Roast Turkey Breast, 165
  Easy Turkey Burgers, 166
  Fiesta Beef Fajitas, 181
  Greek-Style Beef or Bison Burgers, 182
  In-a-Hurry No-Prep Stir-Fry, 151–152
  Kale Salad with Turkey, 170
  Louisiana Creole Jambalaya, 153
  Middle Eastern Meatballs, 167
  One-Skillet Zucchini Pasta with
    Sausage, 162
  Orange-Rosemary Chicken Salad, 161
  Poke Bowl, 192–193
  Pork Tenderloin with Apples and
    Onions, 183
  Quick and Easy Lox, 134
  Rich and Hearty Turkey Chili, 168
  Roasted Salmon Gremolata, 185
  Seared Scallops, 194
  Shrimp Ceviche, 190–191
  Slow Cooker Southwest Pulled Pork,
    180
  Spicy Chicken Drumsticks or Thighs,
    154
  Tuna-Stuffed Tomatoes, 195
  Turkey Meatloaf Loaded with
    Vegetables, 169
  Turkey or Chicken Chorizo, 164
  Turkey or Chicken Italian Sausage, 163
  Turkey or Chicken Savory Sausage, 163
  Turkey Taco Salad, 171
  Zesty Salmon Patties, 195

M

Mac and Cheese recipe, 233
Magnesium, 35
Marinara Sauce recipe, 259
Mary's Hot-and-Sour Soup recipe, 212
Massages, 346–347
Meal Plans, 291–297
Measurement tracker, 371
Meat, processed, elimination of, 48
Meditation, 341–344
Mediterranean Peasant Salad recipe, 232
Mediterranean Quinoa Salad recipe, 307
Mediterranean Scramble recipe, 132
Medium-chain triglycerides (MCTs), 71

Metabolic syndrome, 14
Metabolism, stress and, 341
Microbiomes, gut, 326–328
Middle Eastern Meatballs recipe, 167
Miley, Stephanie, 43
Mocktails
    Blueberry Mojito Mocktail, 279
    Cucumber Gimlet Mocktail, 280
    Lemon-Basil Spritzer, 281
    Salted Thyme and Meyer Lemon
        Mocktail, 282
Moist-heat cooking methods, 199
Mushroom Pâté recipe, 290
Mushrooms
    Asian Chicken Bone Broth, 108
    Asparagus and Mushroom Crustless
        Quiche, 124
    Beef, Egg, and Mushroom Breakfast,
        127
    Braised Chicken with Leeks and
        Mushrooms, 159
    Chicken Stir-Fry, 157–158
    Cream of Wild Mushroom Soup, 201
    Creamy Chicken and Mushrooms,
        305–306
    Mary's Hot-and-Sour Soup, 212
    Mediterranean Scramble, 132
    Mushroom Pâté, 290
    Ratatouille, 230
    Roasted Portobello Burger "Buns," 229
    Shiitake Mushroom Soup, 213
    Turkey Meatloaf Loaded with
        Vegetables, 169
My Favorite Marinade recipe, 265

N

Napa Slaw with Creamy Ginger Dressing
    recipe, 227
Noodles, varieties of, 312–313

O

One-Skillet Zucchini Pasta with Sausage
    recipe, 162
Onions
    Beef, Egg, and Mushroom Breakfast,
        127
    Beef Bone Broth, 100
    Bolognese, 174–175
    Chicken Bone Broth recipe, 98
    Chicken Shawarma, 148

Fiesta Beef Fajitas, 181
fish bone broth, 103
French Onion Beef Bone Broth, 109
Hearty Beef and Vegetable Soup, 203
Herb-Infused Chicken Soup, 204
In-a-Hurry No-Prep Stir-Fry, 151–152
Louisiana Creole Jambalaya, 153
Pico de Gallo (Salsa Fresca), 267
Pork Tenderloin with Apples and
    Onions, 183
Ratatouille, 230
Red Bell Pepper Soup, 214
Roasted Sweet Onions, 229
Rotisserie Chicken Bone Broth, 101
Santa Fe Sauce, 270–271
Savory Vegetable Waffles, 137
Spicy Chicken Soup, 208
as super-cleansers, 336
Tomato, Basil, and Italian Sausage
    Soup, 209
Turkey Bone Broth, 99
Turkey Meatloaf Loaded with
    Vegetables, 169
Vegetarian Potassium-Rich Broth, 105
Orange-Rosemary Chicken Salad recipe,
    161
Orange Vinaigrette recipe, 257
Oven-Steamed Winter Squash recipe, 244
Overnight Breakfast Parfait recipe, 308
Oxidative stress, 41

P

Panna Cotta with Balsamic-Soaked
    Strawberries recipe, 284
Parsnip noodles, 313
Peppers
    Chicken Cutlets with French Herbs and
        Creamy Roasted Red Pepper
        Sauce, 146–147
    Chicken Salad with Crunch, 160
    Chicken Stir-Fry, 157–158
    Creamy Chicken Curry, 145
    Fiesta Beef Fajitas, 181
    Greek-Style Beef or Bison Burgers, 182
    Herb-Infused Chicken Soup, 204
    Louisiana Creole Jambalaya, 153
    Red Bell Pepper Soup, 214
    Rich and Hearty Turkey Chili, 168
    Roasted Red Pepper and Basil Egg Bites,
        135
    Roasted Red Pepper Hummus, 249

Roasted Red Pepper Sauce, 268
Santa Fe Sauce, 270–271
Southwest Breakfast Scramble, 139
Sweet and Savory Breakfast Hash, 140
Turkey Meatloaf Loaded with
    Vegetables, 169
Tuscan Seafood Soup, 210
uses of, 313
Periodization, 320
Pesto recipe, 267
Phosphorus, 35
Pico de Gallo (Salsa Fresca) recipe, 267
Piperline, 107
Poached Pears recipe, 274
Poke Bowl recipe, 192–193
Pork
    Balsamic Roast Pork Loin, 184
    Bolognese, 174–175
    Breakfast Meatballs, 129
    Louisiana Creole Jambalaya, 153
    Pork and Eggs, 133
    Pork Tenderloin with Apples and
        Onions, 183
    Slow Cooker Southwest Pulled Pork,
        180
Pork and Eggs recipe, 133
Pork Tenderloin with Apples and Onions
    recipe, 183
Portion control, 72–73, 120–123
Portuguese Kale and Sweet Potato Soup
    recipe, 206
Posture, 366
Prebiotics, 82, 327
Probert, Lora, 8
Probiotics, 82, 314, 327, 362
Processed fats, 47
Processed meats, 48
Proline, 36
Proteins, benefits of, 121

Q

Quick and Easy Lox recipe, 134
Quick Egg Drop Soup, Grab-and-Go, 196

R

Raspberries, carbohydrates within, 85
Ratatouille recipe, 230
Red Bell Pepper Soup recipe, 214
Rich and Hearty Turkey Chili, Grab-
    and-Go, 196

Rich and Hearty Turkey Chili recipe, 168,
    171
Roasted Cauliflower Hummus recipe,
    248
Roasted Curry Cauliflower recipe, 228
Roasted Garlic recipe, 263
Roasted Kohlrabi recipe, 240
roasted marrow bones recipe, 102
Roasted Portobello Burger "Buns" recipe,
    229
Roasted Red Pepper and Basil Egg Bites
    recipe, 135
Roasted Red Pepper Hummus recipe, 249
Roasted Red Pepper Mayo recipe, 260
Roasted Red Pepper Sauce recipe, 268
Roasted Salmon Gremolata recipe, 185
Roasted Salsa Verde (Green Tomatillo
    Salsa) recipe, 269
Roasted Sweet Onions recipe, 229
Roasted Winter Squash recipe, 244
Roasting vegetables, 224–225
Roast Turkey Breast, Grab-and-Go, 197
Rotisserie Chicken Bone Broth recipe,
    101–102

S

Salads
    Asian Sesame Noodle Salad, 234
    Avocado Egg Salad, Grab-and-Go, 196
    Brussels Sprouts Salad with a Sweet and
        Tangy Vinaigrette, 237
    Chicken Salad with Crunch, 160
    Chopped Balsamic Chicken Salad, 156
    entrée, 118
    Gazpacho Molded Salad, 286
    Instant Salad, Grab-and-Go, 196–197
    Kale Salad with Turkey, 170
    Lemony Cucumber Salad, 226
    Mediterranean Peasant Salad, 232
    Mediterranean Quinoa Salad, 307
    Orange-Rosemary Chicken Salad, 161
    selections for, 117
    Turkey Taco Salad, 171
Salmon
    benefits of, 219
    Buttery Salmon and Asparagus, 189
    Eggs and Salmon, Grab-and-Go, 196
    Roasted Salmon Gremolata, 185
    Salmon and Leek Chowder, 220
    Salmon Mousse, 285
    Smoked Salmon and Eggs, 138

Salmon (cont.)
  Tuna or Salmon, Grab-and-Go, 197
  Zesty Salmon Patties, 195
Salmon and Leek Chowder recipe, 220
Salmon Mousse recipe, 285
Salted Thyme and Meyer Lemon Mocktail
    recipe, 282
Santa Fe Sauce recipe, 270–271
Sauces
  Cheese Sauce, 233
  Chicken Cutlets with French Herbs and
    Creamy Roasted Red Pepper
    Sauce, 146–147
  Chicken with Orange-Rosemary Sauce,
    155
  Cocktail Sauce, 258
  Creamy Avocado Sauce or Salad
    Dressing, 253
  In-a-Hurry No-Prep Stir-Fry, 151–152
  Marinara Sauce, 259
  Roasted Red Pepper Sauce, 268
  Santa Fe Sauce, 270–271
  Tonnato Sauce, 251
Saunas, 347–348
Sausage and Apple Frittata recipe, 136
Sautéing vegetables, 224–225
Savory Vegetable Waffles recipe, 137
Scallions
  Asian Chicken Bone Broth, 108
  Asian Sesame Noodle Salad, 234
  Asian Turkey Burgers, 172
  Baked Egg Cups with Spinach, 125
  Bone Broth Egg Drop Soup, 207
  Chicken Stir-Fry, 157–158
  Cool and Creamy Avocado-Pumpkin
    Soup, 215
  Kale Salad with Turkey, 170
  Mediterranean Quinoa Salad, 307
  Napa Slaw with Creamy Ginger
    Dressing, 227
  Sweet Potato Latke Waffles, 310
  Vegetable Frittata, 141
  Watercress Soup, 216
Seafood
  Air Fryer Fish and Zucchini "Fries,"
    186–188
  Buttery Salmon and Asparagus, 189
  Louisiana Creole Jambalaya, 153
  Poke Bowl, 192–193
  Roasted Salmon Gremolata, 185
  Salmon and Leek Chowder, 220
  Salmon Mousse, 285
  Seared Scallops, 194
  Shrimp Ceviche, 190–191
  Smoked Salmon and Eggs, 138
  Tuna or Salmon, Grab-and-Go, 197
  Tuna-Stuffed Tomatoes, 195
  Tuscan Seafood Soup, 210
  Zesty Salmon Patties, 195
Seared Scallops recipe, 194
Seasonings/spices, 114–115
Seaweed, as super-cleanser, 336
Seed oils, dangers of, 58–59
Self-love, 346–347
Shakes
  Baked Apple Shake, 275
  Blue and Green Shake, 278
  Do-It-Yourself, 276
  Green Goddess Shake, 277
  Strawberry Shake, 277
Sheet Pan Chicken Dinner recipe, 309
Shiitake Mushroom Soup recipe, 213
Shirataki noodles (konjac), 312
Shortcuts, cooking, 176–178
Shrimp Ceviche recipe, 190–191
SIRT3, 41
Skin, 32, 63, 217–219, 381–382. See also
    Wrinkles, erasing
Sleep, 332–333
Slow cookers, 199
Slow Cooker Southwest Pulled Pork recipe,
    180
Smoked Salmon and Eggs recipe, 138
Smoky Chipotle Salsa recipe, 272
Snacks, for intermittent fasting, 110–113
Soda, 48, 51
Soups
  Bone Broth Egg Drop Soup, 207
  Bone Broth Soup, Grab-and-Go, 197
  Call-to-Action Soups
    Cool and Creamy Avocado-Pumpkin
      Soup, 215
    Mary's Hot-and-Sour Soup, 212
    Red Bell Pepper Soup, 214
    Salmon and Leek Chowder, 220
    Shiitake Mushroom Soup, 213
    Watercress Soup, 216
  Coconut Curried Chicken Soup, 200
  Cream of Wild Mushroom Soup, 201
  Greek-Style Lemony Chicken Soup,
    202
  Hearty Beef and Vegetable Soup, 203
  Herb-Infused Chicken Soup, 204
  Italian Wedding Soup, 205

Portuguese Kale and Sweet Potato Soup, 206
Quick Egg Drop Soup, Grab-and-Go, 196
Spicy Chicken Soup, 208
Tomato, Basil, and Italian Sausage Soup, 209
Tuscan Seafood Soup, 210
Southwest Breakfast Scramble recipe, 139
Soy, 9, 47, 55–57
Spicy Chicken Drumsticks or Thighs recipe, 154
Spicy Chicken Soup recipe, 208
Spicy Lime Vinaigrette recipe, 247
Spinach
  Baked Egg Cups with Spinach, 125
  Blue and Green Shake, 278
  Bone Broth Egg Drop Soup, 207
  Green Goddess Shake, 277
  Mediterranean Scramble, 132
  Pesto, 267
  Salmon and Leek Chowder, 220
  Vegetarian Potassium-Rich Broth, 105
  Watercress Soup, 216
Starchy Vegetables
  Baked or Mashed Sweet Potatoes, 243
  Oven-Steamed Winter Squash, 244
  Roasted Winter Squash, 244
  Sweet and Spicy Roasted Sweet Potatoes, 246
Steaming vegetables, 245
Strawberries with a Balsamic Reduction recipe, 274
Strawberry Shake recipe, 277
Stress, 339–349, 353–354
Stress hormones, 13
Sugar, 13–14, 46, 48, 49–50, 51
Super-cleansers, 336–337
Sweet and Savory Breakfast Hash recipe, 140
Sweet and Spicy Roasted Sweet Potatoes recipe, 246
Sweet Black Cherry Gummies recipe, 283
Sweet Potatoes
  Baked or Mashed Sweet Potatoes, 243
  Creamy Chicken Curry, 145
  noodles, 312
  Portuguese Kale and Sweet Potato Soup, 206
  Sweet and Spicy Roasted Sweet Potatoes, 246
  Sweet Potato Latke Waffles, 310
Sweet Potato Latke Waffles recipe, 310

T

Thanksgiving Turkey Bone Broth recipe, 106
Thousand Island Dressing recipe, 250
Thrive Market, 289
Thyroid, 56
Tomato, Basil, and Italian Sausage Soup recipe, 209
Tomatoes
  Breakfast Egg Muffins with Italian Sausage, 128
  Chicken Bone Broth recipe, 98
  Cocktail Sauce, 258
  Creamy Chicken Curry, 145
  Egg and Tomato Skillet, 131
  Gazpacho Molded Salad, 286
  Hearty Beef and Vegetable Soup, 203
  Ketchup, 262
  Louisiana Creole Jambalaya, 153
  Marinara Sauce, 259
  Mediterranean Peasant Salad, 232
  Mediterranean Scramble, 132
  One-Skillet Zucchini Pasta with Sausage, 162
  Pico de Gallo (Salsa Fresca), 267
  Quick and Easy Lox, 134
  Ratatouille, 230
  Rich and Hearty Turkey Chili, 168
  Santa Fe Sauce, 270–271
  Shrimp Ceviche, 190–191
  Smoked Salmon and Eggs, 138
  Smoky Chipotle Salsa, 272
  Southwest Breakfast Scramble, 139
  Spicy Chicken Soup, 208
  Tomato, Basil, and Italian Sausage Soup, 209
  Tuna-Stuffed Tomatoes, 195
  Turkey Bone Broth, 99
  Tuscan Seafood Soup, 210
  Vegetable Frittata, 141
  Vegetarian Potassium-Rich Broth, 105
Tonnato Sauce recipe, 251
Townsend-Gamblin, Denise, 27
Troubleshooting, 75–76
Tumeric, 107
Tuna or Salmon, Grab-and-Go, 197
Tuna-Stuffed Tomatoes recipe, 195
Turkey
  Asian Turkey Burgers, 172
  Baked Scotch Eggs, 126

Turkey *(cont.)*
  Breakfast Egg Muffins with Italian
      Sausage, 128
  Breakfast Meatballs, 129
  Easy Roast Turkey Breast, 165
  Easy Turkey Burgers, 166
  Herb-Infused Chicken Soup, 204
  Italian Wedding Soup, 205
  Kale Salad with Turkey, 170
  Middle Eastern Meatballs, 167
  One-Skillet Zucchini Pasta with
      Sausage, 162
  Portuguese Kale and Sweet Potato Soup,
      206
  Rich and Hearty Turkey Chili, 168
  Roast Turkey Breast, Grab-and-Go,
      197
  Sausage and Apple Frittata, 136
  Sweet and Savory Breakfast Hash, 140
  Tomato, Basil, and Italian Sausage
      Soup, 209
  Turkey Meatloaf Loaded with
      Vegetables, 169
  Turkey or Chicken Chorizo, 164
  Turkey or Chicken Italian Sausage, 163
  Turkey or Chicken Savory Sausage, 163
  Turkey Taco Salad, 171
Turkey Bone Broth, 94, 99, 216
Turkey Meatloaf, Grab-and-Go, 196
Turkey Meatloaf Loaded with Vegetables
    recipe, 169
Turkey or Chicken Chorizo recipe, 164
Turkey or Chicken Italian Sausage recipe,
    163
Turkey or Chicken Savory Sausage recipe,
    163
Turkey Taco Salad recipe, 171
Tuscan Seafood Soup recipe, 210
Tzatziki recipe, 311

V

Vegetable Frittata recipe, 141
Vegetables
  within the 80/20 system, 81
  batch-preparation of, 299–301
  Chicken Salad with Crunch, 160
  Chicken Stir-Fry, 157–158
  Chopped Balsamic Chicken Salad,
      156
  Gazpacho Molded Salad, 286

Hearty Beef and Vegetable Soup, 203
  In-a-Hurry No-Prep Stir-Fry, 151–152
  Kale Salad with Turkey, 170
  Mary's Hot-and-Sour Soup, 212
  Orange-Rosemary Chicken Salad, 161
  Poke Bowl, 192–193
  portions of, 120
  Rich and Hearty Turkey Chili, 168
  roasting, 224–225
  Salmon and Leek Chowder, 220
  sautéing, 224–225
  Savory Vegetable Waffles, 137
  steaming, 245
  as super-cleansers, 336
  Turkey Meatloaf Loaded with
      Vegetables, 169
  Vegetable Frittata, 141
Vegetables, Low-Carb
  Asian Sesame Noodle Salad, 234
  Balsamic Roasted Brussels Sprouts, 235
  Broccoli Salad with Creamy Poppyseed
      Dressing, 236
  Brussels Sprouts Salad with a Sweet and
      Tangy Vinaigrette, 237
  Buffalo Cauliflower, 238
  Cauliflower Rice, 222
  Dairy-Free Creamy Ranch Dressing,
      239
  Garlic Mashed Cauliflower "Potatoes,"
      223
  Lemon-Roasted Asparagus, 226
  Lemony Cucumber Salad, 226
  Mac and Cheese, 233
  Mediterranean Peasant Salad, 232
  Napa Slaw with Creamy Ginger
      Dressing, 227
  Ratatouille, 230
  Roasted Curry Cauliflower, 228
  Roasted Kohlrabi, 240
  Roasted Portobello Burger "Buns," 229
  Roasted Sweet Onions, 229
  Zucchini Fritters, 241–242
  Zucchini Wide-Cut Pasta, 231
Vegetables, Starchy
  Baked or Mashed Sweet Potatoes, 243
  Oven-Steamed Winter Squash, 244
  Roasted Winter Squash, 244
  Sweet and Spicy Roasted Sweet Potatoes,
      246
Vegetarian Potassium-Rich Broth recipe,
    105

W

Walking, 321–323
Water, 70–72, 362–363
Watercress Soup recipe, 216
Whey protein, 121–122
Wrinkles, erasing, 17–18, 32, 365–366

Y

Yeses, strategizing, 353–354
Yogurt, 313–314

Z

Zesty Salmon Patties recipe, 195
Zesty Salmon Patty, Grab-and-Go, 196

Zucchini
    Air Fryer Fish and Zucchini "Fries,"
       186–188
    One-Skillet Zucchini Pasta with
       Sausage, 162
    Savory Vegetable Waffles, 137
    Vegetarian Potassium-Rich Broth,
       105
    Zucchini Breakfast Cakes, 142
    Zucchini Fritters, 241–242
    Zucchini noodles, 312
    Zucchini Wide-Cut Pasta, 231
Zucchini Breakfast Cakes recipe,
    142
Zucchini Fritters recipe, 241–242
Zucchini Wide-Cut Pasta recipe,
    231

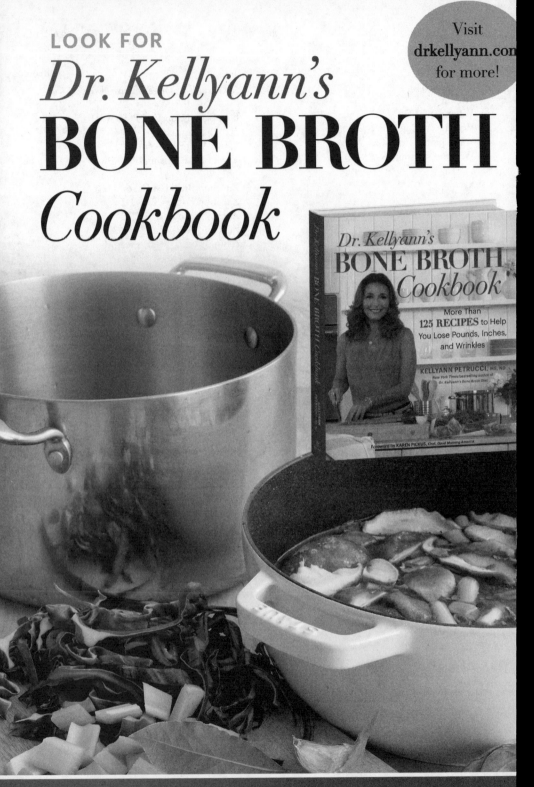